D1519194

THE HEALTH CARE DILEMMA

A Comparison of Health Care Systems in
Three European Countries and the US

THE HEALTH CARE DILEMMA

A Comparison of Health Care Systems in Three European Countries and the US

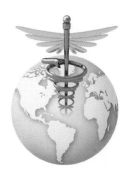

Elizabeth G Armstrong
Harvard Medical School, USA

Martin R Fischer
Witten/Herdecke University, Germany

Ramin W Parsa-Parsi
German Medical Association, Germany

Miriam S Wetzel
Harvard Medical School, USA

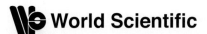
World Scientific

NEW JERSEY · LONDON · SINGAPORE · BEIJING · SHANGHAI · HONG KONG · TAIPEI · CHENNAI

Published by

World Scientific Publishing Co. Pte. Ltd.

5 Toh Tuck Link, Singapore 596224

USA office: 27 Warren Street, Suite 401-402, Hackensack, NJ 07601

UK office: 57 Shelton Street, Covent Garden, London WC2H 9HE

British Library Cataloguing-in-Publication Data
A catalogue record for this book is available from the British Library.

ISBN-13 978-981-4313-96-4
ISBN-10 981-4313-96-3
ISBN-13 978-981-4313-97-1 (pbk)
ISBN-10 981-4313-97-1 (pbk)

Typeset by Stallion Press
Email: enquiries@stallionpress.com

Printed in Singapore by Mainland Press Pte Ltd.

All royalties derived from the sale of this book
are contributed to the Harvard Macy Institute in support of
the worldwide community of health care
professionals innovating through education.

Praise for The Health Care Dilemma: A Comparison of Health Care Systems in Three European Countries and the US

The world of health and healthcare comes alive through its stories. This innovative book gives voice to patients' stories from different countries. It helps readers gain a better understanding of the meaning of health care in the context of local beliefs, culture and practices.

Professor Stephen Field, CBE, MMEd, DUniv, FHEA, FRCP, FRCGP
Chairman of Council
Royal College of General Practitioners, United Kingdom

Finally! A cultural map of real patients' experiences with vital health care systems and their delivery. A must read for every politician, physician and patient.

Larry Weber
Chairman,
Founder and CEO of W2 Group, a global marketingservices company

Provincialism is notoriously dangerous in all social policy debates and debates about health policy are no exception. This book is fortuitously well timed to inform current controversies in the United States, but is likely to be useful to those concerned with health policy everywhere. The insights about and lessons to be learned from the health systems in Denmark, Germany and Sweden described in this book will surely influence debates and decision making for some time.

Peter Williams, JD, PhD
Vice Dean, Academic Affairs
State University of New York at Stony Brook

The grassroots patient care experiences described in this book go a long way toward providing meaningful insights into the diverse challenges faced by future generations of health care professionals.

Eugene C. Corbett, Jr. MD, FACP
Bernard B. and Anne L. Brodie Professor of Medicine
Professor of Nursing
Assistant Dean for Clinical Skills Education
University of Virginia School of Medicine

This is a fascinating book! It puts together comprehensive cases from four countries: by increasing the understanding of foreign health care systems you improve the understanding of your own.

Professor Martin Reincke, MD
Dean of Students
Ludwig Maximilian University School of Medicine
Munich, Germany

Real patient cases provide windows through which the reader gains a view on national health care systems. On opposite sides of the Atlantic, these stories unfold in dramatically different ways.

Quentin Eichbaum, MD, PhD, MPH, MFA, FCAP
College Master
Associate Professor of Pathology, Microbiology and Immunology
Paul L. Foster School of Medicine
Texas Tech University Health Sciences Center

The opportunity to participate in the US-EU Medical Education Exchange was a highlight of my medical school experience. My patient's story was more than a case report — it was a window into the beliefs, attitudes, history and culture of an entire nation and its people. Through these stories, the reader has an opportunity to participate as we did, and to experience the hopes and challenges that are inherent in seeking and providing health care, all from the enriching perspective of the patient.

Aliyah R. Sohani, MD
Massachusetts General Hospital

Contents

Preface

Student-author Jon Duke wrote, "The world of health care is a world of stories; patient stories, doctor stories, nurse stories, student stories, family stories, and even baby stories. Thousands are created every day in the offices, hospitals, and clinics of a nation. And while exploration of government, economics, education, and technology is essential to the analysis of a health care system, it is the personal stories that transform fact and statistics into three-dimensional experience." It is this three-dimensional experience that we endeavor to bring to life in this collection of patient stories and descriptive chapters.

The patient stories in this book represent a window on the health care systems of three European countries and the United States as captured by senior level medical students in a student exchange program entitled "The United States-Europe Medical Education Exchange" (US-EU-MEE). This project was designed by Elizabeth Armstrong and Martin Fischer to develop a more complete understanding of three broadly contrasting health care systems: the single-payer socialized medicine model of Scandinavia, the government-legislated Statutory Health Insurance system of Germany, and the variety of public and private health care providers in the United States.

Surprisingly, the authors found, through a survey of students that very little is taught in medical schools about health care delivery systems. They conceived the plan for a multinational student exchange program that placed advanced medical students in the target countries as participant-observers.

With fresh perspectives, the students were able to take on the role of ethnographers. The observations reflected in these stories will be of special interest to all health care faculties, policy and decision makers and perhaps most importantly to the voting public who are concerned with achieving patient-centric care.

The Consortium

The long-time educational alliance between Harvard Medical School and the Ludwig Maximilians University in Munich, Germany provided the original impetus for the US-EU-MEE project under the leadership of Drs. Elizabeth Armstrong and Martin Fischer between 1999–2005. Each of the two schools enlisted two other medical schools on their respective continents to join the consortium: in Europe the University of Copenhagen, Denmark and the University of Lund, Sweden, and in the United States the Weill Medical College of Cornell University and Dartmouth Medical School. One student from Vanderbilt University School of Medicine participated. The project was supported by grants from the United States Fund for the Improvement of Post Secondary Education (FIPSE), Decision Resources Foundation, and DG XXII of the European Commission.[1,2]

The US-EU-MEE Program

Each student was assigned to follow one patient's journey in the health care system of his or her exchange country for a month under the guidance of a faculty member (clinical preceptor) at the host institution. Students from the United States went to Denmark, Germany, and Sweden and students from those countries came to the United States. The students were assigned to write an interdisciplinary case study that offered a window into the health care system of their host country and an opportunity to compare it with the system in their own country. These are neither classic medical case write-ups, nor problem-based learning cases such as those used in medical school tutorials but are intended to tell the patient's story as he or she experienced it and as it illustrates the workings of the particular health care system.

The patient stories are rich and varied. We meet Hacim, a typical 21-year-old enjoying the nightlife of Copenhagen when he becomes seriously ill, is subsequently diagnosed with tuberculosis and becomes Brian Chang's assigned "patient." There is Lara, the young German mother, whose struggle with recurring breast cancer and the care of her young son is followed by Anne Chiang. Swedish student, Kim Gosai, learns about health care in the United States through the contrasting experiences of Mrs. Kline and Mr. Montero in New York City and Danish student, Jacob Thyssen meets an unusual patient in an unusual hospital in Boston.

While increasing their own personal knowledge base about health care issues, students were instructed to pay particular attention to costs, organization and delivery of health care, quality and outcomes of care, and political, cultural and ethical influences on care. They were given a thorough orientation to the goals of the program before visiting their exchange country. Pre- and post-exchange questionnaires assessed the growth of their knowledge and their perception of the clinical environment in their exchange country.[2]

The cases in this book are written in a variety of essay styles, relatively free of medical technology and jargon. Although all of the student authors were competent in English, those for whom English is their first language naturally tended to write longer and more descriptive cases. The content of the cases is drawn from interviews with the patient, the patient's family, and health care providers involved in the patient's care as well as access to the patient's medical records. The case stories aim to illustrate the workings of the particular health care system as experienced by the patient in a straightforward and factual way.

The date each case was written is listed and reflects the treatment and policy issues at that time. Up-to-date chapters describe the health care systems in Denmark, Germany, Sweden, and the United States and highlight current issues. The student authors have given their permission for the cases to be edited for clarity and readability while retaining their personal reflections.

The Health Care Dilemma

Why is health care a dilemma? Since 1997 health care spending in countries studied by the Organisation for Economic Co-operation and Development (OECD) has accelerated as a percentage of Gross Domestic

Product. By 2020, health care spending is projected to triple in real dollars, consuming 21% of GDP in the U.S. and 15% of GDP in other OECD countries.[3] If this continues, demands on the health care systems threaten to outpace any nation's ability to pay for them. While the United States contemplates ways to provide more government regulated universal across the board coverage, European countries turn toward more private participation to spread the burden of payment and encourage efficiencies.[4]

Emotions run high when it comes to health care. The needs and wants of people in different countries and within countries vary considerably and even the meaning of disease and the treatment of disease are culturally influenced. In spite of high costs and problems of equitable distribution, there are aspects of the health care systems in all of the countries studied that are working well. By listening to patients tell their stories we gain insight into how a particular health care system really works and how its acceptance is viewed by the populace. These patient views represent deep cultural beliefs and expectations in each of the countries represented.

From these observations, individuals, institutions, and ultimately countries can learn from each other and thereby improve their own systems. In these chapters we give voice to patients and to a group of students who are the physicians who will take care of future generations. We hope you find their stories informative and enjoyable.

Acknowledgments

Writing the Acknowledgments is both the most enjoyable task in completing this book and also the most daunting for fear of leaving someone out who supported us at crucial points along the way.

First of all we want to thank the patients in Denmark, Germany, Sweden and the US who allowed their stories to be told anonymously by our thirty medical student-authors. Their real-life experiences lend authenticity and *verismo* to the medical facts of their cases. We have made every effort to protect their privacy.

Our sincere thanks to the students in the United States-Europe Medical Educational Exchange Project (US-EU-MEE) who diligently studied the health care systems of their assigned countries through the care of their patients and wrote a great deal more excellent descriptive material than we could possibly include. We are grateful for their assignment of copyright, which allowed us to work with their patients' stories as they appear in the book. Their student names are given with each of the cases. They are now all fully accredited physicians working in a wide variety of clinical medicine and research positions in many corners of the world. We hope that the experiences they had in capturing these patient stories have enriched their professional lives and the patients and communities they currently serve.

The initial funding to launch the work of the US-EU-MEE project came from the United States Fund for the Improvement of Post Secondary Education (FIPSE) and the DG XXII of the European Commission for which we are grateful. Continued support from Decision Resources and

Samuel C. Fleming made possible the on-going development of these cases. We thank also the consortium member schools listed in the Preface who sent and hosted students. Key contributors to the success of the program at these schools deserve special mention: Knut Aspegren, Lars Kayser, Michael Dall and Marianne Rex Sorensen (University of Copenhagen), Stefan Lindgren, Mona Eriksson and Catarina Andersson Forsman (University of Lund), Klaus Peter, August Konig, Bernadette Aulinger, Daniel Bauer and Frank Christ (Ludwig Maximilians University Munich), Oliver Fein and Carol Storey-Johnson (Weill Medical College of Cornell University), Ellis Rolett, Martha Regan-Smith and Joseph O'Donnell (Dartmouth Medical School), Daniel C. Tosteson, James Sabin, and David Blumenthal, with support from Fred Longenecker and Bernadette Sibuma (Harvard Medical School). Without their dedicated commitment and the participation of many physicians and hospital and staff personnel at each of the institutions, this project would not have been possible.

We were given a tremendous boost in energy and enthusiasm for bringing this project to fruition through a three-day symposium attended by a group of distinguished physicians and medical educators from Denmark, Sweden, Germany, the United Kingdom and the United States, held in Boston, in April 2008. They gave us the benefit of their thinking about the organization of the book and the educational and policy making value of the unique material in the cases. The symposium was made possible by the support of the Harvard Macy Institute and its worldwide community of health care professionals.

We are especially grateful to the national experts who reviewed and offered advice on the chapters addressing their country's health care systems, Marianne Rex Sorensen and Michael Dall in Denmark, and Catarina Andersson Forsman and Stefan Lindgren in Sweden.

Special thanks to Teresa Cushing and Arlene Moniz in Dr. Armstrong's office who managed tasks related to the book along with their day-to-day work, and to Susan Milmoe for valuable professional advice that helped to shape our book proposal. Andrew Jeon and colleagues at Partners Harvard Medical International offered sage advice and generous support on our publication plans for which we are most grateful. Our thanks to Mary Ellis for sharp-eyed proofreading and to Michelle Compton, Executive Director of the Breathing Room organization and Isabel Stenzel Byrnes for permission to use the poems and pictures in Case 21, Chapter 6.

Finally, we are grateful for the assistance of Yubing Zhai, Assistant Vice President, Executive Editor at World Scientific Publishing Company and for the attentive assistance of the Publishing Desk Editor, V.K. Sanjeed.

Elizabeth G. Armstrong, PhD
Martin R. Fischer, MD, MME
Ramin W. Parsa-Parsi, MD, MPH
Miriam S. Wetzel, PhD
Boston, Massachusetts
15 July 2010

Part I

Denmark:
Socially Minded Welfare Policies
and Universal Health Care

Part I

Denmark:
Socially Minded Welfare Policies
and Universal Health Care

1

Danish and US Health Care Systems Compared

Miriam S. Wetzel, PhD

"The first thing I learned is that there is no perfect health care system."

US-EU-MEE medical exchange student[1]

Culture and Politics

For a pleasant walk through the Danish health care system, we can hardly do better than to accompany Jon Duke as he follows his patient, Ellen Konradsen from the care of her General Practitioner through hospitalization for a heart attack and rehabilitation in his story, Experiencing *'hygge'* (see Chapter 2 Case 4). The fundamental premise of health care in Denmark, in the words of the Chief Financial Officer of the Copenhagen Hospital, "is to provide free access to most health services for all people regardless of their economic situation."[2] This reflects the long-standing social political basis of the Danish government.

Danish students coming to the United States do not understand why one of the richest countries in the world does not provide universal health insurance for all of its citizens. After spending time in the US, many see the fundamental difference in philosophy between the strong individualism of a free market society and the deep egalitarianism of a social

3

welfare state, although some still do not agree with it. When Danish student Anne-Marie Dogonowski asked her American patient, Mrs. Hill, if she got any help from the government for daily activities such as shopping, cleaning and cooking, Mrs. Hill replied, "The government does not help you. This is America, you help yourself."[3] However, the 52-year-old Mrs. Hill does receive Supplemental Social Security Income (SSI), and free health care because she is disabled.

Many Americans agree that our modern, urbanized society should do more to equalize access to basic health care. The government has moved in that direction over the years, beginning with the establishment of Medicare and Medicaid in 1965 as part of the Social Security Act amendment.[4] These programs are intended to protect and help the elderly and most needy members of society. Students from both US and European medical schools in the US-EU-MEE project were appalled at the thought of so many Americans who do not have health insurance — currently numbered at 45.7 million, according to US Census Bureau estimates.[5] It is hard to pin down an accurate number, or the exact reasons why so many lack this basic safety net. An estimated 70% of the uninsured are employed, but the remaining 25% likely includes people who work intermittently, as in seasonal work, are self-employed, work for companies that do not offer affordable insurance or choose not to buy insurance.[6]

Organization of the Health Care System — Denmark

Denmark is an industrialized nation of approximately 5.4 million people.[7] It is a constitutional monarchy with a democratically elected parliament and a modern market economy. The country has a history of social welfare minded politics and the government provides many comprehensive public services, including universal health care for its citizens. Since 1970 the government administration was comprised of a national government ("the State"), 14 counties and 273 municipalities, plus the cities of Copenhagen and Frederiksberg, which maintained both county and municipality status.[8]

Health Care Reform

In 2004 this system of counties and municipalities was significantly changed in ways that required considerable restructuring of the health care system. A government proposal called for the counties to be reorganized into five large regions and the municipalities to be reduced to fewer than 100, each with at least 20,000 citizens.[9] This reform was confirmed by the Danish parliament on February 24, 2005 and went into effect on January 1, 2007. The main areas of concern for the five regions are health care and regional development. Their charge is to ensure optimum utilization of resources, and to plan for the future. The local authorities handle tasks directly targeted at the citizen.

The basic role of the central government is to coordinate policy, plan future developments, and advise the local health authorities. In addition to this advisory and regulatory role, the central government is key to the financial support of the health care system. The five regions do not have the power to levy and collect taxes, so they depend on yearly financial agreements with the Ministry of Finance, which sets the agenda and framework for the financial development, and initiatives for the year to come.

For the individual Dane, the new governmental structure is expected to provide "more cohesive treatment across administrative borders and easy and simplified access to prevention, examination, treatment and care of a high professional calibre" according to a report on health and long-term care in Denmark by the Ministry of Interior and Health and the Ministry of Social Affairs.[10]

One of the effects of this change is that the municipalities have a more important role in health care, including the main responsibility for preventive treatment and health promotion. They already administer long-term care, which is free of charge if referred by a General Practitioner (GP), but will have an enhanced role in prevention, rehabilitation not performed in a hospital, dental care for young people under the age of 18, visiting nurse services for new parents, treatment of alcohol and drug abuse, and assistance to people with disabilities. The new regional system furthers the Danish ideal of providing free and equal access to health care for all citizens by equalizing funding across richer and poorer areas of the country. In the simplest terms, this is accomplished by a combination of block grants from the national government, and an "activity-related contribution," paid by the local authorities and calculated according to how much the citizens of that area use the national health service.[11] This provides an incentive to keep costs low.

Since 1973, the National Health Security System (NHSS) has been the health care insurance system for Denmark; the financial administrator of universal health care.[12] This is not likely to change as a result of governmental reorganization. The Ministry of Health and the Ministry of Finance will continue to act as advisory and regulatory bodies at the national level. The State can influence health care delivery and economics to some degree by altering the supply of physicians, as all physician training is at the national level. Under advisement from the Ministry of Health, the number of practitioner licenses may be limited in certain areas to achieve equitable distribution of physicians across Denmark, including rural areas that might otherwise be less attractive locations for physicians.

In the 2007 organizational scheme — as in the old one — there are two sectors. The Primary Sector covers General Practitioners, specialists, visiting nurse services, dental care, and preventive services for children. The Secondary Sector includes the hospitals and psychiatric treatment in a hospital. The GP acts as the gatekeeper between the two, ensuring that patients receive adequate care and are not unnecessarily referred to specialists.[13]

Under the reorganization, both sectors are financed by block grants from the National Health Service and the local activity contribution. Twenty five percent to 60% of the cost of dental services, psychologists, chiropractic, and physical therapy is also expected to be covered by the Primary Sector. The individual citizen pays the difference.

Since 2007 the five regions run the Secondary Sector, including hospitals, GPs, and inpatient psychiatric treatment. Hospital treatment is free but a referral from a General Practitioner is needed for all non-emergency care. The hospitals are charged with examining, treating, and caring for citizens referred from the Primary Sector. They also provide laboratory, x-ray, and other services for the Primary Sector, and Social Psychiatry services, which encompass a network of residential facilities, shelters, and community centers for people who need help in managing everyday life.

Division of Responsibility

A fundamental difference in the practice of medicine in Denmark that surprises American students is the division of responsibilities for the patient between General Practitioners and specialists, and between routine outpatient care and hospital care. This is well illustrated in the case of Ellen Konradsen. When she was admitted to the hospital from the emergency room, her primary care physician, Dr. Jensen, was not notified and there was no further communication about her condition from the hospital physicians. The American student, Jon Duke, bridged this gap by calling Dr. Jensen with news of her recovery from a heart attack. In a previous episode when Ms. Konradsen's diabetes was out of control, she was cared for by hospital physicians and an endocrine consulting physician and Dr. Jensen did not see or hear from her for many months. The only information the General Practitioner routinely receives is a discharge summary that is placed in the patient's computerized record, usually within a few days after discharge.

Another surprise for the American students is the division of responsibility for patients between the "day doctor" and the "night doctor." In Denmark, the government has set a maximum of 37 hours of work per week for all workers including health care personnel; an almost unimaginable concept for American doctors. Dr. Jensen explained to Jon that his workday is from 8 am to 4 pm Monday through Friday and he does not wear a beeper.

Jon asks, "But who does the patient call after hours?"

Dr. Jensen replied that the patient might call the Night Clinic, an office that is staffed by GPs and is open from 4 pm to 8 am or go directly to the hospital emergency room.[14]

It all seems so beautifully simple, but would it work in the US? Americans are accustomed to having access to their own doctors at any time of the day or night. If the doctor must be away, he or she will "sign out" to a colleague. Unless this can be arranged by reciprocal agreement, it may cost the doctor a significant amount of money for coverage. When patients are hospitalized in the US, their own physicians may continue to supervise their care, although there is a growing trend toward "hospitalists" — doctors who work only in the hospital. An important part of their work in the US is to communicate with the patient's primary care doctor.

Wait Time

Perhaps an unintended consequence of the very humane work schedule of Danish physicians is the wait time that is often troublesome to Danish citizens. While an office appointment with a GP is usually available within four to five days, the wait to see a specialist, and the wait for elective surgery sometimes dragged on for weeks or months in the past. The situation has been improved with new policies that allow the patient to seek care outside his or her local area. As we see in Hacim's case (A Foreigner with Tuberculosis),[15] wait time was not a problem because TB patients are seen expeditiously. Waiting for test and x-ray results was a problem, however, for heart transplant patient, Jacob (In the Same Boat).[16] He waited more than 10 days for the result of x-rays while his condition seriously deteriorated, and he did not get the results until he called the physician's office. He then waited more than nine months to be referred to a larger hospital for evaluation for a heart transplant. It is not difficult to see that physicians, nurses, and health care administrative personnel would often find it difficult to keep up with day-to-day tasks when limited to a 37-hour workweek.

Other reasons for dissatisfaction with wait times have to do with the hierarchy of the hospital system. Each year Danish authorities negotiate a budget based on their expected number of patients and the level of care they will need. If a patient, such as Jacob, is transferred from the local hospital, in this case Gentofte, to Rigshospitalet, the county authority would have to pay for his treatment in the larger hospital. With tight budgets, it is understandable that there might be some reluctance to authorize a transfer until it is certain that it is absolutely necessary.

In 1993, in response to lengthy waiting times, the government issued a guarantee that patients waiting longer than two months at their county facility could seek care at any hospital, with their local facility picking up much of the tab.[17] This created competition among the counties and was intended to even out wait times across counties. This policy proved quite problematic, at least in some locales. Instead of improving efficiency or capacity at the hospital, this guarantee — intended primarily to mollify public anger about long waits — exacerbated the funding problems, which themselves contribute to long waits.

In July 2002, this policy was liberalized so that patients waiting more than two months for treatment in a public hospital could be treated at a private hospital with which the county had an agreement in or outside of Denmark. From July 2003 to April 2005, approximately 42,000 patients used this option according to the Ministry of the Interior and Health.[18] About 500 were treated outside of Denmark. Under the 2007 reorganization plan, citizens have the right to go to another hospital if their local hospital cannot accommodate them within *one* month. They will be able to choose any public hospital in Denmark, or any private hospital that has a signed agreement with their county.[19,20] There has also been a change regarding the choice of a GP. Previously the patient must reside within 10 km of the GPs office, but since April 2003, the distance has been increased to 15 km (5 km in the Copenhagen Metropolitan Area).[21]

A lot of attention has been focused on the problem of waiting for elective surgery. Waiting lists for surgery to improve the quality of life of middle aged or elderly people, such as hip and knee replacement and cataract surgery, has long been a source of dissatisfaction.[22] Some progress has been made. From January 1999 to April 2002, waiting times were approximately 105 days. By December 2004, however, the average wait had dropped to 70 days, a decrease of 32%, or more than four weeks.[23] Since the institution of extended choice in October 2007, wait times have decreased by one week each year for typical treatments. Increased resources and activity-based funding have also influenced this improvement.[24]

The challenge will be to see that wait times do not increase as more people with less severe conditions seek treatment. After all, waiting times are a means of rationing health care — a scarce resource, as patients' "wants" outstrip the system's "means." This effect was illustrated in the 1990s when wait times were reduced and suddenly there was a 10-fold increase in cataract surgery in one county, causing the waiting lists to become longer again.[25] Either an alternate way to ration care must be found, or the government, and the citizens, will have to accept the waiting times or face the prospect of increased taxation to pay for more doctors, nurses, and health facilities.

Health Care at the Patient Level — Denmark and the US

In Denmark, basically, primary health care is in the hands of GPs and municipal services. General practitioners are the gatekeepers for all referrals to hospitals or specialists except ophthalmologists and ENT specialists, which can be consulted without a referral. Citizens can choose between two government insurance schemes known as Category 1 and Category 2. Category 1 assigns each person to a general practitioner within 15 km of his or her home, and that physician is the access point for all health services for that individual. All specialty services or hospital stays deemed necessary by the GP are covered in full by the National Health Security System (NHSS). However, if a citizen uses specialty or hospital care without a referral, he or she may be responsible for the costs. In contrast, Category 2 allows GPs and specialists to set their fees without restriction. Patients may see any generalist or specialist at any time, but they must pay out-of-pocket if fees exceed the subsidy to Category 1 patients. Ninety-seven percent of Danes choose Category 1.[26]

In 1998, there were between 1507 and 1610 inhabitants per generalist in all counties except for one (Bornholm, 1317 inhabitants per generalist), which was intended to provide geographic equity in access to health care across Denmark. In the 2007 reforms, the coverage areas among regions and municipalities was carefully recalculated to support better quality of patient care, not only in access to General Practitioners, but also to hospital facilities and specialists.[27] The government also controls licensure of specialists, although there are a small number of specialists who work privately on a fee-for-service basis without NHSS reimbursements.

In contrast to Denmark, geographic equity of medical care is not regulated by the government in the United States and many rural or marginalized urban communities lack access to specialized care or top-of-the-line medical facilities. Federal programs that fund medical training in exchange for service in underserved communities attempt to remedy these inequities. Notable examples are the Indian Health Service, designed to promote the health and wellbeing of Native Americans, and the National Health Service Corps, a branch of the Department of Health and Human Services that places doctors in needy areas.[28] Some non-governmental initiatives, such as the Frontier Nursing Service in Kentucky, also provide health services to underserved rural areas.[29]

In the US, as in Denmark, patients are generally admitted to the hospital on recommendation of their doctors, or directly from a hospital emergency room. In Denmark, municipalities administer the portion of primary care that is not covered by GPs, including nursing care, home nursing visits, dentistry for children and disabled people, and school nursing services. GPs now do childhood vaccinations. The areas in which consumers must contribute out-of-pocket payments include partial cost for physiotherapists, dental care, outpatient pharmaceuticals, some assisted reproduction, the full cost of glasses (unless extremely poor vision is demonstrated), alternative treatments, and elective cosmetic surgery. In the US these services lie outside many basic insurance plans also, and have to be paid for out-of-pocket. There are notable exceptions and wide differences among the states in some of these areas. For example, the state of Massachusetts is among the states having the most aggressive laws requiring insurance companies to cover infertility treatment.[30]

Screening and Health Promotion — Denmark and the US

Both the US and Denmark lack an emphasis on screening and health promotion programs. The US has had some success with anti-smoking campaigns, including the "Great American Smoke-out" sponsored by the American Cancer Society every year on the Thursday before Thanksgiving. Statistics from the Centers for Disease Control indicate that there has been a gradual reduction in the number of American men and women who smoke.[31] Seat belt use and bicycle helmets are promoted in safety campaigns, and every American infant rides in a safety car seat, under penalty of law. There are also seat belt and car seat laws for older children, but they vary from state to state.[32] Abundant government-sponsored and privately produced information is available on the value of exercise, stress reduction, and good nutrition.

Still, it is strange that neither Denmark nor the United States has widespread, government-sponsored screening for markers of cardiovascular disease, such as high blood pressure. Hypertension is now the Number 1 diagnosis in the world, with 1.5 *billion* people or approximately 25% of the world's population affected.[33,34] It seems this would be precisely the type of program that would be valued by any country interested in reducing the burden of chronic disease. Beyond financial issues, however, there are ethical aspects to debate and concern for the validity of screening methods.[35]

Screening for breast cancer is an area where there is considerable difference between Denmark and the US. Although the Danish parliament approved coverage of biannual screening mammograms for women over age 50 in 2000,[36] this is not legally binding and its implementation depends on local availability and expenditure of health care funds. According to OECD data, breast cancer mortality in Denmark was 33.4 per 100,000 women, the highest of the 22 countries reporting.[37] Cancer mortality in the US was 22.4 per 100,000 women in the same study. The link between screening and mortality is not straightforward, but it is possible that when there is a low level of screening, women present for treatment at a more advanced stage of the disease and survival is adversely affected.

Ethics

The fundamental ethical concern of the health care system of Denmark is that all citizens have equal and easy access to health services. Although the US does not have government-sponsored universal health care, Medicare and Medicaid and the SCHIP program for children of low income families offer significant help with health care costs and services to those who need them and are unable to pay. Americans also have a strong record of volunteerism and philanthropy. According to the US Bureau of Labor Statistics, in the year ending September 2006, 61.5 million people volunteered for or through an organization.[38] Americans contribute money and time to thousands of organizations that focus on health needs and research not only within the US, but reaching out to other countries. These organizations include the Peace Corps, UNAIDS, Doctors Without Borders, SmileTrain (offering free surgery for children with cleft palate), Project HOPE and many others.

Ethical issues that are similar in the US and Denmark concern patients' rights, including the right to informed consent, privacy, access to one's own medical records, and dignity at the end of life. Active euthanasia is not approved in either country. Patients in Denmark and the US have the right to view their medical records. In Denmark, if a patient requests it, doctors, nurses and health care workers are obliged to interpret their records for them. Doctors in Denmark are required to inform patients of their legal rights and not to misinform them about available treatments or side effects and potential complications. Signed consent forms are not a part of standard practice in Denmark, unlike the stringent requirement in the US. In Denmark as in the US, "living wills" are used to state a patient's wishes regarding pain treatment, resuscitation, and prolongation of life.[39]

In the late 1970s a system of Scientific Ethics Committees was established in Denmark. The task of these committees (one Central Scientific Ethical Committee and seven regional committees) is to assess and approve, from an ethical perspective, biomedical research projects involving human subjects as well as human biological materials such as fertilized eggs, deceased persons and human embryonic tissue. They review about 3,000 research projects a year. The Central Committee coordinates the regional committees and formulates common guidelines for assessing appeals by researchers when they disagree with the decisions.[40]

Another committee established in Denmark in 1988, the Danish Council of Ethics, functions to provide advice and information to the Parliament and to inform the public about ethical problems raised by developments within the National Health Service and the field of biomedicine. In particular, they provide information and encourage debate on both sides of an issue.[41] For example, Quentin Eichbaum's patient, Jacob, thought there should be more debate about organ transplantation to make the public aware of the need for more available organs for transplant.[42]

Malpractice

Malpractice is much less an issue in Denmark than it is in the US. Doctors in Denmark do not carry malpractice insurance to the extent they do in the US. In the US, malpractice insurance costs physicians and other health care practitioners millions of dollars and contributes to the high cost of medical care. Some states have set up insurance risk pools to reduce pressure on malpractice insurance premiums. In other states, malpractice insurance rates continue to climb especially for specialists who treat high-risk patients.[43]

Patients in Denmark who are victims of malpractice can present grievances to a Patients' Complaints Board, which may reprimand the provider or recommend litigation to the public prosecutor. In 1992, the government established the Patient Insurance Scheme, which allows patients who experience an unfortunate outcome or error in the course of a procedure or treatment to receive monetary compensation for lost wages, permanent disability and pain and suffering without the physician having to admit error or negligence. In Denmark the five regions are obligated to pay damage claims within the limits of the law, either through an insurance company or by self-insuring.[44]

Denmark has had its problems with mistakes in medical care, as have other countries. One report estimated that half of these errors could be prevented and expressed a call for a better reporting system.[45] Similar concern was raised in the US by the 1999 Institute of Medicine report, *To Err is Human: Building a Safer Health System*.[46] Both nations have made a sincere effort to address the problem of medical errors, in Denmark by requiring more stringent documentation and a risk-free error reporting system for physicians, and in the US by close examination and correction of system failure that produces errors.[47]

Medical Education

Students in Denmark enter medical school directly after secondary school and follow a six-year program. The three medical schools at Copenhagen, Aarhus, and Odense have a uniform curriculum prescribed by the government. The Faculty of Health Sciences at the University of Copenhagen welcomes many international students each year and advertises a friendly environment where teachers and students interact freely and questioning and debate are positively encouraged.

There is no cost to the Danish students; education at schools of medicine, law, mathematics, science, and economics is all paid for by taxes. There is some small-group problem-based learning, but mostly the format is large lecture.[48] The clinical years are spent in the hospitals, but unlike the US, students are not part of a medical team. One student termed it "boring." He said they go to the hospital all day but are only allowed to watch.[49] Competition for further specialty training is highly competitive.

Costs

What does health care cost and how is it paid for? In the US as in Denmark, income, property and corporate taxes are the source of governmental funding for health care. In addition to Medicare and Medicaid, the US Department of Veterans Affairs provides patient care and federal benefits to veterans and their dependents. Individuals in the US with no, or low income are eligible for the highest level of free health care but sometimes the complexity of the distribution system is daunting. The cost of prescription drugs is a significant issue in both countries.

How can the Danish government provide free universal health care when it has been nothing but a distant dream in the United States? The short answer is: taxes and the will of the people. In 2005 in Denmark the state, county, and municipal taxes averaged 56% of earned and capital income.[50] Would Americans tolerate paying more than half of their income in taxes? The aging of the population in both countries makes it increasingly difficult, with fewer young workers to support a growing number of older citizens. Under the 2007 government reorganization, Denmark replaced the three-tier national, regional, and local system of taxation with a two-tier system, since the five regions are not authorized to levy taxes.[51] The individual tax burden is based on a progressive income scale.

Denmark–United States Comparison

	Denmark	United States
Population (millions)	5.4	300
Percent of GDP spent on health	7.3%	15.3%
Public (Government) expenditure on health in millions US$ PPP	14,159	854,744
Private expenditure on health in millions US$ PPP	2,677	1,072,447
Total per capita expenditure on health US$ PPP	3,108	6,401
Government expenditure on health as % of total government expenditure	14.4%	18.8%

OECD Health Data 2007. Data from 2004–2005.[52] US$ PPP = Purchasing Power Parity in US$.

Private Insurance in Denmark

To supplement the universal health care coverage in Denmark, there are certain out-of-pocket payments for medical goods or services, and citizens can voluntarily purchase private supplementary health insurance to cover these costs. Most of this insurance is purchased to cover items not included under the government insurance and not to "jump the lines" and escape waiting lists. For example, Kirsten Anderson (see The Silent Killer)[53] pays 1000 DKK (about $169 in 2004) per year for supplementary health insurance to help cover pharmaceutical and general dentistry costs that are not covered by government insurance. The use of private supplementary insurance has become increasingly popular in Denmark in recent years and is expected to grow in spite of the government guarantee of treatment within one month for certain diseases and surgical procedures. If the patient's local or regional hospital cannot perform the needed service, the government will pay for it at a private hospital. Still it is important to note that public expenditures to private hospitals only amount to 1.5% of the total budget.[54]

Interestingly, in Denmark the private insurance market is dominated by one non-profit company called Sygeforsikringen Danmark, in contrast to the large number of insurance companies in the US. According to Danmark information, near the end of 2006, they insured 1.9 million members, or approximately 29% of the population. The insurance is described as "health insurance as a supplement to the Danish National Health Service." Quarterly premium for Category 1 in 2006 (basic supplemental for co-pays, glasses, chiropractic) is DKK 590 ($98). Category 2 gives greater freedom of choice of physicians and specialists for DKK 793 ($132). There is a cheaper rate, "primarily for younger people who do not need much health care." To be accepted by Danmark you must not have been ill or needed medicine for the prior year and you cannot join after age 60.[55]

The increasing trend towards private insurance in Denmark is hotly debated by some who fear that it will siphon off the best physicians in the public sector and that it erodes the ideals of the welfare state. It is true that almost every country that has had universal coverage is finding it more and more difficult to afford and is turning more toward private insurance.[56] One possible reason for the increase in private insurance, specifically policies that cover the use of private hospitals, is waning confidence in the Danish health care system. As patient Kristen Anderson commented, "there has been a backslide in Danish health care" (The Silent Killer).[57] For now, however, the government system remains firmly entrenched as the dominant provider in Denmark.

Holding Down Costs

Bulk purchasing

One method of reducing pharmaceutical expenditures is bulk purchasing. Most Danish hospitals save money through membership in Amgros,[58] an organization that has been owned by several counties and leverages purchasing power for hospitals. Amgros negotiates the price of drugs and other medical equipment resulting in bulk discounts.

Prescription drug coverage

Currently, the Danish government reimbursement for outpatient pharmaceuticals works according to an expenditure-based scale. Below 500 DKK (approximately $83 in 2006) annual drug expense, there is no reimbursement. As total expenditures increase, the percentage of reimbursement increases to a maximum of 85%. Chronically ill patients with permanent drug needs and low-income patients can apply for full reimbursement.[59]

The "G-scheme"

The government has passed legislation to limit pharmaceutical expenditure, including temporary price freezes and cuts, tying drug prices to European averages, and mandatory generic substitutions. In 1991 the Danish Medicines Agency established the "G-scheme," a policy that guarantees generic substitutions unless a brand is prescribed specifically by a physician, though patients may refuse substitutions if they are willing to pay more out of pocket.[60] Substitution practices are similar in the United States. Overall, generics occupy a substantial and growing percentage of total pharmaceutical expenditures in Denmark, from 46% of total expenditures in 1996 to 49% in 1999. A new drug reimbursement structure implemented in 2000 was projected to save approximately 325 million DKK per year by limiting maximum reimbursements for a drug to the average of the two cheapest market prices of the drug.[61]

Practice guidelines

Danish government-issued practice guidelines and outreach programs seek to educate physicians on optimal prescribing practices to improve outcomes and minimize costs. The Institute for Rational Pharmacotherapy is the branch of government that generates practice guidelines. Given the decentralized nature of the health care system, many regions have audits to assess practitioner adherence to guidelines, although penalties for non-adherence are not enforced. The reason Denmark's expenditures on pharmaceuticals ranks among the lowest in Western European countries may be the result of determined efforts to limit drug costs, or it may be at least in part attributable to a less favorable attitude of its citizens towards medications. An American student who spent an entire year in Denmark remarked on the hesitation of the Danish people to rely on drugs. Her host family frowned even on over-the-counter remedies such as cough syrup and people had to be really ill before they would consider taking prescription drugs.[62] TV and print advertisements for prescription drugs are prohibited because of an EU Directive, so Danish citizens are not constantly bombarded with commercials for these products as is the case in the US.

GP gatekeepers

The gatekeeper role of General Practitioners is the key systematic control on costs in Denmark. Based on the analysis of Kirsten Anderson's work-up (The Silent Killer),[63] one way to control costs for newly diagnosed hypertensive patients is to limit expensive supplementary testing unless absolutely necessary. In reality, not every patient who develops hypertension undergoes extra tests; many are treated empirically, and are followed with office exams over time. As there is no additional cost to patients per office visit, there is no incentive to limit such follow-up visits.

Cost sharing

Although office visits to GPs and specialists remain free of co-pays, other medical expenses have been increasingly shared with the patient. From 1980 to 1999 private expenditure as a proportion of total expenditure on health care rose from 12.2% to 17.8%.[64] Most co-payments apply to dental care for adults and pharmaceuticals. As we have seen (**Prescription drug coverage**) there is an annual cap on pharmaceutical expenses and certain chronically ill and low-income patients qualify for total reimbursement. Still, Denmark and other countries with universal health coverage have had to turn increasingly to cost sharing even though it contradicts the principle of equal care for all regardless of ability to pay.

In the United States, many private insurers have attempted to limit the number of visits per patient by adding co-pay fees in addition to substantial baseline insurance premiums. Co-pays for GP visits by patients who subscribe to a standard coverage plan from Blue Cross-Blue Shield, one of the largest private insurers in the United States, are typically $10 to $20, or approximately 10–20% of the total visit fee. In theory, co-pays should offer incentives to patients to reduce unnecessary GP visits, though it is not likely that monitoring hypertension or other chronic diseases by infrequent GP visits would save money in the long run if patients go on to develop more complications and more serious disease.

Limiting tests and reducing hospital stays

Brian Chan, American student in Denmark, pointed out that a striking comparison between the Danish and American health systems is the balance between ordering tests and procedures and saving money. For example, in Denmark, only three sputum samples are required from patients suspected of TB, such as his patient, Hacim (A Foreigner with Tuberculosis in Denmark),[65] while Danish student, Jacob Thyssen, found six specimens routinely collected from his TB patient in the US (A Doctor as Patient at Lemuel Shattuck Hospital).[66] The economies may not be as apparent in the US, but in fact both countries are trying to keep costs down without adversely affecting health care quality. Shorter hospital stays and reducing the number of hospital beds have been used in both countries to cut costs. From 1990 to 2004, Denmark saw the number of acute care hospital beds decrease from 4.1 to 3.3 per thousand population and the US had a reduction from 3.7 to 2.8 per thousand population during the same period.[67] Outpatient visits and admissions to rehabilitation facilities have increased dramatically in both countries.

Market forces

In addition to saving costs by closing facilities and programs, such as the lung clinic in Hvidovre, Denmark has resorted to market pressures to reduce costs. As we have noted, more health costs have been passed on to the patients in the form of co-pays as a means of avoiding a higher tax burden. Market forces have also had a negative effect in Denmark's nursing shortage. Nurses are leaving the public sector because of low pay and poor working conditions and going to work in the private sector.[68] In turn, hospital administrators are forced to hire private nurses at higher salaries. At times there has been a shortage of other health care personnel, including specialists. Another example of the use of market forces is the practice of making a certain percentage of a hospital's budget contingent on efficiency and usage goals. At least in theory, this should provide incentives for hospitals to be efficient and serve more patients to justify the money they receive.[69]

To aid in controlling costs, the system of diagnosis-related group (DRG) payments was gradually introduced in Denmark starting in 2000. This activity-based plan pays hospitals an established fee per patient based on an analysis of costs associated with a patient's diagnosis. This type of funding was seen as a tool to boost internal productivity and distribute cost reduction among all hospitals. At first it applied only to patients who chose to be treated in hospitals outside of their own home county but in 2002 it was expanded nationwide.[70]

Physician compensation

It is difficult to compare physicians' pay in two countries that are as different as Denmark and the US. Cost of living, cultural and social expectations and lifestyle strongly influence what is acceptable. Then there is the mandatory 37-hour workweek to consider. American doctors ordinarily work many more hours. Danish salaries are also subject to the greater than 50% tax bite.

Although salary figures for Danish doctors are difficult to find, there is a great deal of information about their work and their method of compensation in the OECD Working Paper Number 21, "The Supplies of

Physician Services in OECD Countries."[71] This paper describes the payment methods in use in twenty-one OECD countries. The three main methods are: fee-for-service (a fee for each item or unit of care provided), capitation (a set amount of money per patient to cover all care within a given period of time), and salary (lump-sum payment for a specified number of hours per week or month).

In Denmark, primary care physicians are paid by a mix of capitation and fee-for-service. This blended method of payment is thought to result in efficient and cost-effective health care. Medical associations participate in the bargaining process, but physicians have not always approved of the agreements reached. Doctors have many different titles, depending on their function such as "Consultant," "Specialty Consultant," "Hospital Doctor (General)," or "Hospital Doctor (Specialist)." Their salaries vary somewhat depending on their seniority and role in the health care system.

Sustainability

In the *Economic Survey of Denmark, 2005*, The Organisation for Economic Co-operation and Development (OECD) warned that with an aging population, Denmark's welfare system will not be affordable in the coming years without further policy reforms. Raising taxes is not an attractive option because "high taxes have already driven down working hours by making work unattractive relative to leisure."[72] The point is that the work force is expected to become a smaller percentage of the total population in the next few years. Admittedly, it would be difficult to cut back on benefits provided by the welfare state since people have become accustomed and dependent on them. Realistically, costs will continue to rise as new medicines and technologies are developed. The report recommends a "pre-saving strategy" so the necessary funds will be available when the present working generation reaches retirement age and needs more health services.

The US also faces sustainability problems. Officials estimate that Medicare hospital insurance reserves will be exhausted by the year 2019 and Social Security reserves by 2041. Current annual surplus of tax income over expenditures will soon decline and then rapidly become deficits as the "baby boomer" generation retires. Americans have been worrying about the depletion of Social Security funds but actually Medicare (including Medicaid) is in greater financial difficulty. These funds could be brought into balance over the next 75 years by an immediate 16% increase in payroll tax revenue or a reduction of 13% in benefits, but neither measure would be popular with the American people. To ensure that the system remains sustainable beyond 75 years will require even more substantial changes.[73]

Most Americans would like to see all citizens have access to basic health care but not everyone is enthusiastic about being forced by the government to pay for health insurance through taxes and to accept the health care the government chooses to provide. A plan put forth during the Clinton administration in 1993 failed to gain approval by congress and was not supported by the medical community nor well-understood by the average American.[74] Many people think that it may be better to fix what is wrong with the current system than to adopt universal coverage when other countries are finding such plans to be unsustainable and turning more toward a cost sharing system.[75]

Medical Outcomes: How Do Denmark and the US Compare?

The quality of health care systems based on outcomes has been difficult to calculate accurately because of differences in methods of data collection across countries. The OECD has been at work since 2001 through the Health Care Quality Indicators Project to correct this problem.[76] One measure that has been frequently used, in spite of inherent inaccuracies, is life expectancy. Between 1970 and 1996, life expectancy increased in all 15 nations of the European Union and Norway, but Denmark ranked last in its increase, improving the average lifespan by only 2.0 years (to 72.8 years) for males and 2.1 years (to 78.0 years) for females. In comparison, Norway's life expectancy increased by 4.4 years for men and 3.6 years for women, and Sweden's increased 4.3 years for men and 4.4 years for women.[77]

Although part of the difference in increase could be attributed to Denmark's relatively high life expectancies in 1970 — it's hard to show a gain when you are near the top of the list — this concerned the Danish Ministry of Health and they convened a Life Expectancy Committee

(LEC) to uncover the causes of Denmark's relatively poorer gain. The LEC found that Denmark experienced an inordinate amount of "excess mortality," or premature deaths before age 65, largely as a result of high rates of cancers (predominantly lung, breast, and gastrointestinal), cardiovascular diseases, bronchitis, accidents, suicide, and infant mortality. Over the ensuing years, programs were aimed at lifestyle changes to improve these statistics, particularly at smoking cessation and alcohol use.[78]

According to official US longevity statistics, in 1970 overall life expectancy at birth was 70.9 years.[79] By 1995, using OECD data, total life expectancy in the US was 75.7 years. The most recent OECD total life expectancy figures available for Denmark and the US are almost identical: Denmark 77.6; US 77.5. Neither country can claim distinction as a world leader in life expectancy. The top spot now belongs to Japan.

Life Expectancy at Birth in Years

	Denmark			United States			Japan		
	Male	Female	Total	Male	Female	Total	Male	Female	Total
1995	72.7	77.8	75.3	72.5	78.9	75.7	76.4	82.9	79.6
2004	75.2	79.9	77.6	74.8	80.1	77.5	78.6	85.6	82.1

OECD in Figures OECD Observer 2006/Supplement 1[80]

A Final Comparison

The health care systems in the US and Denmark share the problems of an aging population, rising health care costs, and a shrinking workforce. Satisfaction with the universal health care system in Denmark has suffered some erosion caused by long waits, nursing shortages, and increasing out-of-pocket expenses but the Danish people remain largely satisfied with the health care they get.[81]

While in the US we tend to think that most European countries enjoy total government-provided health care, in fact most countries have found their universal health coverage increasingly unsustainable and have gradually moved to a system shared between public and private payment. No health care system can serve every citizen completely equally. Both Danish and US residents in rural areas have less access to specialists, x-ray facilities, and other specialized care inspite of government efforts. Although the Danish system ensures access to basic care with the assignment of GPs to specific geographical areas, Danes are still dependent on the gatekeeper function of the GPs to move on to a higher level of specialist care. As we see in the case of Jacob (In the Same Boat),[82] this role was only circumvented when his mother obtained the help of a cardiologist friend to make use of a special medical-legal directive that resulted in his being seen by a specialist in a tertiary care hospital and immediately placed on the heart transplant list.

Students in the US-EU-MEE program wrote thoughtful comparisons of the health care systems of Denmark and the United States. Jacob Thyssen, Danish student, and colleagues, summarized many of their thoughts in the published paper, USEUMEE — A comparison of the Danish and American health care systems.[83] He writes, "All students believed the American system was modern, ambitious, and well-functioning for insured or wealthy people, whereas the Danish system tended to be fair, with free and equal access, but also economically and technically under-prioritized. They (the students) preferred a health care system with components from both nations — more resourceful than the Danish, but less expensive than the American."

Many people would agree that neither health care system is ideal but each reflects the culture, history, and politics of its own country and each is continually striving to meet the needs of its citizens with the resources available.

Acknowledgments

We gratefully acknowledge the contribution of the work of US-EU-MEE students Brian Chan, Peter Chin, Anne-Marie Dogonowski, Jon Duke, Quentin Eichbaum, Diana Feldman, Robert Garza, Douglas Krakower, and Jacob Thyssen in the preparation of this chapter.

We are also grateful for advice and encouragement from Michael Dall, M.D., Board Member & Chairman of the Danish Medical Association Research and Education Committee and to Marianne Rex Sørensen of the Danish Medical Association for a final reading of the Denmark chapter.

2

Cases Written by US Students in Denmark

Case 1: A Foreigner with Tuberculosis*

Brian Chan

Hacim's Story

Hacim's night had been going well. Just like any other 21-year-old in Copenhagen, he was out at the bars with his friends, enjoying some drinks. And like many other youths in Denmark, he was never without his trusty pack of cigarettes. Trouble is, for the last six months, the cigarettes had been giving him a nasty cough, or so he surmised. He had been thinking about cutting down. "I'm a little young to be getting smokers' lung," he thought. But maybe… he would start cutting down tomorrow.

He took another drag off his Marlboro and brought his beer to his lips. Then he coughed. And coughed again.

He couldn't stop coughing.

And then he noticed a trickle of red extending from the head of the beer to the rim of the glass at his lips.

A saltiness filled his mouth, and he began to spit bright red into a napkin. "Am I vomiting blood?" he asked himself. His mind began to swim. He was almost never sick, but this truly frightened him.

The next day, he paid a visit to a person he hadn't seen for years — not since he had broken his arm playing football. It was his general

---

*This case study was written by Brian Chan when he was a student at Harvard Medical School and participated in the US-EU-MEE exchange at the University of Copenhagen, Denmark, in the spring of 2003.

practitioner (GP), Dr. Ericson. She had been taking care of him and his entire family as long as he could remember, and had done a great job for them ever since Hacim's father and mother had moved to a working-class neighborhood in Copenhagen from their native Macedonia more than twenty years ago. Dr. Ericson was there for Hacim and his brother since their births, helping them grow into healthy young Danes. But being the seemingly healthy young man that he now was, he hadn't been to see her in a while. "I'm always afraid to go the doctor, because they might tell you you're dying or something," laughs Hacim. "Why not enjoy your last few months?"

Dr. Ericson greeted Hacim warmly, but noting his worried expression, told him to sit down and tell his story. Hacim recounted his six months of coughing, how his coughing was worse in the morning, and how the powerful fits of coughing in the shower made his chest hurt. And, of course, he described the blood. She asked about weight loss, and yes, he had lost about five kilograms, which on his thin frame seemed rather significant. She brought out her stethoscope and listened intently to his chest.

Calmly, Dr. Ericson removed the stethoscope from her ears, looked directly at Hacim and said, "Tuberculosis."

"Tuberculosis?" thought Hacim when he heard her say this. The only thing he knew about tuberculosis was that it was pretty uncommon in Denmark. "Where could I have gotten tuberculosis?"

Immediately, Hacim's mind raced back to London, where he had spent a year studying and from where he had returned just three months ago. He thought of the unkempt, odoriferous, and perpetually hacking Brazilian student with whom he had lived for two weeks before deciding he would go crazy if he did not move. Realizing that his roommate may have left him an unwanted souvenir of their time together, Hacim swore at him (in his mind).

With this potential source of infection, Dr. Ericson was confident that Hacim had TB. But, if this were the case, she herself would not be the one to make the final diagnosis or treat him. She drafted a referral form for Hacim to be seen at Gentofte Hospital.

Gentofte Amtssygehus (*Amtssygehus* means "county hospital") resembles a country villa more than a health care facility, as it is a sprawling, low-rise building complete with meticulously groomed gardens, set in the pleasant northern suburb of Hellerup. Gentofte serves as the primary TB hospital in the county, which includes Copenhagen. All TB cases in the area are referred to doctors at Gentofte, although there is also a clinic in the southern half of the county affiliated with the team in Gentofte that can also evaluate patients who potentially have TB.

After a General Practitioner (GP) or a doctor at an outside hospital has suspected TB and made a referral, everything starts and ends at Gentofte: initial evaluation, diagnostic studies, and most importantly, follow-up. There are some exceptions, notably patients with extrapulmonary TB or patients with coexisting HIV infection, although the latter will often be sent to Gentofte after a few days of initial therapy. One reason for the exception is that doctors-in-training at the main university hospital need experience treating patients with TB.

It was a little over a week after his appointment with Dr. Ericson that Hacim found himself at Gentofte. There is no wait to see a doctor if you have TB, unlike the wait for other specialists, which can take months. After checking in with the *Lungemedicinsk* (pulmonary medicine) nurses, Hacim went to the radiology department and got "scanned," that is, he underwent a chest x-ray.

After being handed his x-ray, Hacim returned to the *Lungemedicinsk* floor where he first met Dr. Axel Kok-Jensen. Although you would never hear it from his own lips, Dr. Kok-Jensen has been called "Mr. Tuberculosis" or "Dr. Tuberculosis" by more than one of his colleagues. His expertise is unquestioned, as calls from doctors around the country seeking advice on their own TB patients stream into his office every day. His devotion to his patients and to the goal of eradicating TB in Denmark is legendary and he puts in extra hours every week at the hospital as well as, on occasion, his own vacation time. Perhaps most importantly, his warm "bedside manner" and his ability to relate to his patients regardless of social status have allowed him to reach even the most difficult patients.

Hacim's x-ray revealed white fluffs of infiltrate and a thick ring with a pool of fluid — a cavitation with an air-fluid level — obscuring in his lungs what should have been a dark sky with only light wisps. One look at this x-ray told Kok-Jensen that Dr. Ericson's hunch was almost certainly correct. Dr. Kok-Jensen does not typically perform a physical examination on his patients, as he feels that what he hears in the stethoscope does not correlate well with actual disease. Hacim was no exception.

Hearing that he indeed had tuberculosis, Hacim's stomach flipped. On the outside, he maintained his strong and confident demeanor, although Dr. Kok-Jensen was aware that he was shocked. "He thought there was nothing wrong with him, so when he found out, it was a bit overwhelming."

Hacim still was not sure what it meant to have TB. What was his prognosis? Dr. Kok-Jensen reassured him, saying that 99.5% of patients like Hacim would fully recover. On the other hand, Kok-Jensen was careful to spare Hacim the information that if he had waited another one to two months to seek treatment, the damage to his lungs would likely have been permanent.

Armed with Hacim's history and x-ray, Dr. Kok-Jensen decided to prescribe the standard four-drug regimen of isoniazid, pyrazinamide, ethambutol, and rifampin. Dr. Kok-Jensen gave him his first supply of medicines right there at the hospital, as it is the hospital and not pharmacies that are responsible for distributing TB drugs. Luckily, TB drugs, like HIV drugs, have been prioritized by the government and were thus completely free for Hacim. (On the other hand, other important drugs, including cancer chemotherapy medications, do not enjoy such status.)

Fortunately, Hacim did not warrant an inpatient admission. Not only was he not sick enough, but he had a stable social situation and seemed able and willing to take his medications. Dr. Kok-Jensen handed him a kit so he could collect his own sputum samples at home and send them directly to the Statens Serum Institut, where smears and cultures would be made to identify the tuberculosis bacilli.

Before he left, Dr. Kok-Jensen had one more item of business to discuss: blood tests. He wanted a complete blood count (CBC), liver function tests (LFTs), C-reactive protein and an HIV test. "I want you to get it, not because I think you have it, or are at a high risk, but just to have it and say that it is negative," he explained. Hacim consented, and was told he would have the results at his next visit, in one week. In the meantime, Hacim was to take two weeks off from work.

After finishing up with Dr. Kok-Jensen, Hacim went next door to Grete Hansen's office. Hansen is the county's TB nurse, whose responsibility it is to locate and to perform the initial assessment of family members and colleagues of TB patients who may be infected. Hacim explained that he lived with his parents and his brother, and worked in a large room with twenty or so individuals in a telephone company. Hansen jotted down the contact information for Hacim's home and workplace. Hacim would have to tell his family and friends to come in to Gentofte to get tested for exposure to TB and possibly take prophylactic medication in case of exposure. Because there were so many co-workers with whom Hacim was in contact, she would go down to the office in a few weeks and test everyone there. In the meantime, Hacim would need to tell his family, his friends, and his co-workers about his diagnosis and their need to be evaluated medically.

Thus, not only was Hacim in shock about his diagnosis, but now he knew that he would have to tell all his close friends and acquaintances about it, too. When he got the information, it was a bit too much. There were ten to fifteen minutes when he could not figure out in his mind what it meant for his life. All Hacim could think was, "How will my friends and family react to me?"

Over the next two weeks, Hacim came to know Gentofte quite well, as day after day, he brought in his family and friends — fifty in all — to undergo testing for exposure to TB. A large percentage of them showed signs of exposure without actual disease, and were thus started on nine-month prophylactic therapy. Hacim's cousin was the only one unlucky enough to show signs of TB disease, and thus received the same drug regimen as Hacim. "My cousin was one of the last ones to take the test. It was like a formality for him," explains Hacim. "But when he showed up, he had a cough, and he had TB."

As for Hacim himself, as he puts it, the medications were "like magic pills." Nearly immediately, Hacim's coughing slowed in frequency, and eventually ceased. As an added bonus, this meant he could continue smoking all he wanted. At his one-week follow-up appointment, he looked much healthier. He reported no side effects from the medications aside from some barely perceptible, pinpoint spots on his forehead and the brief shock of seeing his urine turn red (a common side effect of rifampin).

After his two week "forced holiday," Hacim returned to work feeling apprehensive about how his co-workers would react. "Some of them were looking at me, like, hey, who is this guy and why does he have this disease? What's wrong with him?" recalls Hacim. "But I'm not very touchy, it didn't affect me too much. I'm not going to feel bad for anyone. What about me?"

Indeed, the most distressing part of his co-workers' reactions was that the young women were no longer flirting with him. Much of their fear had to do with their lack of knowledge about tuberculosis. As difficult as this time was, this ignorance became a source of some amusement for Hacim. "My friends didn't know what was wrong with me. So they thought I was dying," says Hacim. "They would not know how to say it. And then finally they would say, 'Are you dying Hacim?' And I would laugh and say, "No, I am all right." Throughout this time, his closest friends and family were supportive, helping to buffer the few, more distant acquaintances who regarded him with some distrust and resentment.

Hacim settled back into a more-or-less normal work and social life. He had been at work for about a week when Grete Hansen, the TB nurse, came to his workplace for her scheduled TB screening for forty or so of his co-workers. Hansen's day is frequently spent on the road, administering PPD tests (Purified Protein Derivative — a TB skin test) and fielding questions. It is not uncommon to spot her in local pubs or in Christiania (a ramshackle but quaint squatters' village set amidst Copenhagen's canals) — anywhere TB patients have frequented. Hansen also reports to the doctors at Gentofte as well as the public health authorities, and receives reports from other health care facilities.

Another crucial responsibility of Hansen's is to help out the staff on the inpatient ward if they are having a problem with the TB patients, such as abusiveness or other threatening behavior. "I try to make the patients relax. I 'nurse' them a little," says Hansen. "I know a little more about their daily behavior than the nurses who work in the department."

This skill at relaxing and reassuring the nervous and squeamish came in handy on this particular day. Many of Hacim's coworkers were brimming with questions. Some of these questions concerned their prior inoculation with the bacilli Calmette-Guérin (BCG) vaccine and whether that would affect the test. Fortunately, at this time, none of them had any worrisome symptoms. Hansen deftly reassured the nervous and squeamish and planted the PPD tests that would, in three days, reveal whether they showed signs of TB infection.

When Hansen returned after three days, many of Hacim's co-workers frowned nervously. Some of them had been anxiously looking at their arms for some sign that they had been unlucky. Some of them had indeed noticed a red bump where Hansen had injected them. Still others were unhappy because they thought she was going to give them another shot. However, after all of the workers had been assessed, only three of them had indurations of a size significant enough to warrant further investigation. For these three individuals, Hansen explained the meaning of the positive test, and advised them to make an appointment for an x-ray and examination at Gentofte.

Still, one of the unlucky three was so nervous at the thought of his positive test that he left work and made an appointment to be seen that day. Dr. Kok-Jensen was able to accommodate him in his schedule. His chest x-ray seemed to show no disease, but Dr. Kok-Jensen started him on prophylactic therapy. The patient left apparently reassured that his health would be preserved.

Hacim's next appointment at Gentofte was one month after beginning therapy. He was feeling great, taking his medicines religiously, and having no complaints. Dr. Kok-Jensen informed Hacim that the sputum cultures he had initially produced were shown by the Statens Serum Institut to be positive for TB, as they had all expected. Now, it would be up to Hacim to produce monthly sputum cultures until they were negative, a sign of successful treatment.

Looking back, Hacim is still quite bitter toward his ex-roommate ("that motherf***er gave me TB,") but, on the other hand, is worried that this individual might not be getting adequate care in Brazil and "maybe he will get worse and die." Hacim is thankful he is in Denmark, where his care has been excellent, in his opinion. He has received effective medical care without much wait. Hacim appreciates the medical staff's "easy-going" and warm nature, which helped to calm him when he was feeling distressed.

Moreover, Hacim feels that the quality of care he experienced was not affected by his status as a "foreigner." Hacim is quite aware that many native Danes might look at him as foreign despite his being born in Denmark. He recounts stories of customers speaking with him on the phone, and then sounding shocked and "acting different" when he tells them his foreign-sounding name. He also feels that his father and espe-cially his mother, who wears a Muslim headscarf, have been subjected to discrimination. Anti-foreign bias increased when the right-wing Danish Peoples' Party joined the ruling coalition in Parliament, according to Hacim. Even some people whom he considers family friends will say things that exacerbate Hacim's sense of marginalization. "Some people will say to me, you're the good ones, the other foreigners should go," he elaborates.

Hacim believes that in every aspect of society, including the health care sector, some people will always treat people like him differently. In this most recent encounter with the health system, however, Hacim feels that this was not the case. "I think for doctors, most of the time, a life is a life," states Hacim. This is especially true compared to his perception of health care in Macedonia, where "it is all corruption over there. Only the high society can get good care. But here, you do not have to pay to get good health care."

Overall, then, Hacim's experiences with the Danish health system have been very positive. He will continue to follow-up with the staff at Gentofte until his six months of treatment are completed. But, the worst seems to be behind him, and he looks forward to a complete recovery.

Tuberculosis Detection and Treatment in Denmark

As was the case with Hacim, a non-acute patient with tuberculosis will usually access the Danish medical system first through his general practi-tioner (GP). Depending on symptoms, patients can be sent to a private x-ray clinic (e.g. a radiologist) who will look at the x-ray and determine if they need treatment. This is free of charge for Danes, but these private clinics are only in Copenhagen. Otherwise, patients must go to the hospi-tal for the x-ray; frequently, there is a wait and the hospital will call the patient to schedule the session.

In Denmark, three sputum samples are required from patients with suspected pulmonary TB (one sample for those with suspected extrapul-monary TB). This compares to the six samples often obtained in the United States. Dr. Kok-Jensen recognizes that the American custom will result in fewer missed positive samples, as on occasion it takes five or six samples to obtain a positive result. However, he wonders, "How much do you have to pay for your positive results?" The cost-benefit analysis in the Danish system, therefore, has been deemed to argue against the extra samples. This is especially true given that hospitals are charged more by the Statens Serum Institut for positive samples than they are for negative samples, because of the extra work involved with positive samples.

If TB is suspected clinically, Dr. Kok-Jensen will go ahead and treat, even while diagnostic studies are pending. His philosophy regarding when to treat patients is clear: "I would rather treat a few patients too many, than too few. If you wait, then more damage is done to the patient and to others." In other words, treating a non-infected patient with TB is relatively harmless compared to the danger of not treating an infected patient. He has a vivid anecdote supporting his contention. "We had a patient. He was a Greenlander, he was an alcoholic, he was a vagrant," he explains. "It looked like he had TB. But three months, six months, the x-ray didn't change. After three-fourths of a year, they stopped treating him. Then after another two years, he had really bad TB. He had also infected a child, who ended up with TB meningitis. [The original patient] eventually was cured, but the lung damage was done... he was a lung invalid, and he eventually died from this. He should have been treated when it looked like TB. He should have had another culture. He should have been followed up for two to three years."

If a patient is thought to have TB, he is started on standard drug therapy, after having been advised of possible side effects and having had routine blood cultures sent (to monitor for these side effects, which include kidney and liver damage). The patient is told to return in one week, provided that he or she does not require admission to a hospital and is advised not to return to work for two weeks, although Dr. Kok-Jensen admits that such a precaution is probably more for the coworkers' peace of mind rather than an actual great risk of transmission because the patient will already be receiving therapy and therefore will be less infectious. The patient is also asked to inform the workplace (or have the medical authorities do so), although the patient cannot be asked to do so against his will.

Treatment with the standard drug regimen is maintained for at least three weeks, at which point results of sensitivity testing from the Statens Serum Institut should have returned. Overall, the rate of drug resistance in

Denmark is similar to other developed nations. According to Dr. Kok-Jensen, about ten to twenty percent of cases will be "looked at again" based on results from the sensitivity testing, with a smaller percentage actually having a change in treatment because of drug resistance.

To declare the treatment a success, two negative sputum cultures are needed, with one sputum sample taken monthly until a negative result is obtained, and one at the end of six months of treatment as a final check. Notably absent from the Danish approach to TB is the right of doctors to forcibly admit and treat intransigent but psychologically competent patients — a testament to Danish attitudes regarding individual rights. Instead, medical authorities must use other means — including creativity — to assure compliance. "It is understandable that people have problems taking so many pills for so many months," says Kok-Jensen. "We have to figure out how to make patients take them. If someone goes to a bar every-day, then we'll go to the barkeeper and give him the pills so the patient can remember to take them everyday."

Immigrants and Refugees: A Challenge to the Danish Public Health System

Not surprisingly, as a highly developed nation with a sophisticated med-ical system, Denmark has been and remains a country with a low incidence of tuberculosis. However, the incidence rose in the late 1990s with the arrival of Somali refugees, who come from a land with a very high incidence of TB. (Lillebaek *et al.* 2001). As much as two-thirds of all tuberculosis patients in Denmark are immigrants, half of whom are from Somalia (Lillebaek *et al.* 2002). The Somali population in Denmark has a one to two percent overall incidence rate, far higher than native Danes.

Refugees or asylum seekers are encouraged but not forced to undergo a medical exam (which is not specific for TB) at the time of arrival. Other immigrants need not undergo a complete exam but may access the med-ical system as needed. The lack of tests upon arrival to Denmark reflects the nation's emphasis on individual rights, i.e. the right not to be forced to undergo a medical exam. The irony of this stance, however, is that rather than force a medical exam upon immigrants and refugees, Denmark now just keeps them out as immigration and asylum policies have become much more restrictive in the last several years.

Even when able to reach out to Somalis, doctors encountered another problem. "We couldn't convince many of the Somalis to take medicine if they felt healthy," explains Kok-Jensen. "And those who did, when they came back to their communities, everyone would avoid them because they had TB. So they would stop taking the medicine and take off their masks."

In addition to problems in the outpatient setting, the health system inadequately addresses language and cultural barriers that hinder inpatient health care delivery to the foreign-born, according to Grete Hansen. "It is a very big problem, especially with the Somalian patients who are often not good at the Danish language," explains Hansen. "We can do better with the translators, for example. The first time they are admitted, they need a translator. When they are discharged, they also need a translator so they understand the treatment and when to come back. This does not always happen."

Hansen also believes the hospitals need to expand their limited supply of patient education materials written in foreign languages. "We need a paper that explains what is it like to be in a Danish hospital. What is your behavior, what are we expecting of you, what is your routine on the wards." Hansen feels that this would help stop the commonly-held perception of foreign patients as stubborn: "I think many of the problems we have are just misunderstandings."

A professor in the Department of International Health at Copenhagen University sees the plight of immigrants and refugees with TB as one of the most striking examples of continued inequity in the health system. "How could they move the TB hospital from here (Rigshospitalet, the university hospital in central Copenhagen) to Gentofte, where there are no Somalis, and one of the richest areas in Denmark?" he asks, "We are not as equal as we need to be. It is a scandal. They are not doing screening of immigrants. The case finding is not sufficient. Where is the health education for the minority groups? We wonder why Somalis do not present to the doctor. It is because it is worse than anything else to have TB. It is a stigmatizing disease. And now it is worse because we have AIDS on top of it." He also wonders why Denmark has seen improvements in TB control among populations such as drug addicts by implementing steps such as roving street nurses, but has not done the same for foreigners.

Epidemiology of Tuberculosis in Denmark

In light of decreasing incidence of TB, Kok-Jensen questions whether Directly Observed Treatment Short-course therapy (DOTS) would be appropriate in Denmark. "In New York, they were having a big problem with tuberculosis, and the system was in disorder," he states. "They began to implement DOTS, and they saw reductions in the rates of tuberculosis. And they said, 'Look, DOTS works.' But at the same time, there were many other improvements to the system, correcting a lot of things that had been done wrong. So I think it's not clear that DOTS was the only reason that New York had success."

Kok-Jensen defends the current Danish system. "They say DOTS is cost-effective, and I guess over there [in the United States] they are supposed to directly observe all people taking their medicine, especially in the intensive stages, the first two months. But here, I don't think it would be any better than what we are doing now. Right now, we might be having a one, two percent failure rate. When you look at the total number of people we diagnose with TB, that's one or two people out of a hundred, so we're not really affecting the rate of infection in the whole population. Because that's the point of DOTS, not so much treating the patient, but preventing spread to other people."

There are other concerns in the Danish health care system that affect the treatment of TB as well as other public health problems. While the government struggles to maintain the bottom line, facilities are sometimes closed or moved to other locations. Several years ago cost cutting eliminated the social worker at Gentofte who used to work exclusively with the hospital causing them to rely on a regional social worker for their TB patients.

According to Kok-Jensen, the situation continues to get tighter: "The budget given for routine care decreases every year even though the budget is going up overall because of expensive treatments and equipment." He has another theory regarding the money woes. "Much of the deficit is from the waiting line," he explains. "Patients have the right to go to other hospitals, and we have to pay for that. We have a deficit, and they want to cut our budget further. So the wait will be worse."

The cost pressures are causing strain especially among the nurses and the support staff. "People are angry," says Grete Hansen. "There is bad communication between the nurse-in-charge, the doctors in the administration and the nurses. We know we have to save money, but they will just send us a letter saying, 'No more appointments on Thursday.' Then we have so much work, we have to call all the patients and cancel their appointments, and they have been waiting a long time. And we know that if they are closing that clinic today, they may close our hospital in six months."

Meanwhile, one of the wards at Gentofte is cutting the number of beds because of a shortage of nurses. "They have been hiring outside nurses at a higher price. There is less money for the public nurses, so we are making things harder for the public nurses," says Kok-Jensen.

Grete Hansen echoes these sentiments, and feels that they are representative of nursing in Denmark in general: "Nurses here are underpaid compared to their responsibility, compared to other kinds of jobs and compared to the private sector. If it was a private company, we would have been paid a lot more." Hansen also points to an increase in paperwork and administration (a response to concerns over medical errors), which she believes is taking valuable time away from patient contact. She also notes that patients are becoming more demanding, which she attributes to improved patient knowledge, including use of the Internet, causing what little patient time nurses have to be harried and unpleasant. Further, as the patients in Danish hospitals have become, in general, older and sicker than in years past, the work has become harder for nurses.

The combination of low pay and high workload has contributed to a worsening nursing shortage. According to Hansen, nursing schools are increasingly unable to fill available spots, and those students who attend drop out nearly half of the time. She also feels that those students who stay often have their eye not on "traditional" nursing on the wards but on more lucrative positions such as nurse practitioner practice.

Hansen feels that the government has not done enough to rectify the situation. "The government does some advertising to tell us how great the job is, but they're not raising payment," Hansen states. "There are other groups getting similar payments — teachers, police — who would also want more payment."

The Danish system prides itself on providing quality health care for all Danes. Although Hacim has some lingering suspicions about some native Danes' feelings toward foreigners, he does not feel that health care providers in general, and those who administered to him in this particular episode, have treated him differently because of his ethnicity. Perceptions of the public system as being of high quality have been demonstrated by high satisfaction ratings on surveys and low utilization of private hospitals. This may change, however, if the public system continues to suffer from long waits, nursing shortages, and other problems that force consumers toward the private system.

The issue of how to control costs while maintaining high quality universal care without forcing an increase in taxation is the salient issue facing the Danish health system. Viewing the health system through Hacim's experiences helps to elucidate some of the system's most attractive features and serious challenges. How the Danish system responds to these challenges will greatly determine the future health and wellbeing of millions of patients like Hacim.

References

Cegielski JP *et al*. The global tuberculosis situation. *Infectious Disease Clinics of North America* 16(1): 2002.

The Copenhagen Post. In brief: Lung clinic closure. Page 5. May 23, 2003.

Dragsted UB *et al*. Epidemiology of tuberculosis in HIV-infected patients in Denmark. *Scand J Infect Dis* 31(1):57–61, 1999.

Lillebaek T *et al*. Persistent high incidence of tuberculosis in immigrants in a low-incidence country. *Emerg Infect Dis* 8(7):679–684, 2002.

Lillebaek T *et al*. Risk of *Mycobacterium tuberculosis* transmission in a low-incidence country due to immigration from high-incidence areas. *J Clin Microbiol* 39(3): 855–861, 2001.

Ministry of the Interior and Health. *Health Care in Denmark*, 2002.

Ministry of the Interior and Health. *Municipalities and Counties in Denmark — Tasks and Finance*, 2002.

Rigshospitalet website: www.rigshospitalet.dk.

Rosdahl N. Denmark: concerned and yet content with itself. *Euro Observer* 3(1): 7–8, 2001.

Thomsen VO *et al*. Results from 8 yrs of susceptibility testing of clinical *Mycobacterium tuberculosis* isolates in Denmark. *Eur Respir J* 16(2):203–8, 2000.

Vallgarda S, Krasnik A, Vrangbæk K. Health Care Systems in Transition: Denmark. Copenhagen: *European Observatory on Health Care Systems*, 2001.

World Health Organization. The Global Plan to Stop Tuberculosis. Geneva: WHO, 2002.

UN Millenium Development Goal Indicators website: mdgs.un.org/unsd/mdg.

Case 2: The Silent Killer*

Douglas Krakower

Kirsten Anderson

Kirsten Anderson is a 64-year-old, generally healthy Danish woman with newly diagnosed hypertension. I was happy to have Kirsten as "my case" for several reasons. First, the way she discovered she had hypertension is quite typical for Denmark and the United States — on a routine blood pressure check at a general practitioner's office — and the story of her diagnosis will be familiar to many adults in both nations. Second, her hypertension was sufficiently severe to bring her into contact with the most highly specialized and technically advanced care for hypertension in Denmark, allowing for comparisons at the "cutting edge" of medicine between Denmark and the United States. Third, her willingness to have a medical student accompany her in all aspects of her medical care for a period of one month allowed me to have a comprehensive look at her initial journey through the diagnosis and management of her illness. Finally, Kirsten's impressive command of English and cooperative, charming personality ensured fluid communication between us throughout our partnership.

---

*Douglas Krakower wrote this case when he was a student at Harvard Medical School and participated in the US-EU-MEE medical student exchange at the University of Copenhagen, Denmark in the spring of 2004.

Prior to her diagnosis of hypertension, Kirsten had been in general good health. Her only active medical condition was mild psoriasis. In the distant past, she had been diagnosed with cancer of her jawbone (~40 years ago), which was successfully managed with oral and reconstructive surgery, and a self-limited thyroid infection (~20 years ago). She had been to general practitioners now and then for minor illnesses over the past 20 years, but had not been admitted to the hospital or needed any kind of specialty care throughout that time. She took no medicines on a regular basis.

Even though Kirsten had smoked at least a pack of cigarettes per day for many years (with periods of 3 packs per day), she had no smoking-related health problems, as far as she knew. Her diet was typically Danish, with some recent efforts to reduce her intake of fats and sweets. Exercise consisted of daily walks around her neighborhood or in a nearby park, but no dedicated aerobic activity. To the best of her knowledge, her family history was significant only for thyroid infections, as two of her sisters had experienced episodes of thyroid dysfunction similar to Kirsten's. Looking at family portraits of her mother and grandmother, Kirsten thought they may have had osteoporosis. She was unaware of any family history of hypertension.

Kirsten's only knowledge of her own blood pressure was that it had been normal — "something close to 120/80" — at her last blood pressure measurement, which was around ten years ago. Needless to say, when it comes to blood pressure, a lot can change in ten years, as I soon found out.

Attack!

Given her past good health, Kirsten was surprised by a sudden "attack" of pain in the right side of her abdomen on an otherwise unremarkable evening in November 2003. She had never experienced this type of pain before, and had no idea what it could mean. Although she had lived in Copenhagen for five years, she had not visited a doctor or established contact with a general practitioner in the area, so she telephoned "the mobile doctor service," a service that provides medical house calls as needed.

After two hours, a doctor arrived at her apartment to examine her. The doctor was uncertain as to the cause of the pain, but did not think it was anything of immediate, life-threatening concern, such as appendicitis or other surgical emergency. He offered Kirsten two pills to help reduce the pain, and advised her to seek care from a general practitioner in the morning. When the morning came, enough pain remained to merit a second call to the mobile doctors. A different doctor was on duty, and he offered a similar assessment and treatment plan — take two pills for the pain and see a general practitioner if the pain continues to be bothersome — the Danish equivalent of the familiar "take two aspirins and call me in the morning." However, by that afternoon, the pain had improved dramatically, so Kirsten did not seek further care that day.

Two weeks later, Kirsten decided to contact a general practitioner to search for an answer to the cause of her attack and to establish a relationship with a local doctor. Based on recommendations from friends, Kirsten selected Dr. Anja Larsen, a general practitioner in her neighborhood. Kirsten described Dr. Larsen as a "thorough, kind, and somewhat formal woman" and "more inspiring of confidence than my past general practitioners."

Dr. Larsen began the first office visit by asking Kirsten about the events surrounding the attack of pain. The details Kirsten could offer did not suggest a clear cause for the attack, so Dr. Larsen proceeded to perform a basic physical exam, including a blood pressure measurement, as a starting point for her medical assessment. Dr. Larsen checked the blood pressure by auscultation and recorded a pressure that was markedly elevated at 190/110, with 120/80 or lower considered normal. The remainder of the physical exam was normal as far as Kirsten recalls.

The mysterious attack and the elevated blood pressure prompted Dr. Larsen to pursue two lines of investigation. First, she ordered an abdominal and renal ultrasound to search for any gross pathology that could have precipitated the attack. Both test results were normal. Second, she planned to have Kirsten monitor her blood pressure at home for eight days with an automatic sphygmomanometer, the technical term for a blood pressure cuff, to characterize the daily pattern and extremes of her blood pressure. Unfortunately, both of Dr. Larsen's home monitors were in use by other patients, and Kirsten had to wait for more than a month, until the beginning of February, before she could begin her home measurements.

"The long wait is typical of the backslide in Danish healthcare," Kirsten complained. "Over the past decades, the wait has become longer and longer for so many aspects of healthcare here." When Kirsten finally obtained one of the two measuring devices, she began a detailed home measurement protocol recommended by Dr. Larsen. The protocol lasted eight days. For the first seven days, she measured her blood pressure three times a day, morning, midday, and evening, with duplicate measurements each time, and with 10 minutes of rest before each measurement. On the eighth day, she recorded her pressure every hour without resting before the measurements.

Kirsten missed several of the required measurements during the first seven days, so she continued for several extra days until she had completed seven days. The range of her home pressure measurements were as follows:

Range of Blood Pressure during 7 Days of Home Measurements (minimum-maximum systolic/minimum-maximum diastolic)	
Morning	151–196/82–108
Midday	148–199/92–112
Evening	132–192/77–121

The consistently elevated pressures confirmed that Kirsten's first blood pressure reading of 190/110 in Dr. Larsen's office was not an aberrant measurement, and that she almost certainly suffered from severe, chronic hypertension. "I suppose it started sometime in the last five or ten years, since the last time my pressure was checked," she recounted, "but I have no idea exactly how long it has been high." The only chronic symptom she noticed was occasional, self-limited dizziness over the past several months, but she could not recall any other symptoms that often are the hallmark of severe hypertension, such as headaches, fatigue, vision changes, chest pain, or shortness of breath.

Despite the lack of symptoms, because she had markedly elevated blood pressures recorded at home, Dr. Larsen recommended further testing for Kirsten to rule out rare causes of hypertension and to search for any hypertension-related organ damage. An ophthalmologist examined her eyes and found evidence of mild hypertensive changes. The remainder of the testing would take place at the Department of Clinical Physiology and Nuclear Medicine at Frederiksberg Hospital (*Frederiksberg Klinisk Fysiologisk Nuklear Medicinsk Afdelning*) in Copenhagen, one of the premier departments for hypertension-related care and research in Denmark.

At Frederiksberg Hospital, doctors performed a battery of tests preselected by Dr. Larsen to explore Kirsten's hypertension. The first exam was a 24-hour blood pressure study. Kirsten wore a computerized blood pressure monitor that recorded frequent measurements throughout a 24-hour period, allowing for an analysis of daily blood pressure patterns. The examiners concluded that she had abnormally high pressures throughout the day with a particularly high pressure while in the clinic (193/120). This is a phenomenon known as the "white coat effect," whereby patient anxiety about the medical encounter causes a temporary increase in blood pressure. The seven days of home measurements, however, proved that this was not an isolated high reading. Kirsten was diagnosed with grade II hypertension (Systolic BP 160–169, Diastolic BP 100–109), also known as moderate hypertension, as defined by the 2003 European Society of Hypertension-European Society of Cardiology guidelines for the management of hypertension.

Chronic moderate hypertension can cause end-organ damage, so Kirsten was to have additional tests in two weeks to rule out cardiac and renal abnormalities that can cause hypertension, such as vascular disease of the kidneys. She was scheduled for an echocardiogram, a doppler ultrasound analysis of heart structure and function, and a renogram, a nuclear study to measure renal function.

Kirsten's echocardiogram was within normal limits, suggesting that her heart had not yet sustained damage from her untreated hypertension. The echocardiogram involved measurements of cardiac chamber pressures, muscle wall thickness, and valve function. Any abnormal results of these tests can suggest hypertensive changes in the heart. Dr. Niels Wiinberg in the Department of Clinical Physiology at Frederiksberg Hospital supervised the renogram. For this test, a radioactive tracer was given to Kirsten intravenously at the start of the study, and images of tracer distribution throughout the vascular system were taken over the next 21 minutes. Using mathematical formulae, estimates of the glomerular filtration rate (GFR, a measure of kidney function) of each kidney can be created. Differences in the GFR between the two kidneys could indicate renovascular hypertension, a reversible cause of hypertension.

In Kirsten's case, however, the renogram was also reassuring. No evidence of significant kidney damage was detected, indicating a low probability of a renal cause for her high blood pressure. The study was interpreted as "low likelihood of renovascular hypertension," suggesting an alternate cause of her hypertension, most likely essential hypertension. Overall, her studies indicated that she had essential hypertension, or hypertension with no identifiable cause, the most common type of hypertension in the world.

Seven days after the echocardiogram and renography, Dr. Larsen received the test results and called Kirsten to make an appointment to review them. She explained that the normal results suggested that the hypertension had not yet caused any damage to her organs. Dr. Larsen used the remainder of the 20-minute visit to educate Kirsten on a heart-healthy diet that could decrease her risk of future cardiovascular disease. To limit excessive fat and caloric intake, the low-fat diet would allow her only 10 grams of fat per day. Dr. Larsen reviewed a reference chart of the fat and calorie content for common foods in the Danish diet and gave Kirsten a copy to take home. Other recommendations included losing at least 2–5 kilograms of weight and quitting smoking. Kirsten remarked to her doctor that she had lost 2.5 kilos since her first bout of abdominal pain, but would try to lose more.

When Dr. Larsen began her discussion of anti-hypertensive medications, she asked me which medicine I would choose for Kirsten. I thought that there were several reasonable first-line therapies, including thiazide diuretics, calcium channel blockers, beta-blockers, ACE inhibitors, and angiotensin-II receptor blockers (ARBs). However, I was aware that a recent, widely cited study in the United States suggested that thiazides were as effective as other medicines and were much less costly, and should therefore be first-line therapy in most patients.

Dr. Larsen asked me if I had ever taken a thiazide or a beta-blocker, which I had not. She retorted, "Well I have, and they are terrible. The side effects are not worth the cost savings in my mind, and I always start with an angiotensin-II receptor blocker (ARB) unless a patient tells me that they cannot afford it. They have almost no side effects, and they work very well." She prescribed an ARB called Diovan (valsartan is the generic name), 80 milligrams once daily, and booked a follow-up visit with Kirsten in seven days to see how she was tolerating the drug.

When I later recounted Dr. Larsen's prescribing rationale with several of the doctors at the Department of Clinical Physiology, they did not agree with either Dr. Larsen's or my approach. They thought that the widely cited United States study (known as the ALLHAT trial) should not be interpreted as a mandate to use only thiazides as first-line therapy, but rather as a reassurance that thiazides are equally as effective as the more expensive drugs. Overall, they recommended a case-by-case approach to choosing a first-line drug based on practice guidelines, medical literature, and clinician intuition. They disagreed with Dr. Larsen's approach of starting all patients on ARBs solely because of her personal experience with various drugs, and cited her approach as an example of how actual medical practice by Danish GPs and up-to-date practice guidelines often differ.

At the conclusion of Kirsten's visit, I asked Dr. Larsen for any patient-oriented literature on hypertension that she kept handy in her office. She produced a dizzying array of pamphlets in all colors, shapes and sizes. Some were posted in display boxes in her waiting room for any visitor to take, and others were kept in reserve in her office. All of the pamphlets except one were created or sponsored by pharmaceutical companies with cardiovascular drugs on the market. I did not ask Dr. Larsen how she obtained the pamphlets, but presumably, she received them from pharmaceutical representatives. I noticed that one was produced by a non-profit agency.

Directly after the visit, Kirsten and I walked to her neighborhood pharmacy, the government-affiliated *Apoteket*, and filled her Diovan prescription. The cost was 237.45 Danish kroner (DKK — approximately $39.00, using an exchange rate of 6 DKK to $1 US, 2004 calculation) for 28 pills, which would last her for 4 weeks. I asked Kirsten about the financial burden of the medicine for her, and she explained that her income left her with sufficient funds to afford the added 237 DKK per month. She also had elective, private health insurance to supplement her standard government health insurance, and thus would receive a reimbursement for part of the cost of her prescriptions. She did not know the amount of the reimbursement but guessed that it would be around 20% of the total cost. If she were unable to pay for the medicine, she thought she could consult a municipality-sponsored social worker who would evaluate her finances and possibly authorize a need-based increase in her monthly pension. Kirsten felt fortunate that she did not need to request additional funds.

Several days after she began the Diovan, I had lunch with Kirsten. She felt generally well with no major adverse effects. Already, she had altered her dietary habits according to Dr. Larsen's "very helpful" chart of the fat content of Danish foods, and I noticed that I was having much more butter on my bread than she was. She lit a cigarette in her living room after our meal and admitted that she was unprepared to reduce her smoking at this point. "One change at a time," she said. Otherwise, she feared she would become overwhelmed with new restrictions on her lifestyle. By incorporating the changes slowly and steadily over the next year, she hoped to bring her lifestyle in line with good cardiovascular health.

At Kirsten's seven-day follow-up visit with Dr. Larsen, her systolic blood pressure was still greater than 160 mmHg, so Dr. Larsen increased her prescription to 160 mg of Diovan per day. In general, the plan was for Kirsten to return periodically for blood pressure checks and medication adjustments. All the while, she should try to quit smoking and lose weight.

No further visits or significant medical events occurred for Kirsten during my time in Denmark, so the future of her condition is an open book. Like most patients with hypertension, there are few obvious signs of the damage it causes when the condition is first diagnosed, making it difficult to motivate patients to change their behaviors to protect themselves. Yet hypertension is one of the most common medical diagnoses among adults in the entire world, and has far-reaching implications on the mortality of the Danish people. Kirsten illustrates how the Danish health care system addressed this problem in one woman, but how does the system perform on the whole?

Hypertension Treatment in the Danish Health Care System

Hypertension is commonly referred to as "The Silent Killer" in medicine because it is generally a chronic, symptom-free illness, but it causes great morbidity and mortality through its effects on the cardiovascular system.

Hypertension is not a *cause celebre* in medicine or the public eye, although perhaps it should be, given its impact. Compared to diseases that garner public and media support, like cancer or AIDS, there are few, if any, charity runs or fundraising galas for hypertension. Few people would cite hypertension as the cause of a family member's death, although it lurks behind many of the common diseases that are blamed, such as heart attacks or stroke. Information on the health care delivery issues relating to hypertension is often buried within data on other diseases, and the economic and political dilemmas around hypertension are not obvious.

Hypertension is an excellent example of a disease that relies heavily on drug therapy, which brings an enormous political and economic bull into the china shop. The pharmaceutical industry, whose size and power have earned it the colorful moniker "Big Pharma," with its colossal budgets and a vested interest in increasing drug prescriptions, plays a crucial role in the relationship between patients, doctors, and the government in both Denmark and the US.

The Cost of Hypertension Management in Denmark

As hypertension is managed largely with drug therapy, out-of-pocket payment for prescriptions is relevant. Currently, (2004) the Danish government reimbursement on outpatient pharmaceuticals works according to an expenditure-based scale (Table 2.1).

Kirsten illustrates how the reimbursement scheme applies to patients. To fill her Diovan prescription, she will pay the *Apoteket* pharmacy approximately 237 DKK/month × 12 months/year = 2844 DKK/year (about $474).

Table 2.1.   Government reimbursements for outpatient pharmaceuticals (2004).

Personal Annual Drug Expenditure	Percent Reimbursement
Below 500 DKK	No reimbursement
501–1200 DKK	50%
1200–2800	75%
>2800 DKK	85%
Chronically ill patients with permanent drug needs	Can apply for full reimbursement
Low income patients	Can apply for full reimbursement

The government will reimburse her for 85% of the annual cost. However, a portion of that cost will be covered by her private insurance, although she was unsure of how much pharmaceutical coverage her plan provides.

Regardless of the insurance reimbursement, because she is paying 1000 DKK annually for the policy and she only owes 426 DKK to the *Apoteket*, she will not be able to recoup her premium costs with her Diovan insurance reimbursements, rendering the policy financially unwise for Kirsten. Of course, the calculations do not account for any other prescriptions she may need in the future for either high blood pressure or other conditions she may develop, so the insurance policy may, in the long run, be a sound investment for her.

Patients with hypertension may take a variety of routes through the health care system, depending on the severity of their hypertension and the presence of secondary complications, such as heart or kidney damage. One way to gauge costs is to follow the costs of Kirsten's diagnosis and treatment, assuming she is typical of a patient with hypertension.

The cost of the preliminary diagnosis, made during a physical exam performed by her general practitioner, was merely the cost of the medical appointment. At the Department of Clinical Physiology, her evaluation involved 24-hour blood pressure monitoring, echocardiography, and renography. These tests are used to confirm the diagnosis of hypertension, evaluate for cardiac complications of disease, and rule out renal disease as an underlying cause of her high pressures. Each of these procedures has a price that the department charges to the government (see Table 2.2). Finally, Kirsten has ongoing pharmaceutical costs from her Diovan prescription. Table 2.2 estimates the costs associated with Kirsten's care.

Table 2.2 suggests that a new diagnosis and full work-up for moderate hypertension in 2004 costs 6361 DKK, a little over $1000. Interestingly, the physiological testing she received is not standard in the United States, except in cases where unusual causes of hypertension are suspected (e.g., hypertension in young patients, or patients presenting with sudden onset of severe hypertension). With Kirsten's age and diagnosis of Stage II Hypertension, in the US, clinicians would presume that she has age-related essential hypertension and start treatment empirically. However, other tests that were not performed on Kirsten, such as baseline electrocardiograms and urine studies to look for kidney damage, would be standard for new

Table 2.2. Costs of the diagnosis and management of Kirsten's hypertension, 2004.

Service or Product	Price (DKK) charged by provider	Amount paid to provider by government	Reimbursement to Kirsten by private insurance	Amount paid by Kirsten after reimbursements
General practitioner visit	136	136	0	0
24-hour blood pressure monitoring	873	873	0	0
Echocardiography	794	794	0	0
Renography	1714	1714	0	0
Diovan prescription (annually)	2844	2417	0–426	0–426
Total (DKK):	6361	5934	0–426	0–426
Total ($US)	1060	989	0–71	0–71

hypertensive patients in the United States, though they are comparatively inexpensive.

Without Kirsten's thorough evaluation, the cost of her diagnosis would be greatly reduced, inviting an avenue for cost control. However, the cost of missing an important diagnosis like renal vascular disease may be incalculable in terms of a patient's outcomes, so the importance of sound clinical judgment in ordering tests remains clear, and Kirsten's team is certainly justified in completing her testing.

How are Costs Controlled?

The cost of pharmaceuticals is substantial. Most people who begin drug therapy for hypertension remain on the medicines for life. For example, if Kirsten lives to be 78 years old — the average female life expectancy in Denmark — her drug therapy will cost 2844 DKK per year × 14 years = 39,816 DKK = $6636, using 2004 calculations. To complicate matters further, the cost of hospitalization for hypertension-related complications — for example, if she develops heart or renal disease — is not accounted for in any of the above calculations. If the money spent on drugs prevents future hospital stays, then it will save money over the course of Kirsten's lifespan. If she ultimately spends the same number of days in the hospital over the course of her lifetime regardless of her drug therapy, then there are no financial savings associated with drug therapy.

Ironically, the longer people live after their retirement, the more expensive they become, as they draw from the medical system but no longer contribute appreciably to the gross domestic product. So each kroner spent on Diovan to keep Kirsten alive past her retirement age consumes more net kroner. Of course, the goal of healthcare is to promote longer and more enjoyable lives, not penny-pinch at the expense of the peoples' longevity, so it would not be ethically or philosophically permissible to withhold drug therapy to optimize cost efficiency for people like Kirsten.

The Politics and Economics of Patient and Physician Education

The Danish government had in the past become concerned about the overall health and declining life expectancy of its citizens. A Life Expectancy Committee (LEC) convened by the Ministry of Health recommended public education programs aimed at reducing alcohol consumption and smoking. This spoke directly to Kirsten, a longstanding smoker. She may have the best drug therapy, physiology testing, and GP follow-up, but if she continues to smoke, she will remain at high risk for premature death. The recognition of harmful behaviors like smoking as major factors in health outcomes highlights the importance of patient education and motivation in both Denmark and the US.

Education of patients and health care workers through government and industry-sponsored campaigns is commonplace in Denmark. As mentioned, in the waiting room of Kirsten's GP, there were numerous patient oriented pamphlets about hypertension. They come in all sizes and colors, and are typically full of glossy photos of attractive people. Each brochure explains the basic medical concepts involved in hypertensive disease, the importance of good blood pressure control, and how lifestyle changes and medical therapies may help. Most of them have links to Web sites where readers can learn about hypertension in detail. Pharmaceutical companies created all the brochures that I gathered at the GPs office except for one, and they all incorporated the message that drug therapy is often necessary to control blood pressure adequately.

Admittedly, many patients will need drug therapy to achieve blood pressure goals, although the official stance of the European Society of Hypertension is to emphasize lifestyle changes first in all but the most severe cases. The prevalence of hypertension makes it a high yield avenue for drug sponsored patient and physician marketing and education. The substantial economic gains at stake in the sale of anti-hypertensive medicines invite the question; can patients and physicians trust the information in these pamphlets? Caution is clearly warranted.

To assess the expertise behind these media, I investigated the authorship of several pamphlets. For example, one Pfizer sponsored pamphlet entitled *"Forhojet blodtryck* (Elevated Blood Pressure)" indicates its authorship *"Af speciallaege Bent Sterndorff* (By specialist Bent Sterndorf)." However, Bent Sterndorf's credentials are listed only as *"Dansk Medicinsk Forlag"* (Danish Medical Publishing), a group with no easily discernable medical authority or impartiality, detracting from the trustworthiness of his message.

In fairness to Pfizer, similar brochures were sponsored by Aventis, Alfred Benzon Pharma A/S, Boehringer Ingelheim, and Novartis, among others, and the one brochure from *Dansk Hypertensionsselskab* (The Danish Hypertension Society), a non-profit, government recognized organization, did not differ significantly in its format or message.

Conclusion

Denmark's health care system manages to provide quality care for every Danish citizen regardless of financial means or geographic locale, an impressive accomplishment that is conspicuously absent in the United States. Like Kirsten Anderson, every Dane with hypertension can undergo the studies and treatment that is the national standard of care. Yet the national life expectancy remains sub par compared to similar nations owing to a combination of harmful behaviors, like smoking and poor diet, and a lack of screening programs to capture diseases like hypertension early. Economically, the system is sustainable, given cost controls managed by GPs, but the specter of expensive testing and pharmaceutical influence on patients and physicians leaves the national nest egg vulnerable.

I am grateful to Kirsten for teaching me about the Danish health care system through her kindness and cooperation. I hope she stops smoking, stays on a reasonable diet, and works with her doctor to maintain safe blood pressure, all of which can be done at a very reasonable price in Denmark. That is the best way for her to improve the quantity and quality of her life. On a larger scale, I hope that her story will help me and other medical providers take a look at how we can improve the systems in both countries to optimize the health of citizens on both sides of the Atlantic.

Case 3: A Preemie in Denmark*

Peter Chin

Lise Sorensen had been pregnant for 30 weeks and a day, ten weeks shy of her due date. She beamed with excitement about the approaching birth of her first baby, a living expression of the love between her and Tim, her American boyfriend. Up to this point Lise's pregnancy had progressed smoothly thanks to a regular schedule of prenatal visits to her primary care physician and a hospital-based midwife. A uterine ultrasound performed previously at 20 weeks gestational age and laboratory tests to date revealed a healthy fetus.

On this particular day, however, Lise felt ill. She complained of fever and fatigue for nearly forty-eight hours.

She thought, "I probably have the flu. After all, it is winter."

That same morning she had seen a nurse at her district hospital, the Rigshospitalet, who said the baby was fine and she was okay too. Lise returned home reassured that she probably had a self-limiting viral infection. But that evening at approximately 6:30 she developed sudden lower abdominal pain, severe and unrelenting. She had no nausea or vomiting or other gastrointestinal symptoms; no uterine contractions as far as she could tell; no vaginal bleeding — only constant pain.

---

*Peter Chin wrote this case when he was a student at Dartmouth Medical School and participated in the US-EU-MEE program at the University of Copenhagen, Denmark in 1999.

Lise called the *lægevagten* — the after hours service — for a "night doctor" to make a house call, but she was told the waiting time would be two to three hours. She could not wait that long in so much pain. She could have called for an ambulance but didn't think she was sick enough to warrant that. She never could stand people who winced or whined at the slightest twinge. Instead Lise called for a taxi to take her to the Rigshospitalet, the University of Copenhagen teaching hospital, which also serves as the local community hospital.

Lise went directly to the Emergency Room. Because she was pregnant and in such severe pain, literally screaming at times, Lise was triaged immediately to an examination room. After a short wait and a brief history and physical, the ER staff rapidly sent her upstairs to the obstetrical floor where a uterine ultrasound revealed "placental løsning" — a partial placental abruption or detachment from the wall of the uterus. Moreover, the fetus was tachycardic; the rapid heart beat indicating circulatory compromise. This baby had to be delivered as soon as possible.

Lise underwent an emergency Caesarian section. The operating room (OR) suite on the obstetrical floor was modern, sterile, fully staffed and equipped. The surgeons worked earnestly and, as usual, pediatricians stood by in the OR to evaluate the 30 + 1 week-old preemie right away. Tine Sorensen was born at 7:55 on December 2, 1999, two and a half months before her expected arrival.

Unhappy Birthday

Tine weighed only 1660 grams at birth, about three and a half pounds. At 30 weeks gestational age she suffered from some degree of pulmonary immaturity. There had been no time to administer corticosteroids to Lise, which could have speeded up the development of the baby's lungs. To make things worse, the placental abruption had compromised Tine's cardiorespiratory status *in utero*. She was diagnosed with "*asphyxia neonatalis gravis.*" Finally, Tine was septic at birth with B-hemolytic streptococcus. Not surprisingly, the baby also had a whopping case of Respiratory Distress Syndrome (RDS) at birth. Her APGAR scores on the scale used to assess the viability of infants at birth were 3 at one minute, 3 at five minutes, and 3 at ten minutes on a scale of 1–10. Lise got only a quick look at her tiny daughter.

The neonatal team acted quickly. Luckily, Dr. Jensen, the neonatology *overlæge* — supervising professor — happened to be on call. He intubated Tine within minutes; she would remain on mechanical ventilation for the next twelve days, a long time for any neonate. An arterial line was inserted and blood was sent to the lab to measure blood gases. The team administered surfactant. They transfused the baby and infused pressors — dopamine and norepinephrine — to boost her cardiac function. She was started on a course of ampicillin and gentamycin for her sepsis.

Over the next several days Tine's condition remained precarious. On December 3, her second day of life, an echocardiogram revealed a patent ductus arteriosus (PDA) with significant right to left shunting which contributed to her poor cardiopulmonary status. Still more problems were on the way. On day four Tine suffered a grade III intraventricular hemorrhage. She subsequently developed hydrocephalus and underwent frequent lumbar punctures, as well as direct ventricular punctures through the lambdoid suture, to reduce intracranial pressure. She began to have transient motor symptoms — eye and limb movements — but an EEG proved unremarkable and her motor symptoms resolved spontaneously within a few days. Tim and Lise, now fully recovered, hovered anxiously.

After failed attempts to induce PDA closure with indomethacin, Tine underwent cardiothoracic surgery to repair the "hole in her heart" on December 12. On a positive note, Tine was extubated two days later and began receiving oxygen via nasal C-PAP. Her cardiorespiratory status improved gradually, though the hydrocephalus persisted. The lumbar and ventricular cerebrospinal fluid (CSF) taps continued. Tine remained in the neonatal unit for weeks, gradually gaining weight and maturing.

New Troubles

At about six weeks of age the consultant neurosurgeons recommended placement of a ventricular drain with an Omaya reservoir so that Tine wouldn't have to undergo such invasive CSF aspirations. Instead fluid could be drawn directly from the reservoir as frequently as needed without harming the baby. A ventriculo-peritoneal shunt was not indicated yet because the baby was still too small and her CSF protein levels were too high in the aftermath of her ventricular bleed. The drain would be a reasonable alternative until these contraindications resolved. Both of the baby's parents hated seeing Tine's head repeatedly poked by needles, so they consented to the ventriculostomy, which was performed on January 14.

Unfortunately, about one week later Tine's mental status deteriorated. She became less active, less responsive. Culture of her CSF indicated a staph epidermidis meningitis and ventriculitis, an unfortunate complication caused by her medical treatment. This delivered a severe blow to Tine's improving health. Even with intrathecal vancomycin Tine would not reach her usual level of activity again for several weeks. In fact, she may have suffered some degree of permanent brain damage from the infection.

About a month later, at approximately ten weeks of age, Tine was finally released on "home leave." If she had been referred from another part of the country, home leave would not have been possible. Being able to take her home was a huge milestone for Lise and Tim. Not formally discharged from the hospital, though, they had to take her back every two to three days for intracranial pressure relief. Cab fare was reimbursed by the social welfare system.

These regular visits continued until Tine was about five months old, by which time she had gained enough weight for a ventriculo-peritoneal shunt to be considered; by then her CSF protein levels had diminished as well. On April 4 the neonatal team wheeled her down to the OR suite, where she underwent the procedure which immediately relieved her intracranial pressure. Her cranial vault softened and cranial suture lines approached one another for the first time. By post-op day one she rested comfortably without analgesia. Tine went home on post-op day two.

A Second Beginning

Now, nearly six months old, Tine has been eating well and has gained weight. Lise notes that since the V-P shunt was placed, her baby sleeps on a more regular schedule and seems to eat more. She has bonded well with her mother. There have been no further medical complications thus far, and Lise is quite pleased with the outcome. At this point Tine doesn't appear to have any physical deficits. "Her head has gotten a lot smaller," says Lise. "She's really doing a lot better."

Both parents understand that Tine has a long way to go toward recovery and that her final outcome has yet to be determined. They realize that their child may be disabled mentally, physically, or both. They understand that it will take extra care and effort to raise her. Tine will face many obstacles in the years ahead but between her loving parents and the current Danish social welfare system, she will receive much support. Still, her future remains quite uncertain.

Jante's Law

Tine's case certainly raises many questions regarding medical and social issues. But any discussion regarding the Danish health care system first requires knowing some of the guiding principles of Danish society. Built on equality and equity, their traditional philosophy of Jante's Law as expressed by novelist Axel Sandemose, asserts that sameness is a good thing and that no one should seek nor receive special attention. Flaunting wealth or excessive displays of personal ambition are heavily frowned upon. This all-for-one mentality is the foundation of the social welfare system, of which health care is a large part.

A very high rate of taxation finances the social welfare system in Denmark. Eighty to eighty-five percent of all health care costs are financed directly through tax revenue. Health care is provided for all by the social welfare system, as are retirement communities, dental care for children, disability, and maternity and paternity leave. The truly impoverished are of course not taxed, and the wealthy are very highly taxed. However, the majority of the tax burden falls on the large Danish middle class.

The Danish health system provides universal access to all citizens. Everyone is guaranteed the same level of care. The universal medical plan includes pre-natal care, neonatal home nursing visits, vaccinations and dental care for children, family physician care, emergency care, and all hospital services. Outpatient medications and dental care for adults are partially subsidized.

Generally, the Danes appear comfortable with the universality of their health care system. Everybody receives the health care the government provides and generally it has met their expectations. However, criticism of the system has been growing in recent years. Few days pass without a major newspaper publishing a negative article about health care. The largest source of resentment stems from long waits for elective surgeries and other technical diagnostic and therapeutic procedures, though there is no wait for emergency care as in Lise's case. Based on public opinion data, the General Practitioner (GP) system is regarded as average while prenatal education and care is rated as excellent.

Lise's Access to Care

Within the universal access framework for Danish health care, Lise had no difficulty initiating care throughout the course of her pregnancy. She was seen by her GP initially when she suspected her pregnancy and subsequently was referred to her midwife at 12 weeks. When she went into labor prematurely, she considered a couple of options. First, she called the "night doctor" or *lægevagten* — an on-call physician who makes house calls for the acutely ill. As in Lise's case, there is often a waiting time of two to four hours before a doctor can arrive at the patient's home; occasionally there is very little waiting time. For individuals in less critical situations, the on-call night doctor system works well and potentially keeps health care costs down by reducing hospital ER traffic. However, if the after hours service is unavailable or the patient's symptoms are more severe, he or she can call for an ambulance. Lise used a third option and called for a taxi.

Once in the ER, Lise was triaged immediately to an exam room and only waited five to ten minutes before being seen. In the ER people with less serious illness or injuries generally wait much longer. Lise notes, "Here in Denmark you could sit in the emergency room for a whole day." Her partner Tim, a professional athlete in Europe, has had several such experiences in the past with orthopedic injuries. In Lise's case, however, a definite course of action was determined quickly, and she was triaged from the ER directly to the Obstetrics Department where the diagnosis of placental abruption was made and rapidly led to the emergency surgery.

Tine was delivered by an uncomplicated Caesarian section but had numerous complications in the perinatal period. Fortunately, her family's district community hospital happened to be the Rigshospitalet, which is the largest referral hospital in Denmark and has the best equipped neonatology service in the country. Also fortunately for her, Dr. Jensen happened to be in the hospital at the time of her delivery.

Care of Premature Infants in Denmark

The Rigshospitalet employs some 8,000 people including approximately 830 physicians, of which a quarter are senior physicians. In the neonatology department, the staff of physicians, nurses, nursing assistants and ancillary staff are divided into three teams. As of 1998, the physician staff included two *overlæger* — supervising professors, six *afdelinglæger* — staff neonatologists, and seven *reservelæger* who may or may not be pediatric specialists but are not neonatal specialists. Each of the three neonatal teams also has a chief nurse who supervises about thirty-five nurses. In addition, each team has a laboratory technician who performs both phlebotomy and biochemical laboratory tests. Neonatology staff are generally satisfied with the team arrangement and most note good communication and efficiency with the current system.

According to Dr. Jensen — the neonatology *overlæger* or supervising clinical professor — general management of premature infants in Denmark is undertaken with a "minimal invasiveness" approach, especially with the later pre-term infants. The technology available for care of pre-term infants at the Rigshospitalet is advanced, but the fear of doing too little is balanced with the fear of inducing complications by too much intervention. Thus, the level of aggressiveness in treating pre-term infants is left to the discretion of the clinicians. There are no legal limits placed on clinical decision-making regarding pre-term infants. The law does not determine a gestational age limit below which care is withheld, nor does it dictate an age of prematurity above which care must be administered. The Danish parliament has discussed the issue of age limits in the past, however, with very little support in favor of legislating such limits.

If there is clearly no chance of the infant's survival, a physician may withhold or withdraw care in accordance with legal standards. If survival is possible but a "bad outcome" is anticipated, i.e. disability, the law is less clear. In this setting it is the both the right and the duty of the physician to decide the course of action, provided the parents are not adamantly opposed. In practice, babies born under 24 weeks gestational age are very unlikely to survive hospitalization regardless of the efforts to save them. Only one such infant under 24 weeks' gestational age has ever left the Rigshospitalet, only to die shortly thereafter of other medical complications.

Of note, Tine was the first baby in Denmark to be placed on a newly acquired state-of-the-art respirator — a high frequency oscillator. Delivering very small tidal volumes at a rapid rate, such a ventilator maintains minute ventilation while reducing the risk of barotrauma and/or expansile trauma when compared with conventional ventilators. The equipment had been requested the previous year, but because of the equipment approval process the respirator had not been acquired until the year Tine was born. It had not been used yet because staff had not been fully instructed on its use, and also because there had not been a situation where it was clearly indicated — at least not until Tine was born. Says Lise, "The good thing was that Dr. Jensen got that new respirator. If it hadn't been for that she wouldn't be alive."

Variations in care can occur from hospital to hospital and from county to county where financial resources and personnel may differ. Even within a department in one hospital there is variation in the training level of staff physicians. For example, few positions for neonatal specialization exist; the same is true for all other medical specialties. While candidacy and training for specialties is competitive and long in duration, currently no standard board certification exams exist in any specialty.

Costs of Tine's Hospital Care

Actual costs of care for an inpatient hospitalization are difficult to assess because no billing or financial documentation occurs, and because overhead costs are not identified. In Tine's case, all costs of her inpatient stay were absorbed by the neonatology department's annual budget because she lives in the Rigshospitalet district. Had Tine been referred from another part of the country, her home county would have been charged a previously negotiated rate for all hospital services. Furthermore, her consulting physicians (neurosurgery, cardiothoracic surgery) and other services (radiology, lab chemistry, etc.) did not receive reimbursements of any type. All of these costs were absorbed by their previously determined respective departmental budgets which were established more than a year in advance based on anticipated utilization rates, which are in turn derived from previous years' experience and from current trends including higher costs for new technologies. If a hospital department exceeds its budget, the hospital necessarily absorbs the loss.

Danish hospitals operate under a principle of fixed supply that theoretically matches the calculated needs of their populations, in contrast to the United States where patient demand determines the supply. Each hospital budget in Denmark is established by the county where it is located and is based on previous utilization, anticipated trends and the cost of new technologies. At the Rigshospitalet, approximately 55% of its annual income is fixed and comes directly from the Copenhagen County. The remaining 45% of its income is variable and is derived from other counties; these funds are negotiated on a county-by-county basis according to estimates of patients that will be referred in. Fluctuations and miscalculations in such a system are undesirable but also unavoidable, especially at an institution such as the Rigshospitalet, which is the largest referral center in Denmark with approximately 1200 beds and an annual budget of 3 billion DKK. If the hospital incurs an overall deficit for the year due to a miscalculation of its population's needs, the government necessarily funds the loss. In recent years, many top hospital administrators have been replaced for unsuccessful fiscal management.

One criticism of such a fixed-budget, fixed-supply system is that it may take longer to incorporate costly new technologies and pharmaceuticals. For example, each department at the Rigshospitalet submits an annual request for new equipment, and a central hospital committee evaluates these requests and determines what can and cannot be granted. In practice, each department may request ten or so items but receive only its top one or two requests because of budgetary constraints. Thus, even a clinically proven new technology which may be available in other countries, such as the high frequency oscillator that may have saved Tine's life, could take up to several years to become standard practice in the Danish system.

Similarly, expensive new pharmaceuticals can only be introduced at the expense of other drugs on formulary unless a compelling enough argument can be made to significantly increase a department's overall budget — an unlikely scenario. In the neonatology department, one such dilemma is presented by the use of surfactant, which costs approximately $700 per dose. Currently this one drug comprises thirty percent of the department's drug budget, quite a large figure. In cases of very premature infants with RDS, the saving of hospital costs with the successful use of surfactant more than outweighs the costs of the drugs. However, in cases of extremely premature babies the costs of using surfactant are high due to the increased survival of these very sick infants. Certainly in some cases surfactant may make the difference between survival and death, but its high cost forces the neonatalogy department to ration its use of other pharmaceuticals.

One can approximate the charges for some of the major procedures that Tine underwent, but these figures do not represent actual costs. Rather, these are the charges that would be billed to regional authorities outside of the Copenhagen area for referred patients. For example, a non-intensive neonatology bed in 1998 would have been reimbursed at DKK 4,110 ($603) per night; a neonatal intensive care bed would have been DKK 10,425 ($1531). Tine's patent ductus arteriosus repair would have cost a referring regional authority DKK 33,226 ($4849), and her V-P shunt would have cost DKK 15,253 ($2239). However, charges for patients such as Tine from within the hospital's district are not calculated, estimated or recorded. (Note: conversions of DKK to USD are approximate).

Other day-to-day aspects of Tine's care cannot even be estimated. For example, the cost of Tine's many transcranial ultrasounds prior to ventricular punctures consists of the cost of the machine itself and its maintenance fees divided by the number of times it is used plus the cost of the physician's time. There are no physician fees billed to the patient or the county for performing the imaging procedure, nor are there charges for interpreting the scan. The arrangement is simple — the equipment has already been paid for so it is used as often as needed.

The same principle occurs with radiology, lab chemistries, and other ancillary services. No technical or professional costs are incurred by the patient, by the neonatology department, or by the region. All of the charges are absorbed by the respective departmental budgets, and if budgets are underestimated then they are increased proportionately the following year with cost shifting from department to department if the overall hospital budget is not increased appreciably.

The Patient Perspective

Lise and Tim have differing opinions of the Danish health care system. Lise, born and raised in Denmark, is quite satisfied with the level of care and takes comfort in knowing that all outpatient and inpatient services are paid for. She has grown up with the system and it meets her expectations. Tim on the other hand, born and raised in the United States expresses concerns about the quality of care. He is slower to trust the Danish system, even after living here on and off for two years. "It's different for me. I'm not used to the way they do things," he says. "Even in a hospital the cultures are different."

However, both parents were extremely upset by Tine's hospital acquired meningitis for several reasons. First, they understand that it's a known complication, but they also understand that it was a hospital-caused infection. Probably worse in their minds was the fact that no one communicated the details to them. Rather, the physicians taking care of Tine — a different one nearly every day — neglected to tell the parents that their baby had meningitis. Lise recalls, "I don't think they were direct with us. They just said, 'She has an infection but we don't have to take the tube out.' Two or three days later when Dr. Jensen stopped by to see how things were going he discussed the situation with us, assuming we already knew the details of this development." Tim and Lise were furious that no one had taken the time to have this discussion with them sooner.

"It would be nice to have the same doctor," notes Lise. In Denmark, where doctors' working hours are typically limited to 37 hours a week, continuity of care can be an issue. In intense areas such as neonatology, all of the physicians know virtually all of the patients on the ward because most difficult medical and ethical decisions are arrived at after considerable consultation as a team. Still, reports Lise, "Different doctors tell the story in different ways. Some are direct and not positive. Others are nice and realistic." Lise prefers the latter.

Adds Tim, "Even bad news, if it's realistic, would be okay. It's just a matter of how you do it." He recalls asking one doctor early on if Tine would survive. The doctor just shook his head and said, "I don't know." No explanation, no context, simply, "I don't know." Lise recalls another physician responding to the same question, "Don't think about the future now. We can't think about the future now."

Lise and Tim do recognize that it must be hard for the pediatricians to face so many sick babies and so many bad outcomes in this line of work. They also note that not all of the doctors they encountered were poor communicators. They name several that they like and respect, including Dr. Jensen. But they agree that better continuity would be desirable, and they wish there could have been one doctor to serve as a central contact to update them daily and to consult them on treatment decisions.

Tine's Future

At this point Tine's acute medical issues have been stabilized, but now the need begins for close long term planning and follow up. The family's general practitioner will assume her medical care, and her family will receive considerable support from the social medicine division of the social welfare system, which places a strong emphasis on supportive programs for children and their families.

The interface between the health care system and social welfare in Denmark is the domain of the highly organized social medicine program. Social workers, headed by physicians trained in both clinical expertise as well as social medicine, manage individual cases but also participate in prevention and public education efforts. The goal of social medicine is to assist an individual with specific medical needs as much as possible, including children with social, physical or mental disabilities.

Where possible, children who face such difficulties are integrated into ordinary daycare and schools so that they may interact with non-handicapped peers and undergo as normal a childhood experience as possible. Of note, daycare is a largely utilized program within the domain of social welfare. More than half of all Danish children aged 6 months to 10 years are registered in public daycare facilities. There are also special daycare institutions and schools for disabled children who cannot successfully function in the mainstream programs, although the majority are integrated successfully. Additional staffing and services for children with special needs and their parents are available in areas such as housing, transport, education, counseling and eventual employment. These are provided by the social system under the guiding principle of solidarity — that society is largely responsible for the individual and that it should offer disabled individuals a life as close to the norm as possible.

The extent of Tine's potential physical and/or mental disabilities will probably take several years to become fully evident. However, at six months of age, a social worker has been assigned to her case, and she has already been referred to daycare services with an understanding that she may need special assistance. She will soon meet her primary care physician who will track her developmental progress carefully and make referrals to specialists as needed. Tine will present a challenge to her parents because of the long-term complications of her preterm birth, but at least her mother is confident that the social system in Denmark will provide everything that the family needs. Tine's American father is more reserved in his optimism, but at least for the time being he too is prepared to put his faith in the extensive Danish medical and social support system.

Case 4: Experiencing *'hygge'**

Jon Duke

Ellen Konradsen

I meet Ellen Konradsen for the first time one warm and sunny afternoon in Copenhagen. Arriving at her apartment building just north of Nørrebro station, I locate "Konradsen–Apt 9" on the silver box by the entryway. With the press of a button, a buzz and a click, I am on my way up. And up. It seems Ellen lives on the fourth floor of a building without elevators — quite a daily climb for an 80-year-old woman.

As I reach the fourth floor landing, breathless and beginning to question my own exercise habits, a door swings open. Smile upon her face, dressed in a warm-up suit and stylish Nike tennis visor, Ellen is not quite the little old lady I had imagined. With infectious energy she whisks me into the spacious but lightly decorated living room and seats me by the window.

As she goes off to the kitchen to prepare some tea, my eyes are drawn to the collage of photographs hanging on the wall. Scores of beautiful blond children. Grandchildren? Returning with the tea, she notes my puzzled look. "Oh yes, all mine — eleven grandchildren, seventeen great-grandchildren. Aren't they something?"

---

*Jon Duke wrote the story of this patient when he was a student at Harvard Medical School and participated in the US-EU-MEE program at the University of Copenhagen, Denmark, in April 1999.

Having read the medical record before coming to meet her, I knew something of Ms. Konradsen's life. Born in October 1917, married for a short time then divorced over forty years ago, she never remarried. After raising three daughters, she took a job as a bank assistant and remained for 20 years until her retirement at age 64. Until this time her health had been quite good, with the exception of a few broken bones and an inguinal hernia repair in 1973.

A few years after retirement, however, Ellen began experiencing episodes of vertigo. These led to hospitalization in 1985, which revealed an elevated blood glucose level. She was given advice on diet and exercise regimens, but was unable to control her sugar levels by lifestyle changes alone. Over the past 10 years, a series of oral medicines have been attempted with limited success. Even hospitalization for her diabetes has offered only temporary improvement, with rapid relapse into glucosuria. Fortunately, Ellen has shown no evidence of retinal or kidney disease despite her poor control. In addition to the diabetes she has suffered from a hip fracture, hearing loss, partial retinal vein thrombosis, and continuing vertigo over the past five years.

But Ellen Konradsen's medical record, while true in fact, somehow scarcely resembles the sprightly, energetic woman standing before me. Illness, it seems, has left her resilient and determined rather than angry or discouraged. As she sets the teacups down, her warmth bids us return to the conversation. Seventeen great-grandchildren you say?

"Oh yes, a few are even living in the US, in Utah."

I find out that she has spent considerable time in the United States and even has a doctor she sees when she is there. How perfect! "Well, Ms. Konradsen, I am very interested in hearing your perspectives on health care in Denmark. If you can share some comparisons with the US, that would be terrific as well."

"Oh yes, of course. Dr. Jensen said you were doing a project on medical care in Denmark, is that right? Well I do think you have some wonderful doctors in the United States, no question, but it always costs me a bundle when I have to go see them. Here in Denmark, I haven't paid for a visit to the doctor's in my entire life! I just present my Health Care Reimbursement card to Dr. Jensen or the hospital and the county pays for everything. Some people pay for their own medicines, maybe 25 or 50%

of the cost. But my financial situation being a bit difficult, I receive a special subsidy for this as well."

"Oh, but I tell you even if it cost money, I'd gladly pay 100 kroner to see Dr. Jensen," she continued. "He is such a wonderful man. I go round to see him about once every two months or so, and he listens to my heart and lungs and checks the blood sugar. But he always takes time to talk, to ask about my children and grandchildren. Then there are the days when he visits me here at home. It's very comforting to have him here. I'm told that the doctors in the United States almost never come to the home these days. That's quite a shame, not just for the patients but the doctors too. Couldn't they use a short break in the day with a cup of tea?"

"But I don't want to give you the impression that Dr. Jensen is always sweet-talking me," she says firmly. "In fact, it seems that every time I'm there he tells me I need to exercise more or eat less sugar and fats. Well I am an exerciser — swimming, stationary bike, light gymnastics, at least a daily walk. Oh, but I do have a weakness for chocolate. Always have. My 70-kilo weight right now tells me that the chocolate may be winning over the exercise, but I'll do my best. When Dr. Jensen gives me a hard time about it, I tell him that at least I don't smoke like so many other women I know. I quit 40 years ago and haven't touched a cigarette since. If there's anything else I can help you with, please feel free to ask. And if you're going by to see Dr. Jensen, tell him I said hello."

I thank Ms. Konradsen for her kind hospitality and make my way down to the street. I have 20 minutes before I am scheduled to meet Dr. Jensen at his office, just around the block. Eureka! Across the way I spy a bakery. The smells of the wienerbrød and schweizerkringle are too much to resist. Twelve kroner later, I sit with pastry and coffee in hand, thinking of the encounter with Ellen Konradsen. She seemed very happy with the Danish health care system, perhaps mostly because of her fondness for Dr. Jensen. But she touched on several important points as well.

First among them is the state coverage of medical costs. Denmark is a welfare state, its model based on the principle that "all population groups should enjoy decent living conditions and all citizens should be guaranteed certain fundamental rights in the event of unemployment, sickness or old age." This social contract, financed by taxation rates of almost 60%, charges the government with caring for the health of its people. To this end, it fully finances all primary care visits, specialist visits, hospitalizations, and home nursing. Partial to full subsidies are also available for dentistry, physical therapy, chiropractics, and pharmaceuticals. To carry out these tasks, Denmark spends roughly 6% of its GNP on the health sector (in 1999), representing the lowest percentage expenditure on health care of any Western nation. To maintain such control of medical costs, the government must negotiate physician salaries, hospital reimbursements, lab test and pharmaceutical prices, and many other aspects of the industry. Thus, as we meet the various players in our health care story, we will be certain to explore their respective roles in financing Denmark's health care system.

Dr. Jensen will undoubtedly tell us more about the life of a general practitioner, but there are a few valuable points to be aware of beforehand. The Danish government strictly regulates the number of practicing GPs. Licensing mechanisms are designed to provide one general practitioner for approximately every 1600 Danish residents. But a licensed GP may not simply open a clinic wherever he or she may desire (perhaps on the Strøget in downtown Copenhagen!). Rather, the government regulates the number of clinics per area based on population. Furthermore, only those individuals living within 10 km of a doctor's office (or within 5 km in Copenhagen) may register as a patient, thus tightly regulating a doctor's choice of patients and a patient's choice of doctors. This mechanism is designed to ensure access to care. The necessary proximity also facilitates frequent patient-doctor interactions including occasional house calls.

The General Practitioner

Taking a final sip of coffee, I exit the bakery and head a short distance down Frederikssundsvej to Dr. Jensen's office. Climbing up the stairs, I find a waiting room populated by several adults, children, and infants. My feet follow naturally the curves of the clinic's modern, spacious design and bring me to the open door of Dr. Henrik Jensen, General Practitioner. His secretary is on the telephone but invites me to have a seat as Dr. Jensen finishes with his last patient of the day. Glancing about the office, all seems quite as it would in the United States — computers, fax machines, sleek Ikea furniture.

A patient steps out from a side room and Dr. Jensen appears behind him. "Have a nice day Mr. Vestereng. I'll call you with the results on Tuesday." He turns towards me and smiles broadly. "Ah yes, our American medical student, how nice to finally meet you. Please, come have a seat in my office. Care for something to drink?"

I explain that between Ellen Konradsen's tea and a large coffee at the nearby bakers, I must refuse this final caffeine bolus for the day. He laughs and leans back in his chair.

"So you met with Ms. Konradsen today? A lovely woman she is. If only I could get her to cut down on the sweets! I've known her for 25 years and it's always been the same. But with the difficulty controlling her diabetes, problems with diet and weight can be quite serious. Over the next few months I hope to intensify efforts to control her glucose levels, now ranging 15–20 mmol/l. Some of her other problems, particularly the vertigo, are also quite vexing. She's been seen by both a neurologist and an ENT, neither of whom could offer a substantive explanation for the symptoms."

Amazingly, with nearly 1300 patients in his care, Dr. Jensen was still able to discuss Ellen Konradsen's history with not a single glance at the chart. Perhaps many doctors in the United States have this skill as well, but it is comforting to see that the socializing of medicine need not be synonymous with the decline of the patient-doctor relationship. I ask Dr. Jensen to discuss his life as a GP and his interactions with patients, hospitals, and government.

"The general practitioner in Denmark has a very good life I think. Of course, the training takes many years, as it does in the United States. We enter university following high school and must take 13 semesters of medical school courses to obtain our MD degree. A lottery is then held to select the location for our 18-month internship, which consists of six months each of internal medicine, surgery, and family medicine. Afterwards, trainees spend two to three more years rotating through the hospitals and another six months in a primary care clinic. When their training is complete, they must find an area with an available GP license. This decision often involves relocating from the city to a more rural area, such as Jutland. But wherever a GP may practice, he can be assured that he will receive similar payment for his services."

"Speaking of which, you must be curious as to how we doctors are paid in Denmark. Well, as for the general practitioner living in Copenhagen, we are remunerated through a combination of capitated and fee-for-service plans. One-third of our income is based solely on the number of patients under our care. At the present time we receive 250 DKK ($35) for each person in our practice, with a maximum of 1900 patients. The other two-thirds of our salary is derived from a fee-for-service plan, which is renegotiated with the government every four years."

"Each patient visit, procedure, vaccination, or in-house lab test is compensated according to this Health Care Reimbursement Scheme. By combining fee-for-service with the capitated plan, the government has added some financial incentive to a GP's medical practice."

"You may be wondering how abuses of this system are monitored and controlled. Every year, the GP receives a summary of his individual fee-for-service charges. If his charges are more than 25% above the mean, he will be required to send an explanation for this level of activity. If the excessive spending continues for several years, his license may be in jeopardy. I think such an event is quite rare though, as GPs generally make a fine living, somewhere between the equivalent of $90,000 and $110,000 a year."

"But being a doctor in Denmark or anywhere else should not be about money, of course. It is about the work of doctoring. So let me tell you about how we practice here. This office is shared among three GPs, with one physician-in-training rotating through every 6 months. We each have our own patients of course, but if I am on vacation, my colleagues can cover as necessary."

"The workday for GPs in Denmark is 8 am to 4 pm Monday through Friday. I may do house calls for the first few hours of the day, then begin seeing patients in clinic from 10 am. I usually see approximately 20 patients a day, with appointments lasting between fifteen and thirty minutes each. The average wait time for an appointment is 4–5 days, but we always have one hour per day reserved for same-day consultations (the patient may spend a longer time in the waiting room of course). At 4 pm, the day is done. I have no pager and the office phones block out all incoming calls, so I may finish my paperwork and leave by about 5:00 or 5:30. Such is a fairly typical day I think."

Dr. Jensen pauses a moment, perhaps in response to the increasingly quizzical look on my face. No pager? How do you address patient concerns after hours? Also, there has been no mention of rounding in the hospitals. How do you follow your hospitalized patients? Dr. Jensen raises an eyebrow at this and conjures up a quizzical look of his own. Then with a flicker of realization, he begins to explain.

"Oh, I see your confusion. Yes, in the US the primary care doctors may be involved in the care of a patient at all times and places. Here in Denmark, the divisions are much sharper. After 4 pm I am not available to the patients, so they must address any problems to a special Night Doctor. These doctors are available either by telephone for simple consultations or at the Night Clinic, an office, which is manned by GPs and remains open until 10 pm. After ten, most patients will proceed directly to a hospital emergency room for care."

"In regards to my role *vis-à-vis* hospitalized patients, I have no responsibility or authority over their care for the duration of their time in the hospital. If I send a sick patient to the emergency room, I may call ahead to provide information for the doctors, but that is the full extent of my business there. When the patient is discharged, a summary will be placed in the computerized record for my review. If I am not the one to send the patient to the hospital, no one will contact me. Thus, I might know nothing of my own patient's hospitalization until I receive a discharge summary several weeks later."

"Another point of division between the GP and the hospitals is the hospital specialty clinics. Let's use your patient Ellen Konradsen as an example. She entered the hospital with a hip fracture in November 1995, but she did not return to my care until May 1996. While in-house, her unstable glucose resulted in an endocrinology consultation. This then led to a lengthy outpatient follow-up with the hospitals' endocrine clinic. For several months they managed her diabetes but did not consult me on her status or changing medications. As you can see, the hospitals operate in a world very separate from that of the GP. It unfortunately becomes the patient's responsibility to bridge the chasm."

"Well I've told you much more than you wanted to hear, I imagine. You will undoubtedly learn plenty about the hospitals when you visit them yourself. And please feel free to contact me with any other questions you might have about Ms. Konradsen, life as a GP, or Denmark in general. The summer is a beautiful time to be in Copenhagen — be sure to visit Tivoli Gardens before you go!"

After a warm handshake, I head for the door. Stepping out into the late afternoon sun, I catch a glimpse of the #5 bus coming over the horizon. A sprint to the bus-stop, and soon I am riding east through the distant hum of Nørrebro's shops and restaurants. Dreaming of dinner at an outdoor café along Nyhavn, I settle in for a long ride. Thoughts drift to Dr. Jensen and the broad strokes he has painted on the evolving picture of health care in Denmark. GPs are the centerpiece of the system, similar to the gate-keepers of HMOs in the US. But interestingly, once they have guided their patients into the hospital or specialist's office, they cease to exert an influence on their care. This separation offers the GP a controlled schedule and high quality of life, but must impair continuity of care. Who could know Ellen Konradsen as well as Dr. Jensen? If she were to go into the hospital, his knowledge and presence would be of great value in her treatment and recovery.

Hospital Emergency

During the coming weeks, Ellen notices some changes in her health. A new cough and shortness of breath have appeared, seeming to worsen on the walk up to her apartment. A few days later she first notices a pressure in the center of her chest. Bothersome but not painful, the feeling becomes strongest when she walks or otherwise exerts herself. Two days later, still with the discomfort, Ms. Konradsen calls her general practitioner.

Dr. Jensen is surprised by the call. Ellen has no prior history of angina or dyspnea on exertion. While this may very well be a bronchitis or pneumonia, the complaint of chest pain in a diabetic must be taken very seriously, not only because it is a risk factor for heart disease, but also because the diabetes itself can blunt the sensation of pain from even a significant myocardial infarction. Dr. Jensen suggests that Ellen proceed directly to the Bispebjerg Hospital emergency department for full evaluation.

I receive the call from Dr. Jensen and within 20 minutes have arrived at Bispebjerg, a sprawling complex located three km north of the Panum

Institute (home of the University of Copenhagen's medical school). Bispebjerg Hospital (BBH), one of the two major cardiac centers in Copenhagen, impresses me immediately with its array of late 19th century architecture arising just beyond the main gates. I check the hospital map to determine which of the 40-plus buildings might contain Ms. Konradsen. The Emergency Department is located on the far side of Building 7, up a hill straight ahead. I pass quickly by the statuettes and circular fountains before catching a glimpse of the departing ambulance. Finding the emergency doors, I pass into a long wide hallway, off of which approximately 15 patient rooms are adjoined. I spot Ms. Konradsen in the second room on the left. She appears tired, but not anxious or in distress. A nasal canula for oxygen and an IV in her left arm have already been placed.

"My, a surprise to see you here," she greets me. "I'm afraid I don't feel much like talking today. I've had this pressure in my chest, very unusual. Dr. Jensen was concerned so my daughter drove me in to the hospital. I spoke to the nurse just a few minutes ago and told her about the pain. She placed a small pill under my tongue, and I do feel a bit better. She also gave me an aspirin before going off to call the doctor, who should be here very soon."

Back in the hall, I find the triage nurse, Katharin Nielsen, completing her note on Ms. Konradsen. While we are waiting for the doctor to arrive, she takes a moment to explain how the Emergency Department (ED) operates and what has been done for Ellen thus far.

"The Emergency Department at Bispebjerg consists of two triage nurses, an orthopedist, and a general practitioner," she explains. "The nurses make the decisions as to who will be seen and by whom. A large number of our cases involve simple somatic complaints or accidents, so our two ED attendings can care for these patients and send them home. In cases involving possible hospitalization, we bypass the emergency doctors and contact the appropriate inpatient department. Practically speaking, there are only two medical departments — Cardiology for clear cardiac cases and Internal Medicine for all others. In the case of your patient in Room 2, she may be having some ischemia but her symptoms don't suggest acute myocardial infarction (MI), so she'll be handled by Internal Medicine rather than by Cardiology. Of course, she will receive a standard rule-out MI protocol and I've already given her aspirin, sublingual nitro, and oxygen. If you'll excuse me, I should get the EKG leads placed before the doctor arrives."

With a polite smile, Katharin excuses herself and slips back into the hallway. I gaze around the ED for a moment. It appears well arranged and well equipped, physically very similar to the major Emergency Departments in the US. The differences lie more in the staffing of its physicians. Denmark has no emergency medicine specialists in 1999. Rather, it chooses to rely on skilled nurses and attendings-level orthopedists and GPs for managing basic emergency cases. The dozens of residents that populate the emergency rooms in the US are not found in Denmark. Instead, residents are called to the ED only in cases of a likely admission, and this decision is made by a nurse rather than by a fellow resident.

A white coat dashes by and heads directly for Room 2. I approach the door to find the coat and its wearer, a young blond woman perhaps 25 years old, hurriedly making introductions to Ms. Konradsen and her daughter. She is Anya Oleson, an intern now rotating through a six-month Internal Medicine block at Bispebjerg. As she begins eliciting Ellen's history, I notice the casual dress, jeans and a plain white T-shirt, that she wears beneath her coat. Perhaps she was on-call last night and hasn't had the chance to dress for the day. On the other hand, she looks very focused and well rested — not the face of a post-call intern in the US.

She catches me gazing through the door. I briefly explain my interest in learning about Danish health care and my knowledge of Ellen Konradsen. Anya shrugs, invites me in, and closes the door behind.

Dr. Oleson explains to Ms. Konradsen that they are not sure if she is having a heart attack, but they want her to rest for now and will know more in a few hours. Ellen seems to sink under the information, and she slowly closes her eyes. Hanne, Ms. Konradsen's daughter, gives her hand a squeeze before thanking the doctor. Taking our cue, we leave the two of them to talk and to rest.

Poor Ms. Konradsen, tired and scared. She seems a different person from that charming and enthusiastic character I met earlier. Fortunately, she appears stable for the time being.

Squeaking wheels approach from around the corner. A thin young man has arrived with a gurney to bring Ellen up to the floor. He enters the room, five minutes later exiting with Ellen in the bed and Hanne in tow. They pass through the double doors and out into the cold autumn air. I am surprised to find that the patient floors are located in a building separate from the Emergency Department. A 30-second ambulance ride takes us to Building 12, where we proceed upstairs and stop near the middle of a long yellow corridor. The transport wheels Ellen into a large beige room containing four patient beds, two to a side. The other patients scarcely seem to notice the parade of people that has descended upon the room. A middle-aged, ruddy-faced woman sits engrossed in a romance novel. An elderly lady sleeps soundly through the ruckus, her nasal prongs pulled askance, delivering a steady stream of oxygen to her right ear. Only the patient lying opposite Ellen's bed looks up to give her a smile. Ellen smiles back.

The Resident

An hour later, I spot a resident going through the chart marked Konradsen. We say hello and I inquire as to how things are going.

"Oh, I'm quite well, thank you. Oh, you mean with Ms. Konradsen. Silly me, it's been a long day. Yes, I've been in to see her and her symptoms have actually improved with the nitro. But her EKG here seems to be evolving into a picture of a subendocardial MI. I think we have to call this a myocardial infarction, so she'll have to be transferred to the Cardiology Department."

The resident dictates his note and arranges the transfer to Cardiology (known as the "Y" service). A few minutes later, as I futilely attempt to read a medical textbook in Danish, the resident returns.

"Oh, I apologize for not introducing myself before. I'm Tommi Wegener, a second-year resident in Internal Medicine. Now that we have a few minutes, would you like to get some coffee?"

Tommi leads the way down the stairs and into the staff cafeteria. Taking two coffees with light cream and sugar, we find a corner table by the window. Tommi reaches over and opens the window, letting in a rush of cold air.

"Do you mind if I smoke? He asks as he lights up a cigarette. I know the Americans always think it's terrible when they come over here and see the doctors and patients smoking inside the hospital. But it's Danish culture, difficult to change. But enough about smoking. You say you're interested in learning about health care in Denmark, huh? Well, you've gotta know about the life of a resident then. After all, we're the ones doing all the work! Of course you know that all government employees in Denmark must keep a strict 37-hour workweek. This includes doctors, nurses, technicians, custodians, everybody."

"What? Thirty-seven hours?" I exclaim.

"Oh, you didn't know about that? Yeah, back in 1980 or so, they passed a law reducing everyone's working hours to 37 a week. Some people are even pushing to have it dropped to 36, but I doubt that'll happen. Anyway, they pay us by the hour, so if we end up staying late at the hospital, the government has to pay overtime wages, time-and-a-half. Thus, the higher-ups are very careful to avoid working us beyond the allotted time because it comes out of their budgets. Don't get the wrong impression, we may pull a 50-hour week now and then, but our average over 12 weeks must be at 37, so a 50-hour week will have to be followed by a 24-hour week somewhere in the same three-month period. There were times that I was sent home for an entire week just to balance my schedule."

Jaw agape, I ponder what Tommi has just said. How can a hospital function with residents working only 37 hours a week? How are patients followed? When do they take call? Who ever heard of overtime wages for doctors? I briefly describe the different life of a US resident doctor.

"Ouch! I'm glad I'm in Denmark," Tommi exclaims. "Well, let me explain how the whole thing works here. A typical day for a medical resident is from 8:15 am to 3:15 pm. In the morning we have a meeting with the chief doctors; usually there are two or three in each department. The post-call resident discusses the patients who have come in the previous night and what was done. The chief makes comments and recommendations for the patients' care. Everyone then looks at his shift assignment for the day. One intern will be on ER call, one or two will round on floor patients, one might go to clinic. The more senior residents supervise admissions or assist with situations on the floor. At 1:15 the residents who have seen the ward patients will meet with the chief again to discuss any issues that have risen that day. Following the meeting, they will return to the floor, place new orders for the night, and see any patients who have been admitted by the emergency team. Their work is usually complete by 3:00 or so and they can go home."

"The concept of on-call here is a bit different," Tommi continues. "We have day-call and night-call. The resident on day-call is the ER intern I just mentioned. He will see all new patients who arrive between 8:15 am and 4:00 pm. The night-call intern will arrive and work until 8:15 the following morning. When a senior resident is on call, he is usually in the hospital from 8:15 am to 8:00 pm, then will be available from home for the rest of the night. So our on-call shifts vary between 8 and 16 hours, usually admitting 6–8 patients per 24-hour period. The job assignments change every day and some days you have no assignment and can just stay home. But it is important to remember that the resident who admits the patient from the ER will not necessarily be the one who takes care of her on the floor. And a resident who sees her on the floor one day will not be the one who sees her the next day. Thus we have very little continuity of care with the patients. A test I order on a patient as the floor resident will be followed up by the floor resident the next day, not by me. So it is often hard to see the full course of a patient's illness. I think in America you learn a great deal by following individual patients from beginning to end. Of course, that's why you work a hundred hours a week, right?"

I am not so sure about that, I think silently.

"I think maybe the Danish system lets more people go into medicine without worrying about sacrificing all their time to work," Tommi concludes. "Over 50% of the students in our medical school classes are women, which suggests that people do not see the job of a doctor as compromising their family lives. Of course, the training is still tough. To get specialized in internal medicine, we do 6 ½ years of university, 18 months of internship, two years of introduction to our specialty, then up to four or five years more of advanced specialty training. That is, if we can find a position one after the next. Sometimes we need to do research for a year or two just to gain entrance into the specialty. I know a cardiology doctor who required 13 years of post-graduate training to receive his license. And the salary is not so great during training, and of course, over 50% of that goes to taxes."

I take leave of Bispebjerg Hospital after a very long and eventful day. Ms. Konradsen's myocardial infarction was a surprise, and I wonder if anyone has called Dr. Jensen to let him know about what has happened since this morning. I can call him tomorrow just to be certain. Strolling down Tagensvej, I consider what Tommi has told me about residency in Denmark. How has the American system evolved as it has? Residents working inconceivable hours; even attendings stretching to find time for family and friends. There is an aspect of tradition that runs through American medical training, and residency is its rite of passage. But it must be more than fraternity-style hazing that keeps US resident physicians working as they do. Surely, the patients demand and deserve the time we give them; the system would cease to function without it. Yet, how is it that the Danish system can care well for the health of its people with residents and doctors working such a — dare we say — humane schedule?

The answer, one may argue, is about expectations. Danish citizens are accustomed to state-run services and recognize their inherent inconveniences, including limited working hours. Americans, on the other hand, expect from their doctors not just physical repair, but also time, sensitivity, and personal investment. Simultaneously, the doctors seek to do more than simply fix their patients; they wish to earn their respect, admiration and appreciation as well. So it is with these grandest of ambitions that the American system must grind on, tired and beleaguered though we may be.

The Inpatient

Ms. Konradsen has just started breakfast as I arrive at her room on the acute cardiology wing the next morning. Placing a small bouquet of flowers by her bedside, I sit and inquire how she is feeling.

"Oh, not so bad. The pain in my chest is mostly gone, but I haven't gotten up and walked around yet. I had some trouble sleeping, but I'll get some rest today. The doctors say I shouldn't get out of bed until tomorrow or so."

"How are the doctors treating you?"

"Oh, they're all quite nice, but I think I've had four different doctors in two days. Sometimes I get the feeling they're not even talking to each other. But they were very open with me and my daughter, Hanne, about what was going on, and they told Hanne she could call anytime to ask how I was doing."

The Nurse

I leave Ellen to finish her breakfast and as I step out of the room I am caught by a nurse with a tray full of medicines in small white paper cups. "It's a bit early for visiting hours, I'm afraid. Are you a relative of Ellen's?"

Once again I explain why I am mysteriously wandering around the hospital. She smiles. "Oh, well, you know it's the nurses that really run this place. Why don't I show you around a bit when I finish passing out these medicines."

In a few minutes the nurse, Ilona Christensen, has returned bearing a cup of ginger ale for each of us. She gestures down the hallway, "I've worked this cardiology unit for over 15 years now and I'm still not tired of it. The courage of these patients keeps me feeling strong myself. Up here on the acute floor we have 20 beds with one to four beds per room. You might think that a private room is the preferred option, but studies have found that socializing with one's fellow patients actually speeds recovery. Over here at the central nurses' station, a sophisticated cardiac monitoring system keeps us aware of the status of all our patients. We generally have six nurses working the day shift and four working at night. Each nurse takes three to five patients a shift, but there is no designated primary nurse for each patient. When things are extremely busy, we have nursing helpers to assist with passing out drinks, taking vitals, and so on."

"Nurses and doctors work very closely here in Denmark," she continues. "The relationship is seen as a partnership rather than a hierarchy. We are encouraged to offer our opinions to the doctors and are able to make many decisions independently. Furthermore, department policy allows us to give a wide range of medications before receiving orders from the doctor. This freedom allows us to handle quickly most of the situations that arise in intensive care. And we are allowed to 'push' essentially all medications, from thrombolytics to opiates."

"Another major responsibility of the nurses is to investigate the patient's social supports. If we feel the patient is unable to function without assistance we will contact the Primary Health Service, which arranges home nursing and provides training to the patient's family. If there are issues of poverty, drug abuse, mental disability or other social limitations, we may contact the Social Medicine Department to assist with long term coordination of these issues."

"Well, I hope that's enough information for you. You're always welcome to … Uh-oh, looks like Ms. Johansson in Room 4 just pulled off her leads. I've got to run. Good luck with everything!"

Ilona dashes down the hall and into a four-person room. Interesting, the idea of socializing as a means of therapy. I suspect that the four-patient room would not be a wild success in the United States. Americans do like their privacy. So again it comes down to expectations. Danes focus on community interests, Americans focus on the individual. One particularly interesting issue raised by Ilona is that of nurses being able to "push" all medications and actually offering a number of treatments without doctor's orders, based on departmental standards. In the United States, there are of course circumstances where nurses will give a medication and then ask for the order later but by and large, nurses will page the resident for at least a verbal order before giving any medication. Such behavior is not an indication of poor competence in American nurses, but rather a reflection of the highly charged issue of liability in American hospitals. Doctors must take the final responsibility for decisions not just for medical reasons but for legal ones as well. If nurses could be sued for mistaken dosing, they too would need malpractice insurance. The costs of care would only escalate further.

In Denmark, malpractice suits are a foreign concept. Patients may register complaints with a special court and receive compensation, a maximum of one million DKK ($143,000 in 1999) for loss of private income. But the process is rare and involves no lawyers. While not without value, malpractice suits carry a tremendous cost to the US health care system. The Danish model has been fortunate to escape these tolls.

Rounds

As I stand gazing at the cardiac monitors, trying to remember how to read an EKG, a transport tech stops and asks for the time. "Sure, it's just past 9:00 am."

Oops! I scurry down the stairs and run over to Building 40 just in time for cardiology morning rounds. Sitting around a U-shaped table are two chief doctors flanked by three residents on either side. A row of medical students sit quietly behind them. One chief is wearing an open-collared blue oxford shirt, while the other sports black sweatpants and a dark turtleneck. The residents' outfits generally consist of sandals or sneakers, jeans, and a short-sleeved shirt. The occasional sweater or khaki pants finds its way in among the medical students, but there is not a tie to be seen.

The post-call resident goes through the previous night's admissions — one MI, a pacemaker failure, a new onset a-fib. Then another resident, presumably the floor intern from yesterday, reports on Ms. Konradsen's case.

The chief doctor for the ward, Christian Østergaard, asks to see the EKG. He studies it for a moment then says, "Nice job. These borderline cases can be kind of tricky, but it's clear that this woman has had some kind of ischemic event. In a couple days, let's do an ECHO to get a better picture of how her heart is functioning. I suspect she'll have some areas of akinesis and if her ejection fraction is poor, it'd be best to get her started on an ACE inhibitor. We should also do a myocardial scintigraphy (stress test) to check for perfusion. I suspect she'll need to stay in the hospital at least a week, maybe with some time in geriatric rehabilitation as well. I'll have a look at her later today."

Medical Students

As the meeting concludes, the row of medical students rise from their chairs and funnel one-by-one into an adjacent room. Following them inside, I find the source of their attraction — a large coffee dispenser sitting at the far end of this library/lounge. The medical students pour their cups and sit around discussing last night's revelry at Rust, a popular disco not far from the medical school. A pause in conversation floats along and

I seize the opportunity to ask, "So what is it like being a medical student in Denmark?"

"Boring", says one. "We come in to the hospital every day and basically just watch the residents work. Sometimes we will get to dictate the admission note or visit the ER, but our interaction with the patients doesn't feel very deep."

Another disagrees. "Oh quit your complaining. There's plenty of time with the patients, and why should we do all the residents' work? The big problem with medical school here is all the required reading. Here, look at this pathology text. Over 900 pages and that's just one volume! We must essentially memorize the entire book for our Path exam next year. It's the same way with the medicine and surgery courses. Fortunately, we can miss 20% of our hospital days and still pass a rotation, so by the end everyone's skipping school to hit the books. Kind of ironic, I think."

A third student, avidly leafing through cardiology journals by the side wall, suddenly contributes. "I've actually been to a medical school in the United States. My cousin is a fourth year student at Harvard Medical School in Boston and I met some of his classmates when I was there last year. They seemed to be pretty proud that their university is so old, like established in 1700-something. Ha! I told them that our Faculty of Medicine was founded in 1479! That kept them quiet for a while. But I found some interesting differences between our two schools. First of all has to be the price. Of course we don't pay a single krone to go to a university in Denmark. Schools of medicine, law, math, science, and economics — all paid for by taxes. Perhaps because we have six years dedicated to the study of medicine rather than four, the schools have integrated more social and theoretical courses into our curriculum."

At that point Dr. Østergaard arrives and I follow him into the hallway.

The Specialist

Entering his office I find a compact but impressively adorned room filled with books and journals. "So how are you enjoying your stay in Denmark?" he asks.

"Oh, it's just lovely," I reply.

"I hope you have a chance to travel up to Elsinore Castle. That's where Shakespeare set the story of Hamlet. Apparently he never visited the place, but it's still a great claim to fame."

"So I think that you'll find the practice of cardiology in Denmark very similar to that in the United States. We employ the same technologies and in some areas, such as thrombolysis, we have been far more aggressive than in the United States," he continues. "Cardiology is an explosively popular field with young Danish doctors these days. Part of the explanation is that we once lagged behind other countries in the introduction of invasive coronary catheterization, so now that the technology has taken off, we need to train more and more doctors to perform these procedures. But training young new cardiologists, as I'm sure you've heard, is a lengthy undertaking. To become a licensed doctor requires at least seven years following internship. Most specialists will then take two further years of training to reach the senior doctor level."

"As chief of the department, I am also responsible for coordinating the budget. Each year I must negotiate with the hospital administration to request the amount of money I believe will be necessary to care for our patients. It is always difficult to predict the exact amount. A patient would never be forced from the hospital because budgets are running low; the excess costs are simply absorbed by the system."

"And for all this work, how much do you think we get paid? My American colleagues sometimes laugh when they hear. A new specialist will receive about $55,000 a year, before taxes. A more senior doctor's salary might range between $63,000 and $77,000, while a professor or chief of department will earn perhaps $85,000. With outside grants and research, $100,000 a year is a distant possibility."

"But such is work as a government employee; very different from your fee-for-service system, although I don't imagine many American doctors work 37 hours a week. Actually, I find this limitation to be quite a nuisance. It interferes with the training of our residents and requires that we sacrifice a large part of our professional interests. To learn more about hospital financing in Denmark you should talk to Mr. Niels Gram, chief financial officer of the Copenhagen Hospital Corporation."

"Oh, with regards to Ms. Konradsen, she is still in the early stages of her recovery. We will know more over the next week or so as further studies are completed. Feel free to drop by any time with questions or to go over the results with my residents. And of course, don't forget about Elsinore Castle!"

I call Dr. Jensen at his office just past 10 am. He has heard nothing of Ms. Konradsen since he sent her to the Emergency Department yesterday morning. I give him a brief update and say that it might be a few days before more test results are in. Perhaps contacting Dr. Østergaard would be the best way to keep informed. Later I keep my appointment with Neils Gram and learn more about health care financing in the Danish hospital system.

Experiencing *"hygge"*

A late sunrise filters through the trees as I jog a final circuit of familiar streets the next morning, thinking about home. One indisputable fact about America — it is a nation blessed with abundant riches. Whether those riches have been distributed fairly, been used well, or have taken America's soul and replaced it with Starbuck's and The Gap and Barnes & Noble, is more difficult to answer. But here in Denmark, the feeling of hygge, the uniquely Danish word suggesting coziness, warmth, and good spirit with family and friends soothes me. *Hygge* is the antidote to cold winters. And ironically, *hygge* is the very atmosphere that Starbuck's and Barnes & Noble seek to emulate in their chains of stores. I feel fortunate for having at least once tasted the real thing.

I turn right at the magnificent Rosenborg Castle and head straight for the eastern port. Coming around the Esplanade, I arrive at Copenhagen's landmark statue, *Der Lille Havfrue*, the Little Mermaid. I sit opposite the statue on a wooden bench and gaze upon her as she stares out to sea, thinking deeply, she and I, though I about health care and she about sailors.

My meeting with Niels Gram yesterday has given me much to think about. The fundamental feature of Danish health care financing is that the government is both payer and payee. Health care costs are kept in check because costs are determined on a yearly, not daily, basis as in the US. The radiologist can't start charging more for this forcing the doctors to charge more for that, forcing the insurers to raise their premiums, forcing the employers to drop their health plan and switch to a cheaper HMO. In Denmark, all health care activity is carefully coordinated. Of course, turning all physicians into salaried employees might impair incentive for quality and efficiency. But the sense of community responsibility is a powerful force in Denmark, urging doctors to perform to the best of their abilities. If such a system were instituted in the United States, would community responsibility sustain the quality of care? Would the prosperous American people accept a measure of personal sacrifice to offer a healthy chance to those less fortunate? Yes, is our hope. But for now these answers remain unclear, lost as they are in the dense political fog.

Following Your Heart

Ellen Konradsen was discharged after a full month of geriatric rehabilitation. She spent a total of 51 days in Bispebjerg Hospital and expresses nothing but relief about being free once again. We spoke on the phone yesterday and she suggested we meet here at the cardiac clinic after her appointment today. Just then Ellen emerges from the clinic and enters the waiting room. She is wearing a dark blue sweater with long pants and is holding a small wrapped box in her hands.

"Thanks for coming! I just wanted you to see in person that I am doing much better nowadays, able to walk around by myself with no problem. Life's not perfect of course. I still have trouble with the blood sugars and that vertigo hits me now and then. But it is so nice to be sleeping in my own bed again! Another reason I asked you to meet me here today is that I wanted to see you one last time before your return to America. I truly appreciate all the time you spent with my doctors and me. I think they were careful to take extra-good care of me because you were always there to check on me. Equally important, I hope you learned what you came here to learn and that you will become a wonderful doctor back home in the United States. I got you a small gift to help you remember Denmark. I hope you like it."

Ellen hands me the box and watches anxiously as I open the lid and pull from inside a most charming memento of Denmark — a brightly colored animated "windmill toy" with two workmen chopping wood and the proud red and white Danish flag flying above them.

"Thank you so much!"

"Take good care and best of luck."

Case 5: In the Same Boat*

Quentin Eichbaum

Patient's Story #1: Jacob, Waiting for a Heart

'Jacob,' as I shall call him, is a 32-year-old Danish young man now living with his sister and brother-in-law in Copenhagen. He is over six feet tall with strong Teutonic features and a tousled mop of sunny-blonde hair tumbling into his blue eyes. Lying atop the bed sheets the day I first entered his hospital room, he appeared surprisingly healthy-looking and flashed me a radiant welcoming smile.

Stepping towards him to shake hands, I recall having a fleeting image of him as a modern-day Viking standing on a ship's prow as it ploughed rough seas. He sat up, removed his *Bang and Olufson* earphones and introduced himself. He laughed uproariously when I joked that I had come from Boston to discover whether something was indeed 'rotten in the state of Denmark's' health care system.

This was my introduction to the saga of a resilient young man living at the edge of life in one of the world's most socialized and affluent health care systems. He had been patiently waiting for nine months for a donor heart that he hoped would turn his life around from the precipitous brink

*Quentin Eichbaum wrote the two cases in this chapter when he was a student at Harvard Medical School and participated in the US-EU-MEE program at the University of Copenhagen, Denmark in the spring of 2001.

it was now teetering on, and make it possible for him to return to playing soccer on weekends and to his work as a cargo-loader for Scandinavian Airlines.

Jacob says that before falling ill with his current heart condition, he considered himself to be in 'perfect health.' In Copenhagen, he worked at his strenuous job since age sixteen as a cargo-loader but never experienced any noticeable physical problems with this work. On weekends he played minor league soccer or went sailing on the Baltic. Although he says he has generally been 'quite a sporty person,' he admits that he has always 'tired a little sooner' than his peers during exercise. His mother insists that outside of the 'usual childhood illnesses' he was a normal and healthy child and exhibited no foreboding of heart disease or other serious medical condition.

Jacob's current symptoms first began a few days before a planned vacation with a male friend in the mountains of southern Germany. He began to experience an acute pain in his right shoulder and thought he might have dislocated the joint while lifting heavy objects at work. But, strangely, he could not recall any such specific incident. He made an appointment with his General Practitioner (GP) who sent him for x-rays to a county clinic. Five days later, before he departed on his vacation, he called to see if his GP had received the x-ray results. He had not, and Jacob left on vacation.

In Germany the next day he went with his friend on a walk in the mountains. After walking a while, he began to experience the same sharp pain in his right shoulder, only this time it was accompanied by an uncharacteristic shortness of breath. Indeed, his dyspnea became so acute that, on the walk back to the car, he had to stop every few steps to catch his breath. He had no chest pain or feeling of faintness but experienced a profound weariness and exhaustion.

On the ride back to the hotel, Jacob was unable to sit up straight but found relief only by lying on his right side with his head on his arm. When he awoke the next morning, he noticed his ankles were swollen. He felt 'bloated,' was unable to urinate and did not feel like drinking anything.

Two days later he returned to Copenhagen and called his GP for the results of his x-rays and to report his medical condition. To his distress, his x-rays were still not back and it was now ten days after the images had been taken. His GP was baffled by his condition but suggested they wait for the x-rays. Jacob's condition deteriorated over the next few days until even minimal exertion would exhaust him. He thought of getting a second opinion but was afraid of antagonizing his GP. Instead, he went privately for an evaluation from his brother-in-law Karl, who is a physician.

Karl diagnosed a highly irregular pulse with an alarming diastolic murmur. He immediately called an ambulance to take Jacob to the nearest county hospital for a chest x-ray and a cardiac workup. The x-ray showed that Jacob's heart was dangerously enlarged, with significant pulmonary edema. He was immediately transferred to the larger county hospital at Gentofte for a full cardiac workup including echocardiography, stress testing, a cardiac biopsy, and a nuclear scan to evaluate the pumping function of his ventricles (MUGA scan).

The results confirmed a diagnosis of idiopathic dilated cardiomyopathy with atrial fibrillation but no signs of tissue inflammation. Jacob turned to his brother-in-law for interpretation of this ominous-sounding diagnosis. Karl explained that it meant that Jacob's heart muscle was affected by a disease of unknown origin that was causing his heart to beat irregularly and ineffectively. Jacob wondered how he could have gotten so ill so fast.

Jacob was given diuretics and a beta-blocker among other medications, which he cannot recall. His atrial fibrillation was first treated with medicine but on a number of occasions he underwent electrical cardioversion, which restored a normal heartbeat. Over the past nine months he has been in and out of atrial fibrillation seven times, the longest episode lasting seven days. His condition improved somewhat but he was informed that he might 'at some stage' require a heart transplant. Perplexingly, however, the chief cardiologist at this hospital was reluctant to refer him for transplant evaluation to either of the country's two major transplant centers. Instead, he claimed they could adequately manage Jacob's condition at Gentofte, and that a transplant was not a priority.

At this stage, having some trepidation himself about undergoing heart transplantation, Jacob accepted the chief cardiologist's decision. But when his condition didn't improve after three to four months and this cardiologist was not being forthcoming with him, his mother urged him to seek a second opinion again. Fearing again that such a move might jeopardize his care, he dallied. One of the nurses then hinted to him that financial disincentives might underlie Gentofte's unwillingness to transfer him to Rigshospitalet. Such a transfer would have to be carefully substantiated by Gentofte's cardiology department since the county authority would have to pay for his treatment at Rigshospitalet. It was not clear why Gentofte's cardiology department was uncomfortable about providing substantiating reasons to support his transfer to Rigshospitalet.

Jacob's mother works as an administrator at Rigshospitalet and knew one of its very best cardiologists on a casual basis. She asked whether he would be able to examine her son in his private clinic as a special favor. He agreed and made use of some special medical/legal directive (which he had done only once before in ten years) to see Jacob in his clinic. So it happened that Jacob was subsequently transferred for evaluation at Rigshospitalet. When he examined him, the cardiologist was greatly alarmed at Jacob's condition and stated unequivocally that he would need a heart transplant. Jacob's name was immediately placed on the transplant list.

Jacob believes he lost a valuable three to four months during this period. Had he been evaluated sooner at Rigshospitalet his name might at this stage be higher up on the recipient list. Indeed, a matching donor heart might have been available during this period of unnecessary delay. Being tall, Jacob requires a large heart and this has placed an additional constraint on finding a matching organ. Jacob has considered filing a malpractice complaint to the Danish medical authority concerning Gentofte's reluctance to refer him for transplant evaluation. However, he thinks that the medical complaints system is designed to protect physicians from lawsuits rather than to give patients a fair hearing, so he doubts he would receive any compensation. To the contrary, he is convinced such a move would backfire on him. If other physicians came to hear of his suit he is afraid this could jeopardize his care, so he hasn't pursued the matter.

The condition of Jacob's heart deteriorated from an ejection fraction of 41% in April of 1998 when he was first diagnosed, to 31% in May of 1999, and then to 18% in August of 2000. It has remained at that level since then. Through medical management, his heart rate and blood pressure improved substantially from a rate of 44 beats per minute and a blood pressure of 97/68 in 1998. However, his kidney function has deteriorated and he has had persistently elevated blood urea nitrogen (BUN) and creatinine levels that are complicating factors in preparing him as a recipient of a donor heart. He has been on a variety of diuretics and angiotensin converting enzyme (ACE) inhibitors. Weaning him from these medications has been problematic. His preparedness for a heart transplant thus remains rather precarious. His stage of heart failure is classified as New York Heart Association (NYHA) Class III, meaning that he is comfortable at rest, but mild activity causes fatigue, palpitations, or shortness of breath.

After nine months, Jacob's name was now just fifth on the heart recipient list. The transplant team was becoming increasingly concerned about his deteriorating condition and had begun discussing the possibility of implanting an LVAD (left ventricular assist device). Jacob was resisting this possibility. Not only would such an operation be only a temporizing measure, but it would also make him ineligible for a donor heart for the period of a full month after the placement of the LVAD. His dilemma: what if a donor heart became available during his one month LVAD post-operative period of ineligibility? He also mentioned that he felt somewhat 'powerless' to resist the cardiologists' insistence on an LVAD (an indicator perhaps of a somewhat more paternalistic patient-doctor relationship in the Danish health care system compared with the US).

On the Friday preceding my last week in Copenhagen, Tina, the head nurse in the transplant unit, was spending time with Jacob carefully explaining to him the intricacies of the LVAD. She was drawing on knowledge she had gleaned during a training course attended in Texas. Jacob was still averse to the idea, but he had the weekend 'to think about it.'

When I returned to visit him that Monday afternoon, his room was empty. I was surprised to hear he had been rushed to the operating room for emergency placement of an LVAD. That morning he had suffered two successive cardiac arrests and had to be electrically cardioverted. I visited him in the ICU the next day. He looked weak and very shaken but managed a smile. He was in considerable pain. The LVAD weighs about a kilogram, is bulky and is initially quite uncomfortable. His mother told me that Jacob's near scrapes with death had shaken him deeply. He was despondent about his condition and felt hopeless about ever receiving a donor heart. He had been told an emergency request to other European

Union countries for a donor heart was being considered. So he said he would just keep "waiting and hoping."

That was how I left him, before I departed the next day to fly back to Boston. Jacob managed a wan smile as the nurses struggled to prop him up in a chair that morning. As I shook his hand to say goodbye, he joked in a whisper, "Seems like something really is rotten in the State of Denmark — at least when it comes to heart transplantation!"

Jacob's Insurance, Social Welfare, and Personal Costs

When Jacob's ability to perform his work as a cargo-loader deteriorated he was transferred to successive categories of lighter duty until he was compelled to stop working altogether and accept full welfare support. He has high praise for the compassionate understanding of his employers and for the fairness of the health care system that absorbed virtually all of his costs. Many other seriously ill people have had a 'rougher ride' through the system, he says. Over recent years, a number of checks and balances have been instituted to forestall fraudulent use of the system but these may have complicated matters for regular patients.

An additional piece of financial good fortune for Jacob was that his bank manager had some years earlier advised him to take out some additional 'loss of ability to work' insurance. Jacob's father had apparently failed to do so when he became ill with the sarcoidosis of which he eventually died. This additional insurance has supplemented Jacob's social welfare subsidy by 40%. Indeed, ironically now that he is unemployed he is earning more than he did while working! Social welfare operates on a graded percentage system based on one's capacity to work. Jacob is currently in the highest category, given to patients incapable of working and requiring full support. Payments from his private bank insurance are closely connected with his social welfare status.

While the county and state cover all medical procedures, a default amount of about DKK 500 (about 8 DKK to the US dollar or ~$62.50 in 2001) remains for certain patients to pay for medications. Because Jacob is classified in the highest category of welfare, his default payments are less. Curiously, while the immunosuppressant Imuran (azothioprine) is fully paid by the county authority, Jacob is responsible for payment of about 25% of the cost of his prednisolone. The rationale is not self-evident for why some medications are fully paid by the county authority and others are not. Jacob says his after tax income is currently DKK 95,000 (approximately $11,875).

Organ Donation in Denmark

Denmark's organ donation system is one of Europe's least proactive. Whereas in Germany, Austria, and Switzerland subjects are considered organ donors at birth and have to specifically request to be removed from the state list of donors, in Denmark you become a donor only by carrying an official donor card or by adding your name to a national computer-based donor list. Even then, relatives may nullify a donor's wishes at death and refuse donation. Apparently this occurs rather frequently, much to the disappointment of eager recipients. Spain and Britain also have more proactive organ donation systems than Denmark, with highly effective donor campaigns and with physicians who often directly contact a deceased's relatives to request procurement.

Nonetheless, when organs do become available in Denmark the system is well geared to making effective use of them. Waiting recipients carry cell phones at all times and can be transported with little delay by ambulance or helicopter to a hospital.

Jacob carries such a cell phone. Only family and close friends have the number so he won't miss the much awaited 'transplant call.' He also always notifies his family of his exact whereabouts. He is deeply dissatisfied with Denmark's organ donor system. Had he been living in some other European Union (EU) countries, he believes he would already have a donor heart at this stage. Ethically, he also believes it is justifiable for younger patients like himself to have priority over elderly patients to receive available donated organs. In addition, he considers some patients 'unsuitable' as recipients — alcoholics, smokers, and non-compliant patients. He thinks they should be ineligible for donation since precious organs would be 'wasted' on them.

Jacob also laments that in Denmark there is not enough debate at the national level about the ethics and the general system of organ donation. Such debate he believes would provide incentives for making the system work better. Tina, the head transplant nurse, however, relates how one of the previous heart transplant patients she took care of, a forty-year-old female alcoholic and smoker whom the nurses had considered an unsuitable candidate, actually changed her unhealthy lifestyle quite radically following her transplant and became a well-known national advocate for organ donation. She cites other cases of seemingly 'unsuitable' candidates who radically altered their unhealthy lifestyles following transplantation. She says these remarkable anecdotal cases have added a complicating twist to the ethics of determining which candidates are 'suitable' and deserving as organ recipients.

Patient's Story #2: 'Lief', A Lucky Candidate for a Heart

The story of Lief, as I shall call him, will provide some basis for comparison to Jacob's story. I interviewed Lief towards the end of my stay in Denmark. His story is interesting because his trajectory through Denmark's health care system was very different from that of my first patient, Jacob.

Lief was 11 days *status post* heart transplant when I visited him in the hospital. He was sitting on the window ledge of his room chatting with his wife. He was in very jovial spirits and joked that he would be charging me for the interview. His 'new heart' he said had made him feel like a 'new man,' and his wife chipped in that it had 'given her back her husband'!

Lief is the same age as Jacob, 32 years old. He grew up and still lives and works on a farm on the island of Funen in Denmark. Two years ago he first noticed that he became short of breath while performing manual labor on the farm. At first he thought his symptoms were caused by an episode of 'flu' and decided to 'wait it out.' When he still felt tired and out of breath after more than fourteen days, he made an appointment with his General Practitioner (GP).

His GP was not particularly concerned about Lief's condition and made the diagnosis of 'asthma.' Lief was prescribed a variety of successive asthma medications. He could not recall their names, but they included an inhaler. His condition did not improve, and in addition, he developed a worrisome cough. His GP decided to treat this with a cough suppressant but it did not help. When he was no better after three weeks, he was finally referred to the large county hospital at Odense in Funen.

At the hospital Lief had his first chest x-ray, which indicated significant pulmonary edema with an enlarged heart consistent with dilated cardiomyopathy. He was also diagnosed with atrial fibrillation and was placed on the anticoagulant, warfarin. When he was discharged from the hospital, by mistake his warfarin prescription was not renewed. He developed a blood clot in his left atrium. His condition deteriorated rapidly and he was then re-admitted and started again on warfarin and treated medically with inotropes and ACE inhibitors. He was told he would need a heart transplant.

This came as 'shocking news' to Lief, but he eventually came to grips with it and agreed to have his name placed on the transplant list. His name was ninth in line for a donor heart. He was again discharged from the hospital. Five days later he received an urgent call that a 'perfect' donor heart match was available and that a helicopter would bring him immediately to Rigshospitalet.

Everything 'went so fast' he says he is 'still in a daze' but feeling remarkably better. The entire procedure from beginning to end went so smoothly, he exclaims, that he would any day "rather choose to undergo a heart transplant than a tooth extraction!" He is extraordinarily grateful to the donor whose premature death yielded this heart to him and gave him a new lease on life. He plans upon final discharge to become actively involved in improving the system of organ donation in Denmark.

Lief believes the social support available to him, as a transplant recipient in Denmark is quite generous and certainly more than adequate. The total time period from receiving his diagnosis of dilated cardiomyopathy to receiving his donor heart was only four weeks. From the first appearance of his initial symptoms to receiving his new heart he had a total of only seven physician visits. The GP, he asserts, is the weakest link in the Danish health care system, as it was the GP who initially misdiagnosed him.

Heart Transplantation in Denmark Compared to the US

According to the cardiologists at Rigshospitalet, the median survival of heart transplant patients in Denmark is 8 years and about two thirds of patients are alive after 10 years. The average age of heart transplant patients in Denmark is 43 years compared to 50 years in the US and other parts of the industrialized world. This younger age may in part explain the better survival outcomes of heart transplant patients in Denmark where the 30-day and one-year survival rates slightly exceed those of other countries.

The major medical reason for heart transplantation in Denmark is dilated cardiomyopathy whereas in the US (and most other countries) the major reason for a heart transplant is coronary artery and vascular disease. These differences in underlying etiologies may contribute to the difference in survival outcomes since vascular disease by itself has an overall worse prognosis. In Denmark, the long term complications and causes of death following heart transplant include, as elsewhere, graft versus host disease (GVHD) and cancer resulting from exposure to the toxic immunosuppressants.

Medical Malpractice, Patient Rights and the Patient-Doctor Relationship

Doctors in Denmark are required to inform patients of their legal rights and not to misinform them about available treatments (or their side effects and potential complications). Nonetheless, signed consent forms are not part of standard practice. Medical malpractice litigation occurs only rarely. Instead, the medical council has established its own internal system for addressing patient dissatisfaction and practice irregularities.

The Patients' Board of Complaints is an independent authority with the power to officially reprimand medical staff and even to take them to court. Through the Patient Insurance Scheme of 1992, patients may also claim damages for adverse treatment in public hospitals. Since then, it has also become easier to obtain compensation for disability, loss of pay or economic capacity, as well as 'pain and suffering.' Few cases ever reach the courts. However I was told that some years ago six patients who had received HIV-infected blood via transfusion successfully won a malpractice suite against the relevant health authority. Since then a special 'damages agreement' has been established for compensating those infected through transfusions.

Jacob was of the opinion that the low rate of medical malpractice litigation could be attributed to professional 'protectionism' among physicians and health care workers. Patients, he said, were often concerned that their complaints might be broadcast within the medical community and that this could potentially compromise their long-term care.

In Denmark, patients have the right to view their medical records. If patients request it, doctors, nurses and health care workers are obliged to interpret their records for them. Jacob always requests that physicians and nurses explain all procedures and test results to him and to his mother, who is his health care proxy. He commented on how obliging the staff always was when he requested this service. In Denmark as in the US, 'living wills' are used to state a patient's wishes regarding pain treatment, resuscitation and prolonging life. Nonetheless, with regard to organ donation close relatives can override the patient's wishes.

Jacob is dissatisfied and considers as 'malpractice' the exacerbating delays by both his GP in referring him for specialist care, and by the cardiologists at Gentofte in their delay referring him to Rigshospitalet for transplant evaluation. GPs are compelled to rely on county centers for performing certain tests and procedures such as x-rays. In 2001, results of such tests could take weeks to arrive back at the GP's office. In some cases, momentum towards effective follow up with the patient may be lost. In Jacob's case, even after the x-rays had arrived in his GP's office he was not called about the results and was informed of them only after he specifically inquired.

Comparison of the Cases of Jacob and Lief

The cases of Jacob and Lief provide some thought-provoking contrasts and similarities in their journeys through the Danish health care system. They are two patients of the same age and with a similar diagnosis of dilated cardiomyopathy.

Both patients were initially shocked at the news that they required a heart transplant. Both needed to adapt to the idea of harboring another person's functioning organ inside their bodies. Both, of course, ultimately agreed to the operation. But at this point their trajectories diverge. Whereas Jacob was still waiting after nine months for a donor heart while his condition worsened to the point of requiring an emergency LVAD implant, Lief's perfectly matched heart became available 'so suddenly' that he was still adapting psychologically to being an organ recipient and marveling at his good fortune.

While Lief found the transplant experience less stressful than a tooth extraction, Jacob was deeply shaken by his narrow scrape with death in the week I departed from Copenhagen, and he was profoundly despondent and doubtful that he would receive a donor heart in time.

The contrast in these cases illustrates the pivotal importance of Denmark's infrastructure in regard to organ donation. This may be an obvious conclusion, but it is less obvious that *changes* in this system could have life-saving outcomes for desperate patients like Jacob. It is all too apparent to him that political action is needed concerning this aspect of the health care system.

Both Jacob and Lief agree that the weakest link in the existing system is the GPs. Some of these physicians appear to be inept diagnosticians and are reluctant as gatekeepers to refer patients for essential specialist attention. Both patients, however, expressed their trepidation about the consequences of seeking second opinions on their medical conditions, as they feared reprisals might compromise their long-term care. Be that as it may, both Jacob and Lief were otherwise quite impressed with aspects of the Danish health care system, for instance, the generous financial support and the extensive rehabilitation and social services. Neither expressed the slightest willingness, from what they said they knew of it, to exchange the Danish for the American health care system.

Concluding Impressions and Remarks

Ambling through the wards of the Rigshospitalet, I was struck by how much less 'frenetic' the activity was than that on the wards of American hospitals. Doctors and nurses went about their activities in a calm yet professional manner and appeared to accomplish their tasks at a measured pace and without the apparent "hyperactivity" evident in American hospital wards. The volume of patients may have been less; the hospital stays of patients longer, but also not observed was the laborious note taking and frenzied chart recording which, mostly for legal reasons, has become such an integral part of ward medicine in the US.

Something else I did not see at Rigshospitalet (Denmark's major teaching hospital) were the teams comprised of attending physicians, residents and medical students that are the hallmark of American teaching hospitals. Indeed, in the entire month I spent on the cardiology ward, I never encountered a single student. The attending physicians, a rotating resident or two, and the efficient nursing staff accomplished the daily running of the ward. Attending physicians, rather than medical students, wrote brief progress notes not necessarily every day but usually only when changes in the patient's course of care were made. At Rigshospitalet, charts were all still on paper in 2001 although I was told that moves were afoot to switch to an electronic chart system. Physicians also carried hospital belt phones rather than beepers as in American hospitals, which allowed for immediate communication and circumvented time-consuming pager return calls.

Danish patients seemed considerably more satisfied with, and often proud of, their health care system compared with patients in the US. One reason for the difference in contentment is clearly a consequence of the 'generosity' of the Danish welfare system (admittedly paid for by very high taxes) compared with the privatized system of the US. Other reasons may lie with the HMO-induced stresses of cost-containment in the US, the quicker pace of American medical practice and the evidently higher (and at times outrageous) expectations of American patients. Finally, another stressor on American medical practice lies in its vulnerability to litigation, compared with the "safer" internal handling of malpractice complaints in Denmark.

To conclude, it was interesting for me to reflect that in the course of my Ph.D thesis on rheumatic heart disease I had spent many hours in the same operating room at Groote Schuur Hospital in Cape Town, South Africa, in which the world's first heart transplant had been performed by Dr. Christiaan Barnard in 1967. Indeed, while awaiting specimens of atrial appendage from the cardiac surgeons for the purpose of constructing cDNA genetic libraries of human heart genes, I had spent hours chatting with some of the same nurses and surgeons who had been members of that first heart transplant team many years earlier. The world's first heart transplant patient, Louis Washkansky, survived only five days. In 2001 patients in Denmark not uncommonly live beyond ten years, and for my patient, Lief, the surgery seemed almost routine. It was thus awe-inspiring to reflect on the advances in this complicated surgical operation over the years. Yet even in the sophisticated health care system of the Danish 'welfare' state, there is still one of the original problems of transplantation, namely that of organ donation.

Case 6: Like Father Like Son*

Diana Feldman

When I first met Jan Jacobsen, he was not up to talking to me. He had been admitted to Bispebjerg Hospital after seeing his General Practitioner (GP), Dr. Nils Petersen, two days prior to my visit. On that day Dr. Petersen was called by Mr. Jacobsen's social worker and by his mother. They were most concerned that he had been having bright red blood from his rectum for the past two days. Dr. Petersen decided to make a home visit to evaluate the patient and if need be, refer him to the hospital.

House Call

In Denmark, home visits are not unusual. Since all of the patients live in the region for which the GP is responsible, the furthest the doctor has to travel is about 10km and since the GP does not have hospital responsibilities, there is time allotted in his day to see unscheduled cases in the clinic, or pay a home visit to an acutely ill patient. This is part of the Danish system of separating outpatient and inpatient doctors' responsibilities. It is all part of the Danish social welfare system, which is based on the principle

---

*This case was written by Diana Feldman when she was a student at Weill Medical College, Cornell University and participated in the US-EU-MEE program at the University of Copenhagen, Denmark in the spring of 2002.

that all citizens should be guaranteed care when they encounter social problems such as unemployment, sickness, or dependency.

During his visit, Dr. Petersen found that in addition to the rectal bleeding, Mr. Jacobsen had a great deal of fluid accumulated in his abdomen, swollen ankles, and dilated veins in his legs. He was also running a fever. Clearly, his condition had worsened since the last time Dr. Petersen saw him about two weeks ago. I was given permission to read Mr. Jacobsen's hospital records, which summarize his brief conversation with Dr. Petersen.

"Mr. Jacobsen, I think you should go to the hospital and have some tests done to see what is causing your problems."

"Can't you just give me some medicine? I don't want to go to the hospital again."

"I can't give you medicine until we know what is causing your symptoms. They can make you more comfortable in the hospital."

Dr. Petersen called Bispebjerg Hospital, the local hospital where Mr. Jacobsen had been a patient several times, and gave them his present history.

Hospital Admission

In about an hour and a half an ambulance took Mr. Jacobsen to the hospital's emergency department, where he was interviewed and examined. He had a fever of 40°C, a rapid heartbeat, cough, spider nevi (capillaries showing under the skin in a spiderburst pattern), minimal tremor, and a massive amount of fluid in his abdomen. His skin and the whites of his eyes had a decidedly yellow cast. His rectal exam showed superficial blood but no brisk bleeding. The first set of tests was performed while Mr. Jacobsen was in the emergency department. It was 5 pm on April 2 when the admission note was written. A part of the plan was to do an esophagoscopy in the morning to rule out esophageal varices (enlarged veins in the esophagus).

This plan of treatment differs from the U.S. where the pace of diagnostic evaluation is much quicker, and where an esophagoscopy would be done the same day. I found that it is customary for Danish hospitals to put off procedures and schedule them for the following morning. To save expense, at some hospitals, there are no qualified specialists available at night and no emergency operating rooms running.

The Danish Health Care System

One criticism of the Danish system is the waiting time patients experience for some procedures and even for specialist appointments. This problem originates in the lack of sufficient numbers of personnel and equipment. According to statistics provided by the Ministry of Health, the employment in hospitals has increased at an annual rate of 0.4% over the whole period from 1990 to 1999, yet there is a shortage of personnel in the hospitals.

This problem is complicated by the fact that junior doctors (residents) have a fixed 37-hour workweek. One may think that this is an easy way for the government and the hospitals to save money, but in fact it was one of the achievements of the doctors' union in the 1980s to have a workweek comparable to other professions. Among the main reasons for it was a surplus of physicians and especially residents in the hospitals at that time. These junior doctors could not get as much hands-on experience as they wished because there were too many other eager colleagues "in line." Now, the residents get a base salary for a 37-hour workweek, and even when they work overtime they rarely get extra pay although sometimes they can negotiate extra time off.

Treatment in the Emergency Department

Mr. Jacobsen's doctors in the emergency department did an admission panel of blood tests (including CBC, and electrolytes), electrocardiogram, chest x-ray, liver panel and bilirubin levels, hematology panel, blood cultures, urinalysis and paracentesis. He was started on injections of B-combin (vitamins B1, B2 and riboflavin), thiamin, Losec (proton pump inhibitor) and Risolid (benzodiazepine). The chest x-ray suggested pneumonia, so he was also started on Zinacef and Gentamycin IV.

The next day Mr. Jacobsen was still in the emergency department. The results of his blood culture came back, showing *Streptococci*, so his Zinacef was discontinued and changed to Penicillin IV. He was also worked up for his rapid heartbeat that on the EKG was shown to be an atrial flutter, and he was given Digoxin. The complete blood count revealed leukocytosis and severe anemia, for which he got two units of whole blood. He also had low albumin and high liver function tests (however not as high as before, suggesting that his liver has cirrhosed). Mr. Jacobsen got his own bed in the medicine department of the hospital after spending about 12 hours in the emergency department.

The esophagoscopy was done in the morning of April 4th, on the third day of Mr. Jacobsen's admission. It showed no acute bleeding or esophageal varices (dilated blood vessels). Even though he showed signs of rectal bleeding on digital examination, no further workup for GI bleeding was done. During his hospital stay, Mr. Jacobsen was also found to have an abnormal heart rhythm. He was seen by a cardiology consultant, who suspected endocarditis. I did not see any follow up of this on his chart.

Diuretics were given in an attempt to reduce the ascites (fluid in his abdomen) and ankle swelling but he did not show any significant improvement. He had his ascites drained again on his ninth day in the hospital. Several times throughout the chart it is noted that Mr. Jacobsen has been told about the seriousness of his condition, and that he cannot tolerate any alcohol, and should be under tight control after the discharge. During 10 days of hospitalization, he was seen by 11 different physicians, yet neither Mr. Jacobsen nor his mother knew the prognosis and treatment plan although they tried several times to find out.

When Mr. Jacobsen felt more like talking I was able to meet with him for several pleasant conversations and heard the rest of his story.

Jan Jacobsen's Story

Jan Jacobsen is a 43-year-old man who lives alone in the Nørrebro district of Copenhagen. He was born and grew up in Holte, which is a small town in the country, where he lived with his parents until he was 25 years old. His father held an executive position in a Copenhagen administrative office and was always busy with his work. He was a somewhat distant father, and used to drink a lot, mostly during the multiple meetings at his work, and also at home because of stress. Mr. Jacobsen's mother was a yoga teacher. He has a half-brother whom he has never seen. Mr. Jacobsen's highest education is "common school" for job training after which he acquired an office position as a clerk. He held many jobs, mostly of clerical nature. During his younger years Jan Jacobsen was a drummer, playing rock music. He was also a fan of some rock bands, like Deep Purple, and traveled to other countries to hear them in concerts.

Mr. Jacobsen told me he got married and had a daughter, who is seventeen years old now. About ten years ago, he and his wife separated for multiple reasons. He sees his daughter several times a year, on major holidays. The last time he saw her was on Easter Sunday.

"Do you miss your daughter?" I asked.

"Yes, I would like to see her more often. I love her very much. It is the main reason that I want to get well and keep on living. I want to see her grow up and succeed in life."

"Are your parents still living?"

"My father died of old age in 1996 in a nursing home. I am very close to my mother who is 68 years old now. She lives near me and she is still quite active and takes care of me, although she is complaining of back problems."

From reading Jan Jacobsen's file I learned that according to his General Practitioner, Dr. Nils Petersen, the mother is dominating the patient, who looks for authority, preferring not to take responsibility for his actions, or take part in decisions.

I asked Mr. Jacobsen about his health during childhood.

"I had the common childhood diseases when I was young and I had a lot of infections all through my childhood and up until my adult years. The infections were probably caused by enlarged tonsils. I finally had my tonsils removed when I was 35 years old. It was poor judgment on the part of my doctors that I didn't have them out much sooner."

"Have you always had the same GP (Dr. Petersen)?"

"No. I had another GP but after I separated from my wife, who had the same GP, I decided to change doctors. I first went to Dr. Petersen in 1996."

From Mr. Jacobsen's medical records I learned that his past history included an extensive work-up for acid reflux. Back in 1991, he was admitted to the Ear Nose and Throat Department at Rigshospitalet because of "esophageal cyanosis." In 1993 he had an x-ray of his esophagus because of persistent gastroesophageal reflux, and the doctors found that he had distal esophageal stenosis. In 1995, Mr. Jacobsen had a balloon dilatation of the esophagus performed at Bispebjerg Hospitalet, and was prescribed Losec for three months.

"After I started seeing Dr. Petersen, my symptoms recurred and in 1997, I had another balloon dilatation procedure done at Rigshospitalet," Mr. Jacobson continued. "Both times I had to wait for approximately six months for these procedures after being referred by my doctor. These waiting periods seemed very long since I was having painful symptoms all the time."

"Did you choose to go to Rigshospitalet?"

"No. I was lucky that this was the hospital to which I was assigned and referred to by my GP. I have never chosen a hospital myself although by law, since 1993 Danish citizens can choose to go to any hospital as long as it operates within the Health Care Reimbursement Scheme. There are certain limitations. For instance, you can only receive care at another hospital if your primary hospital has a longer waiting time compared with the other hospital. Of course this applies only to planned admissions. In an emergency the patient cannot choose the hospital."

"Has your medical care been expensive?"

"I have never had to pay for any of my hospitalizations or primary care visits. I could have private (Group 2) insurance but I have never seen the need for it. The only medical expenses I have had are for my medications. It costs me approximately DKK 220, equivalent to about $27 per year (in 2002). The government reimburses the rest of my medication costs."

Drug Costs and Insurance

Looking a little further into the Danish health care system, I found that the drug reimbursement system works in the following way. The patient pays all of the cost up to DKK 500 (about $61) per year. Above that amount, the government reimburses an increasing amount at certain levels of expenditures. Above DKK 2800 (about $341), the government reimburses 85% of the cost (2002 figures).

In spite of the comprehensive public insurance, about 30% of the Danish population also has supplementary private insurance. They get it while they are healthy so they can bypass waiting lists for the public services "just in case" of illness that would require prompt treatment. On the other hand they can still have all the advantages of the public insurance coverage.

Communication

From his medical records I discovered that Mr. Jacobsen suffered from tinnitus (ringing in the ears) and Dr. Petersen decided that it must have been the effects of the loud rock music to which he was constantly exposed when he was a drummer. In 1997, Mr. Jacobsen suffered a fracture of the fifth metatarsal in his right foot during a fall from stairs in a train station. He was conservatively treated. There were no suspicions raised that the patient might have been drunk when the accident occurred.

Mr. Jacobsen told me that there is no tradition of communication between doctors in the hospitals and general practitioners in Denmark. It is very rare that an inpatient attending physician will contact a GP with questions about the patient, or vice versa. Most contact occurs via paperwork. When the patient is referred to a hospital or a clinic, basic history is provided by the GP. When the outpatient treatment is over, the GP receives a "sign-off note" with a brief description of the treatment and copies of lab tests. The GPs very rarely visit their patients when they are hospitalized and if they do, it is not to influence or be involved in the treatment, but more for social reasons.

In case a patient changes his/her general practitioner, depending on what the new general practitioner wants to know and how far back in the patient's history he wants to go, the GP will request a copy of the files from the previous GP (with the permission of the patient of course). When a patient is in the hospital, a different physician may see him or her every day. Thus, it is very easy for patients to lose count of the doctors, get lost in the hospital hierarchy and not know who to speak to if they have questions. In fact, from the patients' point of view, communication between doctors and the patients could be better. This is the most common complaint about the health care in Denmark. Yet, in the first National Survey of patient's views on hospitals' performance in the year 2000, nine out of ten patients were satisfied with the health care system.

An Upsetting Time

I asked Mr. Jacobsen about a visit to his general practitioner in January of 1999.

"I was very close to my grandfather Jacobsen. He died just before Christmas at the age of 81. When I saw Dr. Petersen in January of 1999 I was very upset by my grandfather's death, and I was upset even more by the circumstances surrounding it. I thought he passed away in a very mysterious manner but nobody else in the family wanted to discuss this 'family secret.' I had a lot of trouble concentrating at this time and I had frightening and unusual nightmares that were connected to this whole situation."

"Was Dr. Petersen able to help you?"

"He prescribed a trial of low-dose medication (Truxal) but didn't refer me to a psychiatrist, thank goodness."

I did not ask Mr. Jacobsen why he was happy to escape referral to a psychiatrist, but I did find out that it is not the usual practice in Denmark to refer patients to a psychiatrist for "psychological" problems. Psychiatry is mostly used for "frank" psychiatric diseases, such as schizophrenia, bipolar disorder, and clinical depression. There are also long waiting times for psychiatric specialists. If a patient needs psychological help, he or she may be referred to a psychologist. However, psychologist's visits are only partially covered by public insurance and may be quite expensive. On the other hand, general practitioners in Denmark are trained to help patients with psychological or psychiatric problems.

It is also congruent with the general principle of the Danish health care and social welfare system that an individual's capabilities should be optimized, so for example, the elderly live independently as long as possible, mentally ill live in their own homes with a contact person from the municipality (a social worker) checking up on them, or those who require more intensive assistance live in collective housing. Yet there are not that many special residences available, and some people who require hospitalization wait in line for admission.

In early May of 1999, several people, including Mr. Jacobsen's mother, apparently mentioned to Dr. Petersen that his patient might have a drinking problem. By the use of CAGE questions (see below), the GP found out that Mr. Jacobsen drinks mostly beer, about a 6-pack a day, and wine with meals. At this time he lived with a 35-year-old woman who also consumed a comparable amount of alcohol.

CAGE QUESTIONS
1. Cut — Have you ever felt you ought to cut down on your drinking?
2. Annoyed — Have people annoyed you by criticizing your drinking?
3. Guilt — Have you ever felt bad or guilty about your drinking?
4. Eye Opener — Have you ever had an eye-opener to steady nerves in the morning?

Answering "yes" to 2 questions = strong indication for Alcoholism
Answering "yes" to 3 questions = confirms Alcoholism

Mr. Jacobsen was asked the standard questions when he was hospitalized before. For example, in 1997 his admission history states that the patient drinks one beer per day, but he was not really screened for alcohol abuse. We can only wonder whether his problems could have been prevented if they had been addressed earlier.

In May 1999 Dr. Petersen ordered some blood tests, including a liver panel, which came back with critically high numbers indicating hepatocyte damage and hepatobiliary disease. Mr. Jacobsen was informed of the results, and was strongly advised to quit drinking. Nevertheless, he continued drinking, and in June of the same year, he complained of trembling hands. The liver function tests were repeated, showing similar if not worse results. He was again advised to quit drinking and was offered some social help in houses for alcoholics. He refused this, stating reasons ranging from inconvenient transportation to fears that something would happen to him there. He was also still suffering from acid reflux.

What is the Real Problem?

Mr. Jacobsen was followed in the outpatient GI clinic of Rigshospitalet from November 1998 to March 2000, when he was diagnosed with esophagitis due to alcohol consumption, according to the "sign-off" note in 2000. There were no indications for invasive treatment, and continuation of conservative treatment was recommended. The sign-off note to the GP states that the patient was strongly advised to change life habits, and especially to lose weight and reduce alcohol consumption. He was also offered psychological assistance but he refused it.

Mr. Jacobsen told me that he first started drinking beer when he was 25 years old.

"I don't know why I did it. Everybody drinks beer in Denmark. My father always drank beer. It is easy to get cheap, or even free beer. It was just the thing for a young person to do."

"Have you ever tried to quit?" I asked.

"Dr. Petersen wanted me to go to the program called "The Chain," but I found out it is very expensive and I would have to pay for it myself. There are programs sponsored by Blue Cross and Alcoholics Anonymous, but I think there should be more inpatient hospital treatment programs. Maybe if I had gotten into one of them I could have stopped drinking."

In August of 2000 Mr. Jacobsen's mother called Dr. Petersen and complained that her son could not walk. He also had tingling and numbness in both feet and was seeing double. Dr. Petersen referred him to Bispebjerg Hospitalet and he was admitted in the department of Neurology. He had an MRI to rule out other possibilities, but the diagnosis was: severe alcoholic polyneuropathy. He was treated with Thiamin, B-combin forte (vitamins B1, B2 and riboflavin), and started on Antabuse.

Because he was not able to work, around this time Mr. Jacobsen lost his last job as a clerk and started receiving payments from the union. When he was released from the hospital, his treatment team arranged for him to be assigned to a social agency, "*Københavns Kommune*," which provided a social worker who would visit him several times a week to help with the activities of daily living.

Mr. Jacobsen's condition did not really improve after this hospitalization. Even though he was on Antabuse, he continued drinking, and his doctors decided to discontinue the treatment. Dr. Petersen and Mr. Jacobsen's social worker continued to try and persuade him to enroll in the Blue Cross program for alcoholics or Alcoholics Anonymous, however he refused all of their recommendations.

Mr. Jacobsen's last visit to Dr. Petersen occurred on March 14, 2002. The physical exam revealed ascites, ankle edema, spider nevi and dilated lower extremity veins. Clearly, his condition had worsened. Even though there was no cytological diagnosis, it was clear that he had probably progressed to alcoholic liver cirrhosis.

The last time I saw Mr. Jacobsen in 2002 he was still in the hospital, with plans to be discharged within a few days. His treatment team tried to hammer home the message that he cannot drink alcohol any more. His hospitalization served to stabilize him but did not improve or reverse his condition. Only Mr. Jacobsen could do that.

Case 7: Toughing it Out with Back Pain*

Robert F. Garza

Magnus Pedersen is a man with a very interesting story. At first glance, there appears to be nothing unusual about him. One would think that he is just a normal 64-year-old Danish gentleman. Although he has a slightly slow and stiff gait, he appears to be healthy, even for an elderly man.

Without talking to him, one would also not know that Magnus considers himself a very tough guy. He is not one to complain or ask for help, even when he needs it. He would tell any listener that he is very happy with his life and his health. However, Magnus has been fighting a lifelong struggle with lower back pain. This is his story as he related it to me.

Early Life

I was born and raised in Denmark. At the age of fourteen, my parents decided to get a divorce. Soon afterwards my father passed away. I lived with my mother and two brothers at the time. Because my mother did not make enough money to support us, I decided that I needed to drop out of

---

*Robert F. Garza wrote this case when he was a student at Vanderbilt University School of Medicine and participated in the US-EU-MEE program at the University of Copenhagen, Denmark, in April 2001.

school to help care for my mother and brothers. So, at age fourteen, I left school and began to work. Because I was so young and had no work experience, the only job I could find involved lifting heavy boxes and other items. This was the beginning of my battle with lower back pain. There were many times when I remember being tired and sore after long hours of manual labor.

Over the next ten years I switched jobs many times. By the time I was twenty-four years old I was working for a tire distribution company. The work at this warehouse also included heavy lifting. I had made friends with my boss and I give him credit for setting my life in a new direction.

One day my boss said, "Magnus, if you ever want to do anything else with your life, you need to return to school."

Education and Life Changes

So I began to attend school part-time while working at the tire warehouse. Eventually, I finished my education to the equivalent of a high school diploma in the United States. This enabled me to get better jobs and by age 35 I was working for a liquid gas distribution company. Fortunately, this job included only very minor lifting, but by now the damage to my back had already been done.

As I advanced in this job I worked as a consultant to the clients of the company, and spent most of my time in my automobile, traveling over 100,000 kilometers per year. Unfortunately, this made my back problems even worse. The car provided by the company was not very comfortable. There was no attention paid to ergonomics in those days and the seats were not very friendly to my lumbar region. I would begin to have back pain after driving for a few hours and it became steadily worse.

In 1980, I decided to retire from work. I was really tired of working and especially tired of the endless driving, but a larger part of the decision was that my back was giving me more and more trouble. I took my pension at this time, which is equivalent to disability and retirement pay, and thought I would pursue my interest in politics. I did not last long at this because my back pain continued to get worse.

The Pain Wins

In 1982 I decided to stop being a tough guy and get medical attention for my lower back pain. At this time the pain was so severe that I couldn't move my legs. I was admitted to my local hospital, and the doctors discovered that I had a herniated disk in my lower back. I stayed in the hospital on strict bed rest for six weeks. During this time, I also had massage therapy and physical therapy but neither helped very much. After six weeks of bed rest, I was evaluated by a neurosurgeon, and at this point I was transferred to Rigshospitalet in Copenhagen for further evaluation.

Rigshospitalet is a high level hospital affiliated with the University of Copenhagen academic medical center. You can get some specialist care there that is not available in other areas of Denmark, so I was lucky to end up there in December of 1982. The doctors did a test called a myelogram and decided that I needed surgery to repair a prolapsed disc in my lower back. My hospital records show that I had a partial laminectomy of a herniated disc at L5-S1 in my lumbar spine. Up until this time I was pretty much in the dark about what was going on medically, but I found out that I could ask a nurse to show me my medical records and explain them to me.

Unfortunately, this was not the end of the troubles with my back. I continued to have severe leg pain after the operation, and, two weeks after that first surgery, I was back in the operating room to see what had gone wrong. Afterwards the surgeon told me that the disc at L5 had not herniated a second time, as they had thought, and I did not have any nerve damage. He said they found nothing significant during the operation, and nothing was done. I don't know how this could happen, but fortunately, for whatever reason, I was free of leg pain after this second operation.

I was discharged home from the hospital and did well for several weeks. Then the pain in my back slowly returned and I turned to the doctors again. This time, the pain in my back continued down my left leg all the way to my ankle. My medical records say that I had a positive Lasegue test (straight-leg raise) and some abnormal sensory findings. Late in 1983, I had another myelogram. This showed that the L4-L5 disc in my back had herniated and was compressing the spinal cord in that area. I was referred again to the neurosurgeon and in January 1984, I had my third back operation. The surgeon performed a partial laminectomy of the L4-L5 disc. This time the results were satisfactory. I had a smooth recovery and was free of pain when I was discharged from Rigshospitalet.

My recovery was not permanent, however. Over the next ten years I had plenty of trouble with back pain. Some days it was not there at all but on other days it was so bad that I could not even make it to my part-time job. It was hard for me to keep steady employment because I had to miss so many days out of the year because of the pain. During this time I was a marketing consultant for several firms when I was able to work. Still being a tough guy, I refused to take medicine for my pain during this time unless it was absolutely necessary. I just dealt with it in my own way, trying to live with it and not be a complainer.

More Medical Care

But in 1993 my pain was simply too great to bear. I began once again to seek medical help. By this time I had lost the last job I had because I could not work for six months. I went to several doctors and tried several alternative therapies for my back. Massage therapy and physical therapy did not help. In fact, my pain progressed to the point where I could not even travel to physical therapy and certainly could not do the exercises. In late 1993, my general practitioner again referred me to the neurosurgeon at my local hospital. This doctor examined me and felt that I had no neurologic damage. However, he ordered an x-ray of my lower spine and this showed severe osteoarthritis in my lumbar region, particularly around L4 and L5. Since he thought there was no neurological problem, this neurosurgeon decided to refer me to the orthopedic surgeon at the local hospital for further evaluation. In addition, he thought I needed some titanium instrumentation installed in my lower back by the orthopedic surgeon for structural support.

Waiting for an MRI

I went to see the orthopedic doctor at my local hospital, Hvidovre Hospital. Unfortunately, the procedure that I needed could only be performed at Rigshospitalet, where I had my previous surgeries. But in 1993,

Rigshospitalet was a state hospital to which I could not receive a transfer. I insisted that the State should allow this procedure, but, at that time, patients did not have the option to choose a particular hospital for their care. So, my fight to be admitted to the hospital began. I was put on the long list to receive an MRI scan, and, in 1993, there was only one in the area. This one was at Rigshospitalet, and the waiting time was extraordinarily long.

In the meantime, I was struggling with the pain on a daily basis. I was not employed, so I spent my days at home, keeping myself busy with household chores. I wanted to do exercise and be outdoors, but every time I exerted myself, I would have to lie in bed for a week recovering from the pain so I only went outside to walk about once every three weeks. On some days, the pain was so severe that I could not even dress myself or use the toilet. After one year of dealing with the pain and waiting for an MRI scan, I finally decided it was time to go above being a normal citizen and cry for help. Through my interest in politics I had many opportunities over the years to become friends with politicians at both the local and state level. I wrote a letter to a friend in the Ministry of Health describing my situation, hoping that he could pull some strings to help me move up in line at the MRI scanner. I also needed help getting into Rigshospitalet as a referred patient since the hospital did not accept my transfer in 1993.

During this time, I had a lot of difficulty with the State. Because I was being covered by a pension, I had to meet with a social worker. Often, when I was away at the office of the social worker, the hospital would call and tell me that they could schedule my MRI scan. But since I would not be at home, I would miss the call, and be forced back down the waiting list. This was very irritating. I knew the surgery would not be scheduled until I had the MRI scan. I was in an incredible amount of pain, and I was very frustrated by the process of having to wait to get the medical care I desperately needed.

Finally, in early 1994, I received a letter from my friend in the Ministry of Health that approved my referral to Rigshospitalet. In addition, this letter told me that the hospital was about to receive two new MRI scanners. I am proud to think that my complaint probably had something to do with getting these new scanners.

I saw the orthopedic surgeon, and three months later, in July 1994, I finally received my MRI scan and another myelogram. The surgeon explained that these tests showed that I had spondylosis of the lumbar spine with degenerative compression of the discs at L4-L5 and L5-S1 as well as spondyloarthrosis. The nurse who interpreted my medical records for me explained that this meant that I had stiffening of the joints in this area of my spine and compression of the fibrous, spongy cartilage or discs between the vertebrae in certain areas as well as thickening and inflammation of the bony joints. The orthopedic surgeon felt that it was appropriate to plan for surgery.

A Fourth Operation

In August of 1995, two years after my first visit to my local doctor for leg pain, I was finally admitted to Rigshospitalet for my fourth operation. This time I had a laminectomy at L4-L5 and L5-S1, removal of the hypertrophied facet joints, decompression of the spondylosis, and fusion of the L4, L5, and S1 vertebrae using titanium instrumentation. After the surgery my recovery was swift, and I left the hospital five days later with no leg pain and no complications. I received free transportation home as a service from the State. Since 1995 I continue to have intermittent pain. Some days it is bad, and some days it is not. At least, thank God, it is never as intense or as severe as it was before my operation in 1995.

Those are the facts of my story, but as a medical student from the United States, I am sure you have questions about how satisfied I am with the health care system in Denmark. First of all, I feel very privileged to live in Denmark. I appreciate the free health care I have received. Since my last surgery I feel that I can live a nearly normal life. I have even been able to work part-time after this last operation in 1995. It is true that I pay approximately 70% of my income in taxes but I feel that it is worth it for the quality of life I have in Denmark. The only thing I have had to pay for out-of-pocket is a portion of the cost of my medicines over the years.

The downside is that I would never want to go through the process again. I was very dissatisfied with being shuffled through all aspects of the system. I did not enjoy having to communicate with the social worker on a constant basis and I did not appreciate the wait I had to endure. Two years of constant pain was just too much to bear. It does not make any financial sense to have to wait so long. The pension I was paid by the State during those two years of waiting amounted to more than the total cost of the surgery and all the related tests and office visits. This is inefficient from both a financial and a political perspective. I do not understand why the waiting list has to be so long when the medical resources are available to perform the procedures.

In addition to the inefficiency of the system, there is a negative attitude on the part of the health care providers in general. They have no incentive to treat the patient as a valued customer because they are all salaried workers paid by the State. I often felt like an object rather than a person during my long experience in the health care system. In contrast, I understand that in the free enterprise system in America the patient has more choice of health care plans and physicians. The patient is the focus of care. In this I feel the Danish health care system is somewhat lacking.

A Student's Reflection

This is the end of Magnus Pedersen's story as he related it to me. He has seen the workings of the Danish health care system from a first-hand perspective. He has experienced the disadvantages of the system in terms of the long waiting times and frustrating referral system. But he has also experienced the major advantage to the Danish system, namely, that it is free, despite his paying approximately 70% of his income in taxes.

3

Cases Written by Danish Students in the US

Case 8: A Doctor as Patient*

Jacob Thyssen

The day I went to meet my patient at the Lemuel Shattuck Hospital was bright and sunny. Boston was just emerging from the grunginess of winter with grass turning green and flowering trees ready to burst into bloom.

Clutching my MBTA map, I found my way to the commuter rail station and got off at the Forest Hills Station. My instructions were to look for the Shattuck shuttle van on the Hyde Park side of the station. There was no regular schedule for the van, but I was told that it ran frequently. With no van in sight, and the inviting warmth of the spring sun, I decided to walk to the hospital. It looked like a short distance on the MBTA map, which showed buildings as well as the public transportation route. The hospital seemed to be set in the middle of a park, and I soon saw a sign, "Franklin Park, Jamaica Plain."

As I neared the hospital, I noticed a burly red-haired Boston police-man looking at me quizzically. It was then that I noticed that there were no other pedestrians in the vicinity. At the hospital entrance, two more policemen stood guard. I began to wonder what kind of hospital the Lemuel Shattuck is.

---

*The story of this patient is based on a case written by Jacob Thyssen when he was a student at the Faculty of Health Sciences, University of Copenhagen, Denmark and participated in the US-EU-MEE medical student exchange at Harvard Medical School in March and April 2003.

Inside, I asked directions to my patient's room and was soon shaking hands with Malachi Johnson, a very dark man with very white teeth and a big smile.

He invited me to sit in an overstuffed chair beside his bed and I settled down comfortably. I told him that I had come from Denmark to study health care in the United States, but first I wanted to know a little about his history. I already knew that he was a tuberculosis patient because he was in the TB unit, but I had no more information about him.

"Well, as you might guess, I am not a native of Boston, although I do have relatives living here," he replied. "I was born in Southern Rhodesia, which is now Zimbabwe, but I lived here as a teenager and went to high school here."

"How did you happen to live here as a teenager?"

"My father was a preacher and missionary for a Christian church. His job required a lot of travel and we lived in many places. You know, from Africa we sometimes send missionaries to other parts of the world — they don't always come to us!" He laughed heartily.

"Where else did you live?"

"Oh, in Belgium, Zaire, and Georgia in the United States. I also went to school here in Boston."

"What school did you attend?"

"Boston University," he replied. "I earned my medical degree at BU in 1970 and moved to New York to do my internship year at Harlem Hospital. In 1971 I moved back to Zaire and began my career as a surgeon."

I was pleased to find that my patient was a medical doctor, especially one who had trained in the United States. He should be able to give me lots of insight into the health care system here. I decided to plunge right in and ask his opinion of health care in America.

Mr. Johnson looked around at the clean, cheerful room — very plain but equipped with all the necessities for his comfort. "I am very contented with everything the American health care system has done for me. The doctors and nurses here are top notch. You may wonder what kind of hospital this is, with all the policemen around. Well, they are here because this is a primary site of ambulatory and inpatient services for the Massachusetts Department of Public Health. Prisoners who are sick are taken care of on the fourth floor."

"I see. But tell me more about your career as a surgeon in Zaire."

"Soon after I arrived there, I got married and we started a family. I did thoracic surgery, operating long hours and with very little equipment such as every hospital in the United States has. I operated on many patients with open pulmonary tuberculosis, but there was no money, even for surgical masks, so I often operated without any protection. It was very hard work and I hoped and prayed for a way to bring my family to a better place."

"To make matters worse, there was civil war in the Congo," he continued, "and finally my hospital was forced to shut down and I was left with no way to support my family. God moves in mysterious ways, and in the midst of my despair, there was a sudden ray of light. I received an invitation to a 30th reunion for my class at BU — the class of 1970."

"When was that?" I asked.

"In March, 2000. The reunion was to take place in May. After my initial excitement, I realized that I had no money to buy a plane ticket to Boston. Again, the miraculous happened, and the Christian church my father had served supported me financially and made it possible for me to buy a plane ticket and attend the anniversary party. But I was thinking about more than the party. It was now impossible to make a living in the Congo, so I thought about ways that I could make the trip to Boston more than a brief visit."

"When I got here, I asked the dean of Boston University to allow me to stay and update my medical training in the US. I wanted to learn how to use computers, to see how American doctors work, and become skilled in newer surgical techniques. To my great surprise and delight, the dean approved the plan and gave me the title of Research Associate. He wrote a letter to the US Immigration Service so I could get a visa. Over the years he wrote letters several times to get the visa extended."

"Were you living in the Boston area?" I asked.

"Yes. At first I lived with my cousin and spent time studying and updating myself as I had planned. After a while I started "moonlighting," doing any kind of work I could find for different companies to make a living and send money to my family. As soon as I could afford it, I moved out of my cousin's house and stayed in private rooms. Of course I was working illegally."

"Tell me about your illness. What brought you here to the Shattuck Hospital?"

"In September, 2002 I started to have pain in my lower back. At first I thought it was a muscle pain and I got massages and used over-the-counter pain medicine and took hot showers to relieve it. As time went on, the pain got worse and, as a physician, I thought it could be a herniated disc between L5 and S1. At the time I was working in a supermarket, carrying heavy boxes of meat. It got harder and harder for me to carry the heavy boxes and one day I simply could not stand up straight."

"Did you have any other symptoms?"

"I had numbness for some time but all of a sudden, I was unable to stand. Later that day my cousin took me to the hospital in Framingham. I had no history of alcohol or tobacco abuse and had never stayed in shelters. The only medication I took was aspirin, and the only serious disease I ever had was malaria. The only symptom, other than the pain, was a considerable weight loss over the previous few months."

"At Framingham Hospital I came into my first personal contact with the American medical system. With no insurance, I knew it was best if I went to the Emergency Department. I was familiar with the US law known as EMTALA (Emergency Medical Treatment and Active Labor Act). It is a Federal law that was passed in 1986 and gives everybody the right to emergency care regardless of the ability to pay. It applies to any hospital in the US that participates in Medicare and most hospitals do."

"Under EMTALA I knew I was entitled to screening, emergency care, and transfer to another facility if appropriate. Of course, the ER doctors and nurses at Framingham knew the rules, too, and never asked about my ability to pay. Ironically, I did a clinical rotation at this same hospital more than 30 years earlier, so I knew the place well."

"At Framingham I was diagnosed with tuberculosis of the lower back (Potts Disease). They removed three abscesses along the psoas muscle, started chemotherapy, and gave me a brace for my back. I could not walk and was confined to a wheelchair. I thought I would never walk again. When they had done what they could, they sent me to Lemuel Shattuck Hospital, and that is how I happen to be here."

"Was the care you received at Framingham free?"

"No, not exactly. I did eventually get a bill, and if I ever can, I intend to pay it. Since I am completely indigent, I am now under MassHealth, the Massachusetts Medicaid program."

"You are a lucky person. I hear that there are more than 40 million people in the United States who can't afford medical insurance and cannot get medical care. Do you have any thoughts about that?"

"Well, of course I do feel very sorry for them. I think people who are poor but not completely destitute have the most difficulty. They may be working but do not earn enough to pay for health insurance, or may work "under the table" as I did and not have health insurance from their employer. When I was a student in Boston, I knew plenty of young people who just didn't choose to spend money on health insurance. They preferred to spend it at the pubs and taverns around town, and nobody could force them to buy insurance."

"What did they do when they got sick?"

"If they got really sick, they went to a hospital Emergency Department. It isn't the best care because all they have to do under the EMTALA law is screen and stabilize the patient. Well, actually, because of a recent regulation, they do have to examine you. And a lot of really sick people end up in the Emergency Department. That is what is clogging US Emergency Departments these days. A lot of people who show up do need hospital care, and sometimes there aren't enough rooms to admit them. They end up in the ER or the halls for hours and the crowding interferes with the work of the Emergency Department. When it gets too full, they simply have to turn the ambulances away to another hospital."

"Of course rich Americans can buy all the health care they need," I said.

"True. And more power to them, but look at what the American health care system has done for me — a poor man from another country. I have had excellent medical care with plenty of TLC — Tender Loving Care. I have had surgery and three MRI scans and I am receiving the latest chemotherapy. I have only to reach out my hand and I have all the food and drink I want and the American health care system pays for it all."

"You don't think it's unfair that so many others in this country go without adequate health care?" I asked.

"No, I think if they truly need it they can get it. Medicare and Medicaid programs, SSI (Supplemental Security Income) and state welfare programs are set up to take care of the truly needy and disabled in this country. The paperwork may be a bit daunting, and the process can be frustrating, but the help is there for the neediest people. I thank the health care workers here at the Lemuel Shattuck hospital for giving me back my life. If it were not for them and the American system, I would either be dead by now, or at least unable to walk."

I thanked Mr. Johnson for spending time talking with me and walked out into the spring sunshine marveling at the treatment Malachi Johnson had received in the American health care system and his great satisfaction and gratitude.

The red-haired policeman smiled ever so slightly as I walked to the Hyde Street side of the hospital and waited for the shuttle van.

Case 9: Health Care Contrast in New York*

Anne-Marie Dogonowski

Helen Hill

Mrs. Hill is the first patient I met on the Cardiology Service at New York Presbyterian Hospital, affiliated with Weill Medical College of Cornell University where I was spending a month in a medical student exchange program. She is a 52-year-old African American woman from Queens, New York with a complicated history of heart disease and other ailments. They include coronary artery disease, congestive heart failure, diabetes mellitus, and hypertension. She has also been diagnosed with asthma, glaucoma, and depression. Lately, gastroesophageal reflux disease with a hiatal hernia has been added to the list. To complicate matters, she is seriously overweight, or "morbidly obese" in medical terminology. Mrs. Hill is a widow and lives with one of her adult daughters. She has not worked for most of her life and has recently been designated as disabled.

Mrs. Hill has many risk factors for coronary artery disease: high blood cholesterol, high blood pressure, diabetes and obesity (BMI = 53). Body

---

*Anne-Marie Dogonowski wrote these two case studies when she was a student in the Faculty of Health Sciences, University of Copenhagen and participated in the US-EU-MEE exchange at Weill Medical College of Cornell University in New York in August 2003.

Mass Index (BMI) is calculated by dividing weight in kilograms by height in millimeters squared (kg/m^2). Anyone with a BMI over 30 is considered obese.

She smoked 2–3 cigarettes a day for 23 years, although she quit six months ago. Furthermore, she has a family history of heart disease. Her father died of a myocardial infarction (MI) at the age of 51 and her mother also has high cholesterol, hypertension and diabetes. Mrs. Hill does not recall any preventive measures to diminish some of these risk factors, such as counseling about diet, alcohol, physical activity and smoking. She did participate in a support group for diabetic patients as part of her treatment and learned about sugar count, diet and how to take her insulin.

Reading her chart I find that Mrs. Hill experienced her first heart attack in January 2003. After this incident she had difficulty breathing, causing shortness of breath to a degree that she had to pause after walking half a block. Therefore a procedure called percutaneous transluminal coronary angioplasty (PTCA) with a stent was performed in an outpatient setting at New York Presbyterian Hospital, the university hospital of Columbia and Cornell (NYPH) in February 2003. This is a technique in which a balloon is used to dilate or widen narrowed arteries. The stent is a tiny stainless steel mesh tube placed inside the artery to keep it expanded.

During the next few months Mrs. Hill experienced two more serious episodes of shortness of breath (dyspnea) and was again hospitalized, this time at a hospital in Queens. She was given several diagnoses: gastroesophageal reflux disease (GERD) with hiatal hernia, and lung edema. When she got the additional diagnosis of food poisoning it was too much for her.

"I got tired of the hospital in Queens," she told me. "They did not take their time, only pumped me with medications and kept me going back and forth."

In mid-June Mrs. Hill was hospitalized at this same hospital for the third time. Despite the diuretics given, she still had intermittent shortness of breath and swelling of her legs and feet caused by the accumulation of fluid. At a barbeque party on the fourth of July 2003, she experienced chest pain that she described as "pressure or chest tightness." She became concerned because it resembled the pain she had experienced at the time of her heart attack. This time she was brought by ambulance to the Emergency Room at New York Presbyterian Hospital-Weill Cornell Medical Center. She herself chose to be brought to this hospital saying, "I prayed to God and he said come to this other hospital."

I asked her if she made this choice with the specific intention to be hospitalized in NYPH-Weill Cornell Medical Center, to which she defensively replied, "It is my right to go where I want to go."

In the hospital a cardiac catheterization test showed a moderate left ventricular dysfunction with an ejection fraction (EF) of 40% and single vessel obstructive coronary artery disease, thus confirming the diagnosis of congestive heart failure. When I met Mrs. Hill on the seventh day of her hospitalization, the catheterization with PTCA and stent of the occluded artery had been successfully performed and she expected to be discharged in a few days.

More about Mrs. Hill later.

Harry Ferland

My second patient at NYPH-Weill Medical College is Harry Ferland. Mr. Ferland is a 69-year-old Caucasian American man living in the Bronx, New York. He has always regarded himself as being in good health and lives an active life bowling every other day and playing golf. He retired from work at the age of 57 and since the death of his wife he lives alone in an apartment.

With an extensive family history of heart disease and many risk factors, in 1984 Mr. Ferland was not surprised to have his first heart attack at age 50. His mother died at the age of 71 of heart disease. He explained "the wall of her heart was very weak." His father died of an "enlarged heart" at age 61. "He had 26 heart attacks," Mr. Ferland said.

Mr. Ferland has been smoking two to three packs of cigarettes a day since the age of 12, has elevated cholesterol, hypertension and is severely obese with a calculated Body Mass Index of 49. Like Mrs. Hill, Mr. Ferland does not remember much counseling about steps to improve his health except for the recommendation of his cardiologist to lose weight and to do more exercise.

When he had his first heart attack, Mr. Ferland was hospitalized at Einstein Hospital in the Bronx, where he had bypass surgery called CABG or coronary artery bypass grafting. He was sent home with several prescriptions. He is currently taking eight pills a day: "Since the bypass the pills have been changed so many times that I don't know what I am taking them for," Mr. Ferland complained.

Following the CABG, he felt well for the next 18 years until an incident in 2002 when he experienced dizziness and a racing heart. He went to the Emergency Room at the Westchester Square Hospital in the Bronx, and was transferred to NYPH where he received an automatic implantable cardioverter defibrillator (AICD) pacemaker. This is a device that delivers an electric shock to the heart to restore normal rhythm.

In the beginning of July 2003, Mr. Ferland experienced "pressure" in his chest and shortness of breath. He had felt this sensation before but this time it did not go away. He went to the Emergency Room at a community hospital thirty minutes away from New York City, conveniently located near his son's home where he was visiting. His ECG and echocardiography were normal and he was sent home with the message "nothing is wrong with your heart."

A few weeks later, experiencing the same chest pain and shortness of breath, Mr. Ferland went to see his primary care practitioner (PCP). He was told to "take it easy and if the pressure comes back, then go to the ER," Mr. Ferland recalled.

The pressure did come back that same day and he was brought by ambulance to Westchester Square Hospital in the Bronx (a community hospital affiliated with NYPH) and given nitroglycerine. His enzymes (creatine kinase-MB and troponin-I) were elevated and he received treatment for myocardial infarction — a heart attack. He was transferred to NYPH on July 16, 2003 for cardiac catheterization, since this procedure was not performed in the small local Westchester Square Hospital. The catheterization showed triple vessel coronary artery disease with a new occlusion and severely impaired left ventricular function. During the catheterization a PTCA with stent was performed on the acutely occluded artery.

At the time I met Mr. Ferland he had been hospitalized in NYPH for six days. He was still suffering from shortness of breath but his condition was improving. Before this hospitalization he had gradually felt more fatigued. He was able to walk 10 blocks before becoming short of breath and he was short of breath when lying on his back but not after getting up. During hospitalization he had had nightly incidents of dyspnea at rest and was obviously dyspnaic during our conversation. He had been given the diagnosis of severe congestive heart failure, classified New York Heart Association (NYHA) IV with an Ejection Fraction of 25%. This meant that he had symptoms while at rest that were aggravated by activity. He was waiting for echocardiography to further diagnose his condition and expected to be discharged in a few days.

Health Care Costs for Mrs. Hill and Mr. Ferland

As a Danish medical student in the United States, these are my observations of US health care. The United States is the only industrialized western nation without universal national health insurance. Instead, health care services can be purchased through out-of-pocket payment to insurance companies or are provided by the government-financed programs, Medicare and Medicaid. With the introduction of private insurance a third-party payer (the insurance company) is added to the scenario, thus insurance becomes a dominant feature regardless from where you approach the American health care system.

Mrs. Hill has both Medicaid and Medicare insurance. She has had Medicaid insurance since 1975 because of her low-income situation. Having many concomitant diseases and weak vision, she has been designated disabled by her doctor. She is thus eligible for Medicare insurance without having reached the age of 65. Mrs. Hill demonstrated some uncertainty about the reasons for being entitled to her different insurances. "It is the medical system that has put me on my insurances," she says.

She has no medical expenses at all and does not pay for any of her medications. Mrs. Hill has no idea what her actual expenses are for medical care and prescription medications, but it probably totals upwards of a thousand dollars a month, and with hospitalizations, many thousands a year, which is paid entirely by the government programs.

Mr. Ferland's health care expenses are covered by three types of insurance: an employment-based private group health maintenance organization insurance (HMO), another individual private insurance through Blue Cross and Blue Shield, and Medicare. He worked as an unskilled laborer for the New York City Parks Department for 22 years until he retired in 1991. A great benefit from this work was health insurance covering himself, his wife and their children. "When you are married and have five kids you need that health insurance — that's the most important thing," he told me.

The employment-based group health insurance covers his doctor consultations. He pays $50 every month for this insurance in 2003. "If I had not worked for the City, I would have paid $600 a month — that is why I worked for the city," Mr. Ferland explains. The individual private Blue Cross and Blue Shield insurance covers both HMO and Medicare co-payments.

Being over 65 years old, Mr. Ferland is entitled to Medicare insurance. He automatically has part A and pays an additional $43 a month in 2003 for part B, which is again reimbursed by the City. (Note: this basic payment has risen to $96.40 by 2009, with higher amounts according to income). He has yet another agreement with his union organization for drug coverage, for which he pays $25 a month. In this agreement he has to pay $3 out-of-pocket for every prescription written for a generic drug, and more if a drug is non-generic. Mr. Ferland is a good example of a patient who has several insurance plans to achieve almost comprehensive coverage.

Having a combination of private and government insurance, as Mr. Ferland has, does not mean unrestricted and unlimited access to health services. His HMO puts some restrictions on medical care by requiring that he obtain a referral for any visit to a specialist and his private Blue Cross Blue Shield coverage may not include eye examinations and glasses.

I asked Mr. Ferland if he is satisfied with his health insurance. He replied, "My plan is pretty good compared with other plans but it could be better. Why should we have to pay for insurance to cover the deductibles?"

He mentions dissatisfaction with some of his HMO's restrictions. "I can only go to certain doctors. I do not have a choice or it will cost me more."

Moreover Mr. Ferland finds it difficult to know the extent of his coverage: "You do not know what certain insurance covers. I have millions of books about it. To find out I have to go through these books. They should have a place where you can call and tell them 'this is my plan' and what it covers should be answered by computer. You do not want to find out in the end, that you have to pay for it."

Mrs. Hill's Primary Care, Specialist Care and Follow-up

Since Mrs. Hill had an MI in January 2003 she was followed by five different doctors. She saw an endocrinologist every two weeks for her diabetes, she consulted her two PCPs every two weeks, she visited her cardiologist once a month and occasionally she saw an ophthalmologist for her glaucoma. This is a good illustration of American and modern medicine: each specialist treats a separate part of the body, thus it is not unusual to have five different doctors involved with your health. Under Medicare, Mrs. Hill has the option of choosing her doctors herself. They are all conveniently located less than one-and-a-half miles from her home.

Because of her several serious diseases Mrs. Hill has an extended list of medications. For her congestive heart failure and hypertension she takes Plavix (clopidogrel), aspirin, Imdur (isosorbide mononitrate), Atenolol (chlorthalidone), Lasix (furosemide), Altace (ramipril) and Lipitor (atorvastatin). She also takes Lantus (insulin glargine) and Humalog (insulin lispro) for her diabetes, the antidepressant Zoloft (sertraline), the hypnotic Ambien (zolpidem), and finally an Albuterol inhaler for her asthma. It was unclear to me who adjusts her medicine according to her congestive heart failure symptoms, which I know is not a simple task. She complained to me about her PCP and specialists, "They just gave me pills and sent me home and it was not even the right medication."

After her present hospitalization Mrs. Hill anticipates that she will be followed by a cardiologist at NYPH and will receive physical therapy. I questioned Mrs. Hill about the details of the frequency, location and professionals involved in the follow-up of her congestive heart failure to which she responded, "I have no idea my dear, this is New York." She assumed she would have free transportation back and forth between her home in Queens and the hospital in Manhattan.

Mr. Ferland's Medical Care

Mr. Ferland has both a PCP and a cardiologist near his home. The PCP takes care of all his medical problems and also adjusts his long list of medications for arrhythmia and congestive heart failure: amioderone hydrochloride, Toprol (metoprolol), Lisinopril (ACE-inhibitor), Lasix (furosemide), aspirin, Zocor (simvastatin) and the antidepressant Trazadone. He sees his cardiologist for a periodic stress test, though Mr. Ferland has not consulted him for a few years, saying, "In that doctor's office they do not follow up the treatment." But Mr. Ferland says he is satisfied with both his doctors and their cooperation.

Quality of Care and Patient Satisfaction

Mrs. Hill is very satisfied with her stay in NYPH although she is discontented with the disparity in the quality of treatment received in other hospitals. "No one is doing anything for me — only at NYPH they are more concerned than in Queens. Every hospital does not have the same procedures, they do things differently." I asked Mrs. Hill who she thinks is responsible for her health. She answers, "Myself. Doctors too — they do have to know what they are doing."

In contrast to Denmark and other European countries with national health coverage where waiting time for procedures is a main concern, Mrs. Hill has not experienced any waiting time, either for outpatient consultations or procedures done in a hospital.

Overall, Mr. Ferland expresses satisfaction with the US health care system. As mentioned earlier, he would like to have more transparency in insurance coverage. He would also prefer the insurance company to pay all his bills without any deductibles and to have a free choice of doctors without the need of a referral. He tells me that it is easy to obtain a second opinion in the US, although there are uncertainties. "You do not know who to go to. You do not know who is good and not good. I did not like the second opinion I got. The doctor said if you lose 50 pounds and take your medication, maybe you will be alright."

Mr. Ferland did not experience any waiting for treatment during his illness, either in outpatient or inpatient setting. "You do not wait — you get it (treatment) when you need it. Only in the ER you have to wait all day long," he says.

He is especially pleased by the treatment he has received in the NYPH, which is a renowned university hospital in the upper east side of Manhattan. "This place here is pretty good. They follow up and treat you pretty good."

Lastly I asked Mr. Ferland if he could imagine anything done for him that would normalize his life, to which he answered, "I don't know. It is something I'd have to think about."

I was thinking about help with the activities of daily living and other support systems available in Denmark, but he was not accustomed to thinking of this kind of help as part of his medical care.

Social Implications of Disease

Mrs. Hill has been a widow since 2000 and has two daughters. She lives with the youngest who is 21 years old, unmarried and soon expecting a baby. Both daughters and Mrs. Hill's 78-year-old mother help her with daily activities such as shopping, cleaning and cooking. I asked if she receives any help from the government to which she replies, "The government does not help you – this is America, you help yourself. The government gives you nothing, I live day by day."

However, Mrs. Hill receives income of $576 a month on Social Security (SSI) and her health care expenses are fully covered by Medicare and Medicaid because of her disability status. In spite of having a college degree in psychology she has been unemployed most of her life. She worked full time for four years in a daycare center and recently had a 20-hours per week job in telemarketing, "but the doctors made me stop working because of my heart and eyes." Stress is part of her daily life, she explains, "Bills have to be paid — everyday living is stressful for me. I am taking one day at a time."

Mr. Ferland's Situation

Mr. Ferland lives alone in an apartment since he became a widower three years ago. He pays his rent, health insurance and other necessary expenses from his work pension and SSI, "It is enough to make it run — you always keep your head above the water," Mr. Ferland says.

Until now he has managed to take care of his daily duties such as cleaning and cooking himself. "If I am no better than I am now when I go home from the hospital I will need some help," he says. He does not know if there is a possibility of obtaining home aid.

Following his bypass surgery Mr. Ferland received physiotherapy twice a week for nine weeks with monitored exercise until the insurance company stopped paying for it. He has never received home care aid or any other help with daily activities. During this hospitalization he will meet with a social worker from whom he does not have high expectations. He comments, "What does it mean; it means nothing."

Social Aspects of Medical Treatment in the US

Coming from Denmark, a country where social measures are emphasized along with the medical treatment to normalize the patient's life as much as possible, I asked one of the doctors at NYPH if he thinks enough is done in this respect for patients in America. He answers, "Something is done, but not enough."

He mentions the campaign against smoking to reduce the risk for lung cancer and heart disease, which is regarded as a successful preventive campaign in the US. It is done through strict regulations prohibiting smoking inside public buildings and many restaurants and cafés. Everywhere in front of the tall buildings of Manhattan you see people smoking a cigarette, whereupon they return upstairs — and nobody seems to complain about this law.

I asked this same doctor about the statement often heard that it is possible for anybody to receive good health care by going to an Emergency Room because by law, everybody must be treated. His comment was: "The service received in the ER is not the best, is costly for the hospital and inconvenient for the patient. The patients do not have their own doctor and have no check-ups. In the ER there is obviously no preventive care, no follow-up visit and the patient has to wait for hours before a physician can see him or her. Furthermore the care delivered in the ER is far more expensive than the service of a primary care provider (PCP) and therefore is of great disadvantage in terms of costs. It also completely changes the character of an ER into a primary care center."

I witnessed this myself during an elective as a medical student in the pediatric ER at the NYPH-Weill Cornell Medical Center. Most children came for trivial complaints like viral infections or asthma.

Summary

The United States is the only country in the world that spends the highest percentage of their Gross Domestic Product (GDP) on health care — 18%, compared to Denmark's 13.5% (according to Organisation for Economic Cooperation and Development 2006 data). The drivers of the continual rise in the cost of care are new technologies being developed and taken into use, malpractice insurance and indemnities, an aging population that has to be taken care of, and high administrative costs. Even though Denmark (and Europe on the whole) also faces the costs of new technology and an elderly population it is difficult to compare the United States to a country with such a small (5 million inhabitants) and homogeneous population. The United States is an enormous country with over 270 million people from very diverse ethnic and educational backgrounds.

From the experience of my two patients suffering from congestive heart failure with the American health care system and through conversations with two talented cardiologists, I recognize that the United States can offer the individual patient high quality health care with the newest available technology and medication. It is a system that emphasizes specialist care and by nature provides very competent physicians in their specific fields. The patients do not seem troubled by having five different doctors for each health problem. However the number of uninsured and underinsured people remains an important problem.

It is easy for patients to obtain a second opinion. Patients do not complain about waiting time for any treatment in either inpatient or outpatient settings, which is one of the chief complaints in the Danish health care system (and in other European countries). American patients are very demanding and seem to have high expectations of their health care system. My two patients expressed an overall satisfaction with the final treatment received, yet both commented on the disparity in the quality of treatment between different hospitals.

Compared to Denmark the social measures offered along with the treatment of disease are limited or just adequate in the United States according to the opinions of both of my patients and physicians. The continual rise in health care costs is a main concern and the introduction of managed care has not solved the problem. Exactly what is the optimal way to reimburse providers to encourage both high quality and economical medical practice remains an unanswered question. The issue of malpractice has transformed medical practice into defensive medicine and physicians are leaving high-risk specialties. There is a lack of transparency in the American health care system — no one really seems to have the oversight over this complex system. But despite its problems, the US health care system is capable of providing the individual patient with the best care in the world.

Part II

Germany:
Solidarity and Cradle to Grave
Health Care

Part II

Germany:
Solidarity and Cradle to Grave
Health Care

4

German and US Health Care Systems Compared

Miriam S. Wetzel, PhD and Ramin W. Parsa-Parsi, MD, MPH

Broad Similarities

German health care has the honor of being among the best in the world. It has also been among the most expensive, sharing that distinction with the United States and Switzerland.[1] Germany and the United States also share several common goals and problems related to providing a high level of dependable health care for their citizens. Both countries face major problems of rising costs, aging populations, and increasing expectations of the health care system. Citizens and governments of both Germany and the United States recognize the need for substantial change to address these problems.

There are philosophical differences in the approach to health care in the two countries. Germany is a social market economy based on the fundamental principal of solidarity — the belief that it is desirable and beneficial for a society to provide for the needs of all of its citizens and that the risks of the individual are shared by the entire community.[2] This concept includes cradle-to-grave, comprehensive health care for almost all Germans as well as insurance for unemployment, retirement, and long-term care. Germany has the oldest universal health care system in the world.

The United States is a free-market economy with strong reliance on the initiative of the individual and emphasis on personal freedom.

Government-sponsored Medicare and Medicaid insurance, along with the Veterans Administration and a variety of state-supported free care and welfare programs provide health care for the most needy US citizens.[3] Since the 1940s, a large percentage of health insurance has been provided through the workplace. In spite of the fact that the private insurance industry plays a much larger role in the US than in Germany, public spending for health care in the US is higher than in many leading European and Asian countries.[4]

Common Problems

Ironically, the technology that has brought great gains in the treatment of disease has also contributed to health care's problems. As medical technology has introduced more advanced and effective treatments, the cost has grown exponentially. Sophisticated diagnostic tests require expensive and sophisticated equipment and highly trained specialists. Pharmaceuticals represent a substantial part of the increased cost in both Germany and the US[5] although the argument is made that they can also prevent illness and death and therefore lower costs. The cost of hospital and outpatient care has outpaced the growth in cost of other goods and services and is expected to continue to rise.[6] New developments, from electronic health records to multislice scanners and surgical robots have pushed the cost of health care to new heights.[7]

The proportion of older people in the population of both countries is also increasing, in part because of new health technology and better living conditions. This older segment of the population is generally retired and no longer contributing to the government significantly through payroll taxes. According to US Social Security information, in 2007 3.3 workers in the US were needed to provide for the health care and government services for one retiree. By the year 2032 when many of the "baby boom" generation have retired there will be only 2.1 workers to support each beneficiary.[8] By the year 2050 a similar situation is predicted in Germany.[9]

Although the US has been regularly criticized for having more than 45 million citizens without health insurance,[10] until new laws took effect in 2007 and 2009, Germany also had an estimated 200,000 citizens who were uninsured.[11] As in the US, many of these individuals are self-employed or workers in part-time occupations. Both countries are looking for ways to address this problem. Germany has introduced even more comprehensive compulsory health insurance in the public (since April 2007) and the private sector (since 2009).[12] This should provide coverage for Germany's uninsured.

Health Care Comparisons

Germany, with a landmass of more than 350,000 square kilometers, similar in size to the state of Montana, has a population of 82.6 million people, making it one of the most populous countries in Europe. The Federal Republic of Germany is divided into 16 *Länder* (states) and has a combined system of socialized and private health care that is closely regulated by the government. The United States, with 48 contiguous states plus Alaska and Hawaii, has a landmass of more than 9.8 million square kilometers and a population that passed 302 million in 2007 and reached 309 million in 2009.[13] Health care in the United States is paid for by a combination of public and private organizations, but the private sector represents a much larger proportion than in Germany. The Organisation for Economic Co-operation and Development (OECD) provides data for the comparisons in Tables 4.1 and 4.2.[14] Figures are for 2007, the latest year available.

The total percentage of gross domestic product (GDP) spent on health by both countries has risen since 1993 when Germany spent 9.6% and the US spent 13.6% (see Table 4.3).[15] Both countries have managed at times to slow the growth but not totally halt its inexorable climb. The

Table 4.1. Expenditure on health — Percent Gross Domestic Product — Germany.

Indicator	Value
Total expenditure on health as percent of gross domestic product	10.4
Public expenditure on health as percent of total expenditure on health	76.9
Out-of-pocket expenditure as percent of total expenditure on health	13.1
Private health insurance expenditure as percent of total expenditure on health	9.3
Per capita expenditure in USD Purchasing Power parity	$3588

OECD Health Data 2009 — Version November 2009.

Table 4.2.   Expenditure on health — Percent Gross Domestic Product — US.

Indicator	Value
Total expenditure on health as percent of gross domestic product	16.0
Public expenditure on health as percent of total expenditure on health	45.4
Out-of-pocket expenditure as percent of total expenditure on health	12.2
Private health insurance expenditure as percent of total expenditure on health	36.2
Per capita expenditure in USD Purchasing Power parity	$7290

OECD Health Data 2009 — Version November 2009.

Table 4.3.   Expenditure on health — Percent Gross Domestic Product — Germany and the US 1988–2007.

Year	1988	1989	1990	1991	1992	1993	1994	1995	1996	1997
Germany	8.9	8.3	8.3	*	9.6	9.6	9.8	10.1	10.4	10.2
USA	11.1	11.5	12.2	12.9	13.3	13.6	13.5	13.6	13.5	13.4

Year	1998	1999	2000	2001	2002	2003	2004	2005	2006	2007
Germany	10.2	10.3	10.3	10.4	10.6	10.8	10.6	10.7	10.5	10.4
USA	13.4	13.5	13.6	14.3	15.1	15.6	15.6	15.7	15.8	16.0

OECD Health Data 2009 — Version November 2009.
*German reunification. Break in series.

increase in the US of almost 5 percentage points in GDP spent on health from 1988 to 2007 represents a higher rate of growth than in most other high-income countries. It outstrips the rate of growth in the US economy, causing concern about paying for health care costs in the future should this trend continue.

The general government or public expenditures (including Statutory Health Insurance) as a percentage of total expenditure on health has decreased for Germany from 80.7% in 1993 to 76.9% in 2007, while in the US this figure has increased from 43.0% in 1993 to 45.2% in 2007 (see Table 4.4).[16]

Another comparison is the amount per capita spent on health since 1970, the first year OECD data are available for Germany (see Table 4.5).[17]

These figures clearly show that spending on health per capita in Germany and the US was very similar during the 1970s, but in the 1980s

Table 4.4. Total public expenditure on health — As a percent of total expenditure on health — Germany and US 1988–2007.

Year	1988	1989	1990	1991	1992	1993	1994	1995	1996	1997
Germany	77.2	76.0	76.2	*	81.5	80.7	80.8	81.6	82.2	80.8
USA	39.1	39.1	39.2	40.7	41.9	43.0	44.4	44.9	45.0	44.7

Year	1998	1999	2000	2001	2002	2003	2004	2005	2006	2007
Germany	80.1	79.8	79.7	79.3	79.2	78.7	77.0	77.0	76.8	76.9
USA	43.5	43.1	43.2	44.2	44.1	43.9	44.3	44.4	45.2	45.4

OECD Health Data 2009 — Version November 2009.
*German reunification. Break in series.

these figures began to climb in the US. In 1991–1992 Germany incurred increased expenses related to the reunification of East and West Germany, but by 1993 had returned to modest yearly increases while US expenditures continued to soar. US spending in 2007 is slightly more than twice as much per capita as in Germany.

The German Health Care System

The beginning of the German health care system is usually attributed to Chancellor Otto von Bismarck in 1883, but actually started as early as 1845 when Prussia enacted statutory health insurance for workers of selected occupations.[18] Bismarck deserves credit for offering health insurance to all German citizens by proposing a series of insurance programs during a time of social unrest. One of the goals was to keep workers healthy at low cost. This early system of universal health care was part of a broad social welfare program that included coverage for accident, disability, old age, and unemployment.[19] The structure was based on existing local self-governing social insurance funds known as *Krankenkassen*, or sickness funds, which were responsible for collecting dues and financing the health care expenditures of their members.

The modern Statutory Health Insurance (SHI) system that grew out of that early beginning has remained basically the same over the years and insures approximately 90% of German citizens. SHI covers essentially the cost of all medical care. It is a decentralized system in which government

Table 4.5. Total expenditure on health per capita — USD Purchasing Power Parity — Germany and US 1970–2007.

Year	1970	1971	1972	1973	1974	1975	1976	1977	1978	1979
Germany	269	311	353	409	483	572	638	694	776	857
USA	356	391	432	474	533	601	682	767	852	956

Year	1980	1981	1982	1983	1984	1985	1986	1987	1988	1989
Germany	971	1101	1147	1212	1310	1409	1454	1533	1666	1659
USA	1091	1255	1402	1532	1671	1811	1925	2076	2304	2541

Year	1990	1991	1992	1993	1994	1995	1996	1997	1998	1999
Germany	1768	*	1976	1992	2128	2274	2399	2413	2483	2592
USA	2810	3035	3251	3447	3589	3748	3900	4055	4236	4450

Year	2000	2001	2002	2003	2004	2005	2006	2007
Germany	2671	2808	2937	3088	3160	3348	3464	3588
USA	4704	5053	5453	5851	6194	6558	6933	7290

OECD Health Data 2009 — Version November 2009.

*German reunification. Break in series.

at the *Länder* level and the non-profit sickness funds have maintained a tremendous amount of autonomy. Until January 2009 sickness funds could set their own rate of required contribution from members. This rate had varied from as low as 12.4% to as high as 16.7% of a member's gross salary.[20] However, everybody in the same *Krankenkasse* at the same salary level paid the same amount. Premiums are set according to salary rather than marital status, family size, or health. Since 2009 the government is in the process of setting a universal premium rate, which applies to all SH Insurers. The rate was initially set at 15.5% but was lowered to 14.9% by July 2009 to adjust for the worldwide economic crisis, which hit the German economy, employers and consumers significantly. The newly obtained power of the government over the premium rates could thus be demonstrated. The government contributed tax money to make up for the missing income for the insurance.[21]

Twentieth Century Changes

During the twentieth century, numerous changes and adjustments were made to the German health care system. Since 1994 most geographic and occupational limits to enrollment have been lifted and people have been permitted to join almost any of the *Krankenkassen*. Even prior to this time, many of the smaller funds representing certain professions had consolidated and there was consolidation within *Länder*. This created a certain amount of competition and resulted in a reduction in the number of sickness funds from 1,152 in 1994 to 242 in 2007[22] and further reduction to around 200 in 2009.[23]

With the freedom to choose more freely among funds, there was the possibility that more people would choose sickness funds that required a lower contribution. To distribute risk more evenly, a Risk Structure Compensation (RSC) scheme went into effect in 1996. Funds that had younger, healthier members were required to contribute to a national pool, which then distributed the money among the poorer funds. In 2006 about 15.1 billion Euros were redistributed among sickness funds for risk adjustment.[24]

All workers earning less than €48,600 gross income per year (€4,050 per month), or about $68,600 per year (in June 2009 exchange rate) must enroll in a public insurance fund (with a few exceptions) and contribute a fixed percentage of their gross salary.[25] About half of this contribution is funded by employers and the other half is paid directly by employees. People who make between €400 and €800 a month pay less for their health insurance and there are additional government subsidies for the poor, the elderly, and the unemployed. All funds are required to provide a minimum package of health care benefits that cover most ambulatory, inpatient, and pharmaceutical expenses and a substantial, but decreasing proportion of dental expenses. Spouses and dependent children up to 18 years of age are also covered, provided they do not earn a salary above a fixed ceiling.

State and federal employees, *beamte*, are not covered by Germany's statutory health insurance.[26] Approximately 80% of their health care costs are paid directly by the government through *beihilfe* or "public aid" and they purchase private insurance to cover the rest. When they are hospitalized, privately insured patients, including public servants, might be given single rooms and treated by the head of the department. This was the case with Karl Lieder (*Nie Krank*)[27] who was treated by an *Oberartz* in the hospital because he had private insurance. Later his financial circumstances changed drastically and he turned to the social aid agency, *Verband Deutscher Kriegsversehrter* (VDK) for help. They found a way for him to retire and become eligible to rejoin a public insurance fund, but this is a very rare occurrence.

Workers who earn more than €48,600 per year may enroll in a sickness fund or opt out and purchase private insurance.[28] They are not required to pay into the Statutory Health Insurance system and may choose from among a variety of plans offered by many private insurance firms. In the case of Herr von Walther (*A Ray of Hope*)[29] the expense for his mental illness and lengthy hospitalizations were covered by private insurance. Because Herr von Walther could not work his parents were able to continue to carry him on their *Allianz Versicherung* plan.

The premiums for private insurance are risk-adjusted, hence are higher for individuals who have health problems and insurers may reject applicants.[30] In contrast to the SHI system, every single member of the family has to be individually insured and paid for. Once a person has chosen private insurance, almost without exception, he or she cannot return to the SHI system. In 2009 as in 2006, 10.3% of Germans were enrolled in full private health insurance with one of the 46 private insurers.[31] This includes self-employed individuals, employees above the income level for required SHI insurance and civil servants. In 2006, 18,400,500 contracts were active for supplementary private insurance in Germany (an increase of 7.68% from 2005).[32] In some ways this insurance is similar to the "medigap" policies available in the US, which Americans purchase to cover co-pays and other out-of-pocket health care expenses. In Germany these supplementary insurance plans pay for extra amenities such as a private room during hospitalization or treatment by the chief-of-service. Some plans help to pay for prescription medicines or additional dental coverage.

Contributions for retirees to the public sickness funds are paid by the retirees themselves and by their pension funds. In theory, the contributions of young workers will offset the high medical expenses of the elderly. This has proven to be problematic as the aging population grows larger and a downturn in the German economy keeps the workforce smaller. For unemployed individuals, the sickness fund premiums are paid by the Federal Agency for Employment.[33] This was the situation for Mrs. Baumgartner (Frau Baumgartner's Story)[34] although she must still pay a percentage of her pension to her *Krankenkasse* and pay a modest co-pay for her prescriptions. She was indignant when she was assessed a hefty co-pay for a 20-day stay at a *Kur* (rehabilitation spa). At that time, by law she was entitled to *Kur* visits of three or four weeks every two years, but the effectiveness of these treatments was coming under increasing criticism and they were later phased out of SHI coverage.

The Five Pillars

In January 1995 long-term care was added as a benefit to the statutory health insurance. This completed Germany's "five pillars" of social welfare (see Table 4.6). The federal government governs all five social insurances through the body of federal legislation known as the Social Code Book.[35] The Social Code Book contains information about rights of members in the public insurance program, describes who is eligible and who is excluded, grants authority to local organizations, and details a minimum set of

Table 4.6.   Five Pillars of Germany's Social Welfare.

Five Pillars of Statutory Social Insurance
• Unemployment Insurance
• Pension Insurance
• Health Insurance
• Accident Insurance
• Long-term Care Insurance

benefits that must be provided through the Statutory Health Insurance program. The Ministry of Health and Social Security had general oversight responsibility for the entire health care delivery system until 2005 when government reorganization resulted in the reinstatement of the Ministry of Health separate from the Ministry of Social Affairs.[36]

The German Federal Joint Committee (*Gemeinsamer Bundesausschuss* G-BA) plays a special role in the regulation of the German health care system. It includes representatives of the self-governance bodies of physicians, dentists and statutory health insurers and the German Hospital Federation. Its role can be compared roughly to the US combination of the Federal Drug Administration, the Joint Commission on the Accreditation of Healthcare Organizations, the Institute of Medicine, boards of different health care professionals, and medical specialty boards. Its directives are legally binding but may be subject to complaints in social courts. The G-BA is mainly concerned that benefits and coverage of the Statutory Health Insurance system are "adequate, appropriate, and efficient."[37]

Costs

Over a period of years, the required contribution rates to the *Krankenkassen* steadily increased for German citizens. From 1997 to 2001, members of *Deutsche Angestellten Krankenkasse* (DAK), a large sickness fund, contributed 13.8% of their salaries. In 2002 the premium increased to 14.9%. The range throughout Germany in 2007 was 12.4% to 16.7% with an average of 14.82% up to €42,750 per year. In January 2009 the rate was set at 15.5% by the government and lowered to 14.9% in July 2009.[38]

During the 1980s, as health care costs skyrocketed in the United States, with an annual average rate of growth 33% higher than the national economic growth,[39] West Germany's expenditures held steady at a rate only 3% above overall economic growth. Between 1980 and 1990, West Germany was seen as a model for other countries for continuing to provide health care for all its citizens while holding the increase to only 2%, which was in line with the nation's economic growth.[40]

Germany took strong measures to achieve this enviable rate of slow growth starting in 1977 with the Health Insurance Cost Containment Act. Between 1977 and 1996 the German government introduced 46 major laws, with 6,800 detailed regulations aimed at curbing rising costs.[41] The goal was to limit increases in health care spending to the rate of increase in contributory income. During this time many cost containment measures were passed and rescinded, depending on the political party in power.

Reunification of East and West Germany in 1990 posed a challenge to the SHI system. Very different health care systems existed in the two Germany's. The aim of reunification treaties and legislation was to raise the living and health care standard of the East to that of the West. Indicators of improved health, such as increased life expectancy, a decline in neonatal mortality and falling death rates from diseases such as hypertension, cardiovascular disease and certain cancers have been attributed to better health care under the Statutory Health Insurance system after reunification. These gains came at a cost to the West while the economy of the East was getting up to speed.[42]

Reform Efforts

One of the major efforts at reform and cost cutting as Germany entered the 21st century was former Chancellor Gerhard Schröder's "Agenda 2010" or Modernization Act of 2004. When he became Chancellor he announced a series of reforms to address Germany's high unemployment rate and the burgeoning cost of its social welfare services including health care. His "Agenda 2010" called for plans to trim dental benefits, require a modest co-pay for prescription drugs and charge a fee of €10 for every three-month period in which a person visited a doctor. A "day fare" of €10 would also be charged for hospital stays for a maximum of 28 days.[43] However, exemptions applied when more than 2% of the gross household income per annum or 1% of the income for patients with serious chronic diseases had been spent on co-payments.

The Chancellor's reforms met with criticism, even within his own party but he stood by them saying, "We will have to curtail the work of the state, encourage more individual responsibility, and require greater individual performance from each person."[44] He was accused by some of undermining the philosophy of social responsibility while others felt the reforms were short-term solutions and did not go far enough to effect real change.[45]

The pharmaceutical industry was the object of strong reform efforts and legislative controls during this time. Cost-containment measures such as price freezes, emphasis on generics, reference drug pricing, and mandatory rebates from pharmacies to sickness funds were methods employed. From 2003 to 2004 the compulsory discount on all drugs not included in the reference price system increased from 6% to 16%. Industry spokespersons predicted a loss of €1.5 billion in 2004.[46] For the first time, patients were required to pay a small co-pay for certain drugs, but this could hardly be expected to be a significant cost savings for the government.

The legal requirement that sickness funds must operate within their budget each year was one very simple and consistent cost-containment measure. The *Krankenkassen* are allowed only to spend the revenue from contributions received each year and must not have any surplus or deficit. In the event of either, depending on whether it is a surplus or deficit, the sickness funds must either increase benefits or increase the contribution rate. As the government paid for fewer benefits, out-of-pocket expenditures as a share of total health care expenditures naturally increased. In 1992, they accounted for 10.7% of total expenditures. In 2002, the percentage rose by 1.5% to a level of 12.2% and in 2009 it was 14%.[47] With the change to government set premium rates in 2009, SH Insurers may ask their members for additional payments if they have a deficit and must pay back contributions to their members if they generate a surplus. This new regulation is meant to stimulate competition among SH Insurers.[48]

The most basic problem for Germany's health care system was the shortfall of contributions from workers and employers to fund the benefits. A way had to be found to decrease non-wage labor costs for employers and boost new job creation. In 2005, through a series of adjustments, the contribution of employees was increased by 0.45% and the contribution of employers was decreased by the same amount, thus the longstanding 50-50 ratio of contribution payment by employer and employee was changed. Even at contribution rates close to 14%, funding was falling far short of covering costs with an expected shortfall of €7 billion ($9 billion USD) in 2007. Barbara Marnach, a spokeswoman for the large public health insurance plan, AOK, spoke about this problem. "There have to be different sources of revenue. We've basically said the financing basis has to be broadened."[49] Throughout the spring of 2006 there were heated discussions about how to financially sustain the health care system, and hard lobbying by the public health insurance funds and other interests.

Reform efforts were directed towards the hospitals as well. The number of beds in acute care hospitals had been decreased over the previous decade in part because of shorter hospital stays. There was a corresponding increase in beds in rehabilitation facilities. With an average number of acute hospital beds of 6.4 per 1000 people, Germany was still well above the European Union average of 4.1 in 2004.[50] By federal order, Diagnosis Related Groups (DRGs) was chosen as the main method of hospital reimbursement. Proponents of the system, modeled after Australia's, hoped it would improve hospital utilization and decrease hospital stays.[51]

No area of health care escaped scrutiny. Without a gate keeping system, German citizens could freely choose to visit primary care or specialist physicians. Planners hoped imposing co-pays would discourage excessive use. There were also cost implications in the system of separation of ambulatory and hospital-based care when there was a lack of communication between a patient's outpatient and inpatient doctors and tests were repeated unnecessarily. No doubt the system contributed to these occurrences but there were always specialists and in-hospital physicians who voluntarily followed their patients at all levels of care. For example, Isolde Baumgartner (Frau Baumgartner's Story)[52] was cared for in the hospital Rheumatology Clinic by an *Assistenzartz* who monitored her general health and functioned more like a primary care doctor. At her clinic appointments Mrs. Baumgartner would sometimes wait for two hours so she could see this particular physician.

Under Chancellor Schröder's reforms the SHI funds no longer provided funeral allowances, life-style medications (e.g. Viagra), most over-the-counter drugs and there was a restricted reimbursement for glasses. Popular spa "cures" began to be frowned upon and taxi transportation to doctor's appointments was curtailed. Mr. Schröder expected the results of these reforms to lower the cost of health care from 14.4% of gross wages to 13%. However, the gradual chipping away at basic health care benefits was seen as eroding the original intent to provide universal coverage and pleased no one.[53] Eventually, the need for substantial change became apparent. This task fell to a new Chancellor.

Angela Merkel's Reforms

Angela Merkel, who became Chancellor in November 2005, made health care reform a prime objective of her four-year administration. Her three top goals were to achieve sustainable finances, encourage more competition among public insurance funds, and reduce the non-wage labor costs for health insurance. In February 2006 she first unveiled a plan for comprehensive change,[54] however, it met with disapproval from citizens and health care professionals alike and its implementation was delayed several months until adjustments could be made. The main source of objection by the public was that it raised their required contribution rate while services were cut further.

Physicians and other health care workers demonstrated in the streets and conducted a series of planned strikes for months in 2006. They feared that the changes would result in the loss of as many as 20,000 jobs, according to news releases.[55] The strikes were not necessarily a reaction to the planned health care reforms but were protests of poor working conditions and low salaries for physicians in general. They were organized by the physicians' union (Marburger Bund) and led to new contracts and improvements in working hours and income for physicians, independent of the national health care reforms.

In February 2007, a revised proposal was ready for a vote and was passed by the Upper House of the German Parliament on February 2.[56] The lower house approved it on February 16,[57] although there was still opposition, some of it from Merkel's own Christian Social Democratic coalition. Parts of the law went into effect on April 1, 2007 with other parts delayed until 2009 to allow time for changes in the way the money to fund the program is collected and distributed. With a change in politics in future elections, some critics speculate that certain features of the law may be dismantled before they have a chance to be fully implemented.[58]

Main Points of the 2007 Reform

The main points of the 2007 reform are:[59]

- Private insurance companies must offer so-called "Basic Health Insurance Plans" in addition to their existing plans. These plans should offer basic health care (similar to the SHI benefit package) mostly to currently uninsured self-employed people or employees who have lost their jobs. Applicants cannot be rejected and premiums must not be risk-adjusted.
- The government has set up one large centralized SHI fund. The morbidity-oriented risk-adjustment is done at this level using up to 80 disease groups. Hence, the National Health Fund pays a risk-adjusted lump sum per member to the individual sickness funds.
- The government sets uniform premiums as a percentage of salary, the same for everybody, to be paid into this fund instead of the varying rates previously assessed by the insurance funds.
- SHI funds are allowed to offer special customized insurance plans, which may include bonus programs, plans with varying annual deductibles, and GP-programs.

As the saying goes, "The devil is in the details." And there are many details involved in the revised German health care plan. For example, accumulated accrued reserves may now be transferred to a different company if the individual switches between private insurers, however this is strictly regulated and has many exceptions. The government started collecting uniform premiums in the giant health fund in 2009. From this fund they will pay approximately 200 separate insurance providers a fixed amount per insured person. Insurance funds needing more money to cover their obligations are allowed to raise an additional premium, no more than 1% of household income, directly from their members.[60] On the other hand, efficiently working sickness funds may reimburse their members and hence stimulate competition among insurers. Retired people on low pensions and people who have been unemployed for a long time are exempt from paying extra levies. Anyone enrolled in the state insurance programs may be allowed to switch insurers if they are asked for additional payments.

With these reforms, health insurance became mandatory since April 2007 for all SHI-eligible people and since January 2009 for the entire population. This will provide insurance for the estimated 200,000 uninsured in Germany.[61] These are mostly self-employed and freelance workers. Mandatory health insurance contributions shared by employers and employees were raised an average of 0.5 percentage points in January 2007 to help fund these changes. They are also intended to account for a 3% increase in Value Added Tax (VAT) since January 2007 and wipe out existing debt by 2009.[62]

Children's health care will be funded in a new way by monies from general tax revenue. In 2007 and 2008 the government provided €2.5 billion to cover children's health. This amount will gradually escalate until it reaches €14 billion a year by 2016 to be transferred to the new health fund. Measures to save the government an estimated €500 million a year in drug costs and a proposal to introduce a price-capping system designed to give pharmacies more scope to negotiate prices with drug companies and wholesalers were dropped from the reform package.[63]

Although the new health plan is not pleasing to everybody in all respects, Chancellor Merkel called it a "breakthrough" and Health Minister Ulla Schmidt said it will "reduce bureaucracy, boost competition, and cut costs in a system that swallows around €140 billion a year ($179 billion) and employs 4.2 million people."[64] This is the figure for the SHI sector only in total health care expense for 2007 of around €252 billion. To pay for this universal health care system and other government costs, the German people pay taxes that can add up to 50% or more of their wages — like most Continental Europeans. This includes income tax rates up to 45%, social security taxes of 19.9%, health care payroll taxes of 14.3%, unemployment insurance of 4.2%, and the 19% VAT tax.[65]

On the day the bill passed, Bavarian Prime Minister Edmund Stoiber said in a speech to the upper house in Berlin, "The bill was a compromise as everyone had to lower their sights because the positions of the Social Democrats and Christian Democrats were too different." He concluded, "This reform will, despite all the criticism, guarantee high-quality medical treatment for all in the future, by providing more competition and more flexibility."[66]

Divided Opinion

Opinions are divided as to whether the new health plan leads the country towards more socialism and whether this is good or bad. Not surprisingly, critics say the reform package has not met the goal of lowering the cost of health care premiums for workers and employees; in fact the contribution rate has been raised. They say it will put more power in the government's hands and make it more difficult for the public insurance companies to compete. New procedures and organizations will need to be created to run the large national health fund.[67]

Its supporters say the plan will make the health care system more transparent and market-oriented[68] but Barbara Marnach of the large public insurance fund AOK said, "Instead of cutting bureaucracy, it creates a whole new one. We haven't gotten more authority to act on the free market; rather this reform leads to further socialism. It will simply be less efficient."[69] Walter Hirche, the Free Democrat economy minister in the state of Lower Saxony told the Upper House on February 16, 2007 that the health fund "is even more bureaucratic, opaque and expensive" than the existing fund system.[70]

Representing another point of view, on German public radio, Sophia Schlette, head of health care policy for the Bertelsmann Foundation, said that fears of an overblown bureaucracy are exaggerated. She said, "The countries that do better when it comes to costs and various health care indicators are interestingly enough those countries that have what here is being described as the horror scenario of the single health fund system."[71]

A reported 21,000 health insurance company employees took to the streets in early March 2007, demanding that the government rethink its reform plan. They claimed that they are not fearful about change and fully agree that reform is needed, but not this combination of reforms that not even the members of the coalition government seemed happy about.[72] Marlies Volkmer, a Social Democrat lawmaker who sits on parliament's health committee said in an interview on February 2, 2007, "The [national] health fund won't solve the funding problems. Instead of adopting this compromise, it would've been more honest to say we'll leave things as they are." She abstained in the vote in the lower house.[73]

There is concern among the Free Democrats that the new health plan may hurt Germany's 48 private health insurers financially. Party leader, Guido Westerwelle told parliament before the February 2 vote, "It's like two hikers who reach a swamp and can't agree whether to turn left or right. Instead of turning back, they march straight into it."[74]

All of this debate leaves Germans uncertain about what has happened to their health care system. They tend to be wary about the word "reform" because it seems to indicate that something they have had is about to be taken away from them.[75] Indeed it has been necessary to rein in some of the generous benefits they have enjoyed and to look seriously for ways to cut expenses in a system that has been running up to a €7 billion deficit each year.[76] Germans are quick to criticize their health care system while much of the world has admired the "near universal coverage" they have enjoyed for so many years. In a survey by the Commonwealth Fund, an American health care foundation, 55% of Germans thought the system needed fundamental reform. Only 35% of Germans rated it excellent.[77] "The quality in Germany is not bad at all, even though in looking at the costs, it might be better," Boris Augurzky, head of the health care department at the Rhineland-Westphalia Institute for Economic Research told *Deutsche Welle* reporter Kyle James. "Still, Germans almost never have to put up with long waiting times for treatment like they do in England or Scandinavia."[78]

What do German physicians think of the 2007 and 2009 health care reforms? A first reaction is fear that it will eventually lead to an increasingly state run system, which limits physician autonomy, fuels further hidden rationing and consequently jeopardizes patient care. The health care reforms, including the changes in the physician payment system, also had negative implications on physician salaries in some regions of the country. Time will tell whether the problems that prompted angry demonstrations have been resolved.

Jeanne Arenz, head of the health care department at *Paritätischer Wohlfartsverband,* an umbrella group for German charitable organizations, agrees that the quality of German health care is good. She thinks there will be higher co-payments and more services that will not be covered by insurance plans in the future.

"I think it's because Germans want to feel 100% secure when it comes to health care," she said, "and that's just not possible anymore."[79]

Acknowledgments

We gratefully acknowledge the contributions of US-EU-MEE students S. Elissa Altin, Benedikt Aulinger, Marion Bohatschek, Jack Casey, Anne Chiang, Alden Vincent Chiu, Oliver Fuchs, Corinne Jenderek, Anna Ratiner, Malte Rieken, Christine Hsu Rohde, Gregory Sawicki, Aimee Shu and Charles Wira III in the preparation of this chapter.

5

Cases Written by US Students in Germany

Case 10: An Easter Surprise*

Anne Chiang

April 1997

Lara Steinmeyer, a 31-year-old mother living in a tiny village called Seeg in the Bavarian Alps, discovered a round and smooth surprise on Easter Saturday. Her fingers brushed against it, a small hard knot in her breast, as she toweled off after a shower. "It's nothing, I'm sure," she whispered to the mirror, as her fingers pressed on the lump in small, worrying circles. "I've never been sick a day in my life."

But only six months ago, her partner's mother had undergone an operation for breast cancer. And three years ago, her father had died of colon cancer. No use taking chances. She'd call her "*Hausarzt*" (General Practitioner) on Tuesday, as soon the holiday weekend was over.

Lara was born in Seeg, Germany, a small village of 2,500 inhabitants, the second child in a family of four, two girls and two boys. She was brought up in a warm Bavarian environment with strong Catholic underpinnings. From her parents, she inherited both a practical mindset and a sunny disposition. After her basic schooling in Seeg, she made temporary forays to nearby towns to complete her vocational training in office work and to look for employment.

---

*This case was written by Anne Chiang in 1999 when she was a student at the Weill Medical College of Cornell University and participated in the US-EU-MEE exchange at Ludwig Maximilians University, Munich, Germany.

At age 25, Lara married a quiet, mild-natured man. Too quiet. She left him several years later for another man, with whom she had a son, Thomas. Both the child's father and her ex-husband came from the area around Seeg. All of Lara's close circle of family and friends had settled within a 30 km radius of each other. Her older sister and family bought a nearby farm, while Lara's two younger brothers still lived at home with their mother, a ten-minute drive away. Less than five kilometers in the opposite direction was the home and office of Dr. Bauer, the family doctor. Dr. Bauer had treated her father's colon cancer.

"It's probably nothing, I'm sure," said Dr. Bauer on Tuesday as he examined her breast. "Likely just a result of hormonal variation, common to young women like yourself. We'll check it again after your next menstrual period."

Over the years Dr. Bauer had fulfilled his ambition to become a successful general practitioner (GP), the mainstay of the German health care system. Working at least 12 hours a day, he'd built a thriving, large-sized family practice, which pulled in over 600,000 DM (deutsche marks) a year in 1999. (Note: In 2002 the Euro became the official currency of Germany).

Dr. Bauer's office hours were packed into three afternoons a week; sometimes, he'd scribble out 150 prescriptions in a day. Otherwise, he'd make visits to homebound patients, often visiting ten in one day. Once a week, he'd pop over to the old folk's home for several hours. Even though he netted a healthy 200,000 DM after subtracting costs and taxes, he felt overworked. As the local doctor, he might be called at any hour to calm an anxious patient or revive an unconscious accident victim.

When Lara returned to see Dr. Bauer after her period, the lump was still there. Aside from recommending a mammogram, Dr. Bauer advised no treatment other than watching and waiting. Over the next few weeks, the small lump seemed to grow larger. Finally, Dr. Bauer referred Lara to a gynecology practice in Marktoberdorf, 15 km away, for a lumpectomy. Three doctors who also held operating privileges at the local hospital shared this ambulatory practice. This arrangement was unusual in Germany, since doctors usually decided early in their training to practice either hospital or ambulatory medicine. But Dr. Zimmermann, the youngest member of the gynecology practice, viewed such an arrangement with hospital affiliation as ideal. Not only did cost sharing allow the purchase of better equipment but patients could be seen in the hospital clinic, with direct access to mammography and hospital radiologists. Every week, one doctor would operate at the hospital (routine gynecological operations and obstetrical deliveries) and oversee 25 inpatient beds, while the other two would see clinic patients. The clinic had 150 to 170 patient visits per week.

"Most likely the lump will be benign, Lara, since you are so young," said Dr. Zimmermann, reassuringly. "If the pathology comes back showing cancerous cells, I'd recommend an immediate mastectomy. Chances are against it, but you should decide now what you'd like us to do in that case."

Lara was stunned but agreed with Dr. Zimmermann, and signed the consent form for an eventual mastectomy.

On May 28, 1997, Lara underwent a lumpectomy in Marktoberdorf. While still a bit foggy from the narcotics, she was told the pathology results — invasive ductal carcinoma. When she woke up next, her right breast and axillary lymph nodes had been removed, along with a tumor the size of a small tangerine. Eight of the 21 lymph nodes contained malignant cells. The tumor cells were poorly differentiated, which made Lara's prognosis even worse.

When Lara could think clearly again, her first concern was for her son, Tommy. Her partner, Tommy's father, Peter, assured her that between him, her mother, her older sister and the many other friends and relatives in the immediate area, they would take good care of Tommy while she recuperated.

After a mastectomy operation in Germany, many patients convalesce for three to four weeks at a rehabilitation clinic. Lara went to the oncological clinic in Oberstaufen, which is affiliated with the university in Munich. Such a stay was recognized as a necessary aspect of a patient's care so one could gain strength, both physically and emotionally and return to work. Patients had time to mull over the past events, to ask questions about prognosis and treatment, and to learn about available social services. Rehabilitation stays were reimbursed by one's *"Rentenversicherung"* or retirement insurance fund.

The Oberstaufen clinic had 250 beds available for cancer patients receiving acute treatment or rehabilitation services. Acute patients paid a higher daily rate than did the rehabilitation patients — 400 DM and 100 DM per day, respectively. A typical acute patient might be a woman with metastatic ovarian cancer who was undergoing chemotherapy. The aim of her care would be palliative, not rehabilitative; thus, the cost of her care was borne by her *"Krankenkasse"* or health insurance fund.

About ninety percent of Germany's population is insured by public employment-based health insurance funds. Together, the employer and wage earner evenly split the contribution to the *Krankenkassen*, which totals 13–15% of the worker's wage (in 1999). In return, the employee and dependents are insured for their health costs, including an exhaustive array of preventive, diagnostic, and therapeutic services, as well as medications. A few high-income individuals opt for private insurance, where risk-based premiums often result in a lower monthly contribution. Lara belonged to a public *Krankenkasse*. With over nine million insured, it was the largest in Germany.

All *Krankenkassen* reimbursed hospitals according to a per diem rate; the hospitals then paid their employees a fixed salary. Ambulatory doctors were directly reimbursed for services through a point system (e.g. a normal delivery for 180 DM — 300 points at 0.6 DM per point). Since the global budget for ambulatory services was capped, the yearly point value would change, according to the total amount of services performed. Dr. Zimmermann compared the global budget to a *"Kuchen"* or cake, "It's the same size whether five or thirty people eat it…the individual pieces just get smaller."

As more doctors performed more services to increase their earnings, the worth of each service sank. For example, a routine cancer prevention work-up, which previously cost 80 DM, was now reimbursed for only 45 DM.

At Oberstaufen, Lara learned arm exercises to reduce lymph accumulation, and got fitted for a special bra. She participated in water gymnastics, massage therapy, and went on a few outings. She met once with a psychotherapist and several times with a self-help group of breast cancer patients. Many of the self-help group members spoke about their experiences with advanced disease, which Lara felt was depressing and 'more than she wanted to know.' Other information provided about social services was more useful. With the help of the Oberstaufen social worker, she applied to the government for 60% handicapped status, which reduced the cost of her telephone service from 24 DM to 9 DM per month. Patients with advanced metastatic breast cancer were eligible for 80% handicapped status, which exempted them from radio/broadcasting fees (30 DM per month) and reduced public transportation fares by 50%. Lara found that she was eligible for household help at home for up to one year during a three-year period. Family members, such as her mother or Peter, could not be reimbursed. She submitted the paperwork to her *Krankenkasse* and received approval for seven hours of outside household help per day.

University doctors from Munich visited Oberstaufen weekly to discuss rare or problematic cases. Lara's case was an unusual one, since the majority of breast cancer patients at Oberstaufen were post-menopausal. Although she could certainly receive chemotherapy in Oberstaufen or even Marktoberdorf, the head oncologist advised her to seek treatment at the university clinic in Munich. There, Lara would have maximum access to clinical studies and the latest research data. Often, pharmaceutical companies donated costly new medications for participants in clinical trials. University hospitals also received public funds and grants, which helped to defray the costs of expensive chemotherapy. Privately owned clinics or practices had to balance their own books without public funds or grants; the subsequent financial pressure was tangible. In Marktoberdorf, for example, the local hospital administration denied one of Dr. Zimmermann's patients, a 67-year-old woman, the use of an expensive chemotherapeutic agent called paclitaxel. At Oberstaufen, patient services and medications were not restricted, but personnel had been cut to make ends meet.

Dr. Zimmermann agreed that the university should handle Lara's chemotherapy, despite the potential time and cost of travel to Munich, two to two-and-a-half hours each way by train. If Lara had been an elderly patient with well-differentiated breast cancer, he'd have started her on routine chemotherapy in Marktoberdorf. All three gynecologists had trained at large university hospitals and were proficient in the entire range of obstetrical/gynecological operations and treatment, including chemotherapy. But as part of care at the local level, they concentrated on simpler "bread and butter" cases, referring more unusual and complex cases to the university.

Since Lara was so young, and her cancer so aggressive, she deserved the most sophisticated treatment to survive. Her travel costs to and from Munich for chemotherapy would total almost 7000 DM over the next two years, but her *Krankenkasse* would approve and reimburse the entire amount. Lara was freed from any travel co-payments (usually 25 DM each way, for the first and last trip of a treatment series) as she earned less than 1764 DM per month. In fact, her only co-payment for health care costs was for hospital stays, a yearly maximum of 238 DM (17 DM/day for two weeks).

In July 1997 Lara started a high dose chemotherapy regimen as part of clinical trials at Grosshadern, the university hospital in a suburb of Munich. She had decided against participating in a double blind study in which half of the patients received high doses and the other half, standard doses. Instead, she enrolled in a trial where all participants received high doses. She traveled to Grosshadern every 14 days until November to receive chemotherapy — three cycles of epirubicin, three cycles of paclitaxel, and finally, three cycles of cyclophosphamide. The drugs were donated by the company co-sponsoring the study — a total cost of around 14,700 DM. Patients could tolerate the high dosages because of the sequential administration of the drugs.

Side effects from the medications ranged from nausea (especially from epirubicin) to hair loss. Paclitaxel irritated the skin on Lara's back and footsoles. After every few steps, her feet would itch maddeningly. "Still, I never felt like an experimental rabbit," said Lara. "I felt I was in the best hands at Grosshadern, especially because of the research there."

To receive chemotherapy at Grosshadern, Lara had to register as a "part-time" inpatient, a patient who would not be admitted for an overnight stay. The daily rate for "part-timers" was 38 DM less than for "full-timers," but the services were identical. Lara usually was admitted to station I4, one of the gynecology wards. Two young resident physicians took turns assisting in the operating room and covering the 30–40 patients. Hurrying from patient to patient, they had little time to answer questions or to develop the doctor-patient relationship. Although an attending physician was responsible for training and supervising the residents, her day was booked up in the operating room. Because nurses were not allowed to administer chemotherapy, Lara spent many hours waiting for the resident to administer her intravenous medications in between their numerous tasks. When no one was available, a doctor from the neighboring station would be recruited to start the infusion. "You have to take the initiative and ask a lot of questions and keep an eye on your own treatment," Lara explained. "If you see the medication has run out, ring the nurse right away to tell the doctor. And patience is important…if I earned my income through waiting, I'd be rich by now."

Lara hated spending so much time away from Tommy and was feeling quite useless to her family by now. In October she applied for an*"Erwerbsunfahigkeit"* or "unfit-for-work" status, which meant that she would receive *"Krankengeld,"* monthly payments from her health insurance fund, for 78 weeks. Although she was not working, her employer could not fire her because of her illness. After the chemotherapy at Grosshadern was finished in November, Lara gradually gained strength. A CT scan done in the spring was normal. She stopped receiving household help, and returned to work in early April 1998.

Before her illness, Lara had worked in the public relations office of a nearby rehabilitation spa/clinic. Her employer sorely missed her during the time she was away; temporary replacements lacked Lara's enthusiasm and efficiency. For a two-week test period, Lara worked part-time, to see if she could withstand the demands of working again. She passed with flying colors. Tommy, now three years old, spent his days in the public pre-school kindergarten and his father and grandmother helped to care for him while Lara regained her strength.

April 1998

Easter Saturday, exactly one year after Lara discovered the first lump in her breast, her fingers felt another small, hard knob underneath the skin, where her right breast had been. This time there was no delay. She called Dr. Zimmermann at the first opportunity and was in his office in less than 48 hours. At first he thought that the hardness might possibly be related to the port tubing for administering chemotherapy inserted in Oberstaufen. He sent Lara to Oberstaufen, where the physician there confirmed that the new lump was independent of the port tubing. A needle biopsy of the lump

was performed; it confirmed the presence of malignant, poorly differentiated cells in the chest wall. The cancer had come back.

Lara then underwent her second operation in Marktoberdorf — exci-
sion of the cancerous tissue in the chest wall. This time, she recuperated
at home, reinstituting outside household help for two weeks only. She then
began 25 daily adjuvant radiation treatments during the week in the
nearby town of Kaufbeuren, and again Peter and her mother took over the
care of Tommy. This series of treatments ended in July 1998. At the same
time, she began hormonal therapy with tamoxifen and a GnRH antagonist.
She tolerated the radiation quite well, with only slight reddening like sun-
burn as evidence of her treatment. During this time, Lara experienced no
significant physical pains or distress, but she was having frequent argu-
ments with Peter. The conflicts seemed to be personality-driven, and did
not relate directly to her illness.

According to Lara, "Every cancer patient has their own theory about
their sickness." She believed that a combination of physical and emotional
stress might have led to her cancer. The year after her father died, she
moved in with Peter, who was then her new boyfriend and became pregnant within one month. Suddenly, she was responsible for a new child and
a new partner, doing all the housework and helping with the farmwork.
Within a year of her son's birth, she started her new public relations job.
Lara was worn down by these factors — relationship stress, guilt at leaving her husband, new responsibilities at home and work — but had no
time to deal with the emotional issues because of the physical demands of
her schedule. When her cancer returned, however, Lara decided to "clean
house" and reduce the amount of stress in her life. As a result, she separated from Peter, reclaimed her maiden name, and moved with her son
into her own apartment, still only 2 km away.

In September 1998, Lara was told that her previous chemotherapy,
radiation and hormone therapy had been ineffective. Radiographic and
nuclear imaging showed new tumor metastases in her spine and possibly
her lungs. What were the options for such a treatment-resistant tumor?
One possibility mentioned by the doctors in Grosshadern was Herceptin,
a new antibody therapy available only in the US. Some breast tumors
over-expressed a gene called *c-erb2*. Clinical progression of these tumors
seemed to be deterred by treatment with Herceptin, an antibody that

bound the product of the *c-erb2* gene. If Lara's tumor showed strong overexpression of *c-erb2*, she would qualify to go to New York City for 6–8 weeks to participate in clinical trials.

Unfortunately, the DNA analysis of the tumor showed only weak *c-erb2* over-expression, barring her from the study. The university doctors decided to start Lara on a different chemotherapy regimen — liposomal doxorubicin and vinorelbine. Lara resumed her travels to Grosshadern for treatment twice a month from October to January, leaving Tommy alternately in the care of either her mother or older sister. She tolerated the medications quite well, with no hair loss. Imaging studies in November confirmed no progression of the bone metastases and no lymph node or pulmonary involvement.

From the beginning of her illness, friends and acquaintances had showered Lara with advice and books on herbal and dietary remedies, cancer nutrition, and alternative medicine. During the initial chemotherapy, Lara drank beet juice daily, which she believed would help raise her platelet levels. She cut down on meat and dairy products, concentrating more on fruits and vegetables. When she asked her doctors in Grosshadern about dietary recommendations or alternative medicine, they answered, "As long as it doesn't hurt you, and you think it might help... go ahead and try it."

Still, it was clear that the medical establishment did not regard the alternative medicine sector very highly. Few studies demonstrated clear efficacy of alternative therapies. Federal agencies did not regulate contents of herbal or alternative medicine supplements. Although some alternative medicine practitioners or *"heilpraktiker"* seemed experienced and qualified, others were considered quacks.

When Lara's tumor resurfaced, her confidence in conventional chemotherapy was somewhat shaken. Upon a friend's recommendation, she drove 70 km to Scheidegg to see Mr. Hahn, a renowned *Heilpraktiker*. Since the age of 17, Mr. Hahn had worked in various capacities in the medical field — as an anesthetist, a lab technician, and a physical therapist. His current practice, shared with five other *Heilpraktiker*, was humming; the waiting list was five to six months. The majority of their clients were cancer patients who had failed chemotherapy.

Some patients flew in from Hamburg, Vienna, and even New York for consultation. His treatment modalities included immune therapy — stabilization of the immune system via substances such as mistletoe, ant serum, one's own blood or *"Eigenblut,"* and snake venom, purported to activate certain enzymes. Other substances helped to attack micrometastases in the blood and in other organs. According to Mr. Hahn, he was the first *Heilpraktiker* in Germany licensed to offer hyperthermic tumor therapy, a technique using radiation to subject tumor tissue to temperatures of 42 degrees Celsius. The costs of Mr. Hahn's therapy were not covered by the *Krankenkasse*, but were occasionally reimbursed by private health insurance companies, according to a price list last amended in 1982.

Lara's initial visit to Mr. Hahn lasted an hour. She signed on for a series of 11 to 12 weekly treatments. Over the course of her treatment, she paid 3,880 DM out of pocket for consultation fees and 2,000 DM for prescribed medications and associated travel costs. She was simultaneously undergoing chemotherapy at Grosshadern, so her travel schedule was exhausting. When Mr. Hahn recommended hyperthermic treatment for her tumor, Lara consulted with Dr. Schmitt, one of the doctors at Grosshadern. He informed Lara that hyperthermic therapy was available (and reimbursable) at the university hospital, but advised her against it for two reasons. First, the temperature elevation would place added stress on her heart, which was already at risk from the high doses of doxorubicin. Secondly, hyperthermic therapy was most effective in wiping out localized tumors, rather than diffuse or micro-metastases. Lara decided to hold off on the hyperthermic therapy, and in fact, discontinued her visits to Scheidegg. The financial burden of Mr. Hahn's therapies was adding up.

Lara retired prematurely on January 1, 1999 at age 33 because of her advanced disease, and received a monthly pension of 1,470 DM. Every month she also received a *"Kindergeld"* payment of 250 DM for her son and a disability payment of 385 DM. Her total income per month was 2,105 DM. Her expenses added up to about 1,250 DM per month, plus food and clothing costs. Her monthly expenses included rent (770 DM), phone bill (70–80 DM), electricity (50 DM), kindergarten (75 DM), automatic bank savings deposit (100 DM), retirement savings deposit (190 DM for 3 months), life insurance (65 DM), health, auto, and accident/damages insurance (20 DM). Lara broke even every month, with a little breathing room. With some previous savings, she could still go out for an occasional dinner with a girlfriend or splurge on a toy for her son.

But as Tommy got older, he would need more clothes and toys, and perhaps a computer.

In a hospital questionnaire dated mid-January 1999, Lara reported her quality of life as "average." She reported no pain, but rather increasing weakness, fatigue, and insomnia. At this time, her liver was examined. The cancer had spread again, this time to several diffuse sites in her liver. Her doctors proposed a combination therapy with Herceptin and low doses of docetaxol. Herceptin had become available in Germany through the international pharmacy, even though it had not been approved for nationwide sales in local pharmacies.

On February 10, 1999 Grosshadern sent a letter to Lara's *Krankenkasse* to request reimbursement for Herceptin therapy. Up until now, the *Krankenkasse* had reimbursed Grosshadern for Lara's care, according to the "part-timer" per diem rate of 338 DM. But Herceptin was just too expensive for the university to cover alone, with a three to four week supply running 4,515 DM. It was up to the *"Medizinische Dienst,"* the medical expert within the insurance company, to review Grosshadern's application. In just over a week, the approval for a three-month trial of Herceptin was faxed back. The first infusion of Herceptin was pumped into Lara's arm three days later.

At the end of February, Lara experienced some strange symptoms — numbness around her lips and chin. The university doctors suspected that the tumor had spread to her brain; a CT scan had shown a thickening of the meningeal layers surrounding the brain. Lara underwent an operation for placement of a port, which would allow chemotherapeutic agents to be injected directly into the brain. At the same time, cerebrospinal fluid (CSF) from within the brain could be easily removed to check for micrometastases. CSF was obtained three times from the port, and twice from the base of Lara's spine via lumbar puncture. Analysis of all of the CSF samples showed no evidence of malignant cells. Yet, Lara was feeling poorly, and had severe bouts of nausea for several weeks after the operation. Since she had used up her quota of household help, she and Tommy moved back home with her mother and brothers. Tommy's father, Peter, still took him on weekends and sometimes on chemotherapy days when Lara traveled to Grosshadern. But being at her mother's house relieved Lara of daily chores such as cooking and cleaning. As her stomach pains subsided over the next weeks, she felt strong enough to return to her own apartment with Tommy.

Lara describes herself as a person who tries to think positively. When she found the first lump, she felt shocked and frightened. But the subsequent diagnoses came one at a time — the lymph nodes, then the second lump, the bone metastases, and the liver metastases — with enough time in between to "work over" and accept the findings in her mind. Lara has never felt that she has been sentenced to death, without hope. She still thinks about breast reconstruction someday, despite knowing that she will "probably never be healed." And she looks forward to meeting a partner with whom she can share her life. Recently she answered a personal ad for the first time and met a very nice man with two children. After learning that his wife recently died of breast cancer, she decided not to see him again. Lara hopes that Herceptin will "hold the cancer in check," so that she can spend as much time as possible with Tommy, who is now four years old. Tommy knows that his mother is sick, but they have never discussed the subject of her possible death. "He is just too young to understand," says Lara. "Maybe when he is older, or if I become sicker... maybe I'll talk to him about it then."

Lara has no idea of the expense of her chemotherapy. A bare-bones estimate of her chemotherapeutic medications at Grosshadern (including Herceptin) tops 67,000 DM. The university has borne the brunt of that cost, with the *Krankenkasse* only reimbursing Grosshadern about 10,000 DM for thirty "part-time" days spent at the hospital receiving chemotherapy and 11,000 DM for Herceptin. However, the *Krankenkasse* has paid for the additional costs of travel (6,100 DM), household help (25,800 DM), radiation therapy (15,000 DM), operations, rehabilitation stays, and *Krankengeld*. All told, the *Krankenkasse* will have shelled out over 100,000 DM in two years for Lara's health care. Most of the correspondence regarding reimbursement occurs directly between Grosshadern and the *Krankenkasse* representative, with young residents writing the requisite letters. The residents must also sign Lara's travel receipts, which she then brings to the local office in Seeg. Up to now, Lara's health care costs have never been questioned. But the *Krankenkasse* has only approved Herceptin for three months. If the cancer in Lara's body fails to respond to treatment and progresses further, she knows that Herceptin will likely be discontinued.

April 1999

"April, April, der weiss nicht, was er will," goes the Bavarian saying, to explain the capricious whims of April's weather.[a] On this Easter Saturday, old man April has remained silent, bestowing no more unwelcome surprises on Lara. She breathes a sigh of relief, and starts to pack her and Tommy's bags for a *"Mutterkindkur"* on the coast of Northern Germany in May, a four week spa visit with activities and services for mothers and their children. The future is a black box for Lara, but she'll take it step by step, struggling to remain healthy, independent, and optimistic for as long as she can.

---

[a] April, April, he knows not what he wants.

Case 11: *Nie Krank**

Christine Hsu Rohde

> *"The life I love is playing music with my friends..."*
>
> *Willie Nelson*

"The thing I remember most was watching my left hand fall on my face and not being able to do anything about it."

Like a slow-motion sequence in an action movie, this image from Karl Lieder's stroke embedded itself in his memory. Lieder had always been healthy, never taking medications and rarely visiting the family doctor. However, his *"Schlaganfall,"* as strokes are called in Germany, completely altered the path of his life.

Born in 1945 in a small town called Eisenerz in Steiermark, a region of Austria, Karl Lieder trained as a locksmith. He remained in his familiar surroundings until he turned twenty, at which point he moved to the Feldmoching area of Munich, Germany. After a few years of working as a locksmith, Lieder grew tired of his occupation and decided to return to school for further training. He graduated as a *"Maschinenbautechniker,"* an engineer who works with metal construction.

---

*Christine Hsu Rohde wrote this case when she was a student at Harvard Medical School and participated in the US-EU-MEE medical student exchange at Ludwig-Maximilians University, Munich, Germany in 2000.

177

Lieder found a job in Munich and met Elsa, who worked as a nurse at Grosshadern, a university hospital nearby. They were married and after a few years had a son, Fabian. Life settled into a comfortable pattern for Lieder and he worked in Munich for the next thirteen years. His special pastime and pleasure was watching his son grow, and playing tunes from his native Austria for him on his *"Steirische Diatonische Harmonika,"* a type of accordion.

During this time Karl had little occasion to think about health care. He was enrolled as a statutory member of *Techniker Krankenkasse*, a sickness fund that provides coverage for a large number of technical employees. He and his employer each paid half of the required premium. As a young man, however, he never got sick and did not require most of the benefits offered by his insurance. His wife, Elsa, received insurance coverage through her employer with BARMER *Krankenkasse*, the largest sickness fund in Germany.

In 1983, Karl decided to go into his own business as the owner of a steel construction company. His years as a *Maschinenbautechniker* had prepared him technically and financially to become self-employed. At this point, a friend advised him to switch to a private insurance plan. Knowing that once he moved out of the public sickness funds, he would not be allowed to return, Karl put a great deal of thought into the decision. His friend persuaded him that it was the best move and he changed his personal insurance to a private plan with *Deutsche Krankenversicherung* AG (DKV). The premiums for a young healthy man were low, and after all, he could afford to have private insurance now. Otherwise, if he remained in the public system, he would have to pay the entire premium because he was self-employed. His wife remained with BARMER because her salary did not enable her to afford private insurance.

Karl continued to be healthy and never saw his family physician (*"Hausarzt"*), Dr. Richter, except for an occasional cold. *"Er war nie krank* (He was never sick)," recalls Elsa. Dental care, eyeglasses, and other medical needs were paid for by DKV and they never had problems with their insurance being unwilling to pay for their few health care needs.

Changing Fortunes

Unfortunately, Karl's business did not perform well and he was forced to sell it in 1995. He then began work as the manager of a construction company in Leipzig in the former East Germany. He found this job stressful, especially the long distance he had to drive every week from Munich to Leipzig, leaving Elsa and Fabian in Munich. After three years, this company had difficulty paying his salary and owed him several months back pay. Tired of the long drives and the financial instability of the company, he quit his job in 1998.

At the beginning of 1998, he took over ownership of a local bar and liquor store named "*Stüberl*" in Feldmoching, back in Munich. Lieder enjoyed the lifestyle of working in his bar. Most of his customers were locals and friends, and his days passed talking, keeping a complete stock of beer, wine, and liquor, and running the business on his own. Still, he worked hard, operating his bar from 7 am until 10 pm everyday. One of the pleasures of owning the bar was that he could spend a great deal of time playing his *Diatonische* to entertain his customers and friends.

Coming from a family that rarely had health problems, Karl never thought very much about taking care of his health. One of his few visits to a doctor was more than ten years ago for general screening for prostate cancer. His wife, Elsa, with her knowledge as a nurse, encouraged him to get his PSA checked when he was 42. He went to an urologist who did a digital rectal exam and PSA test, both of which were normal. However, the physician also ran a battery of blood tests and discovered that Karl's cholesterol was elevated. The urologist suggested that he see his family doctor to discuss the abnormal level, but Karl did not have the time and failed to follow up. His health had never been a source of worry and he continued to be unconcerned.

Changing Health

He was more annoyed than concerned when he began to have headaches over the past two years. He blamed them on "*der Föhn*," a tropical wind that periodically comes across the Alps into Bavaria. These headaches are common in the region, especially among women. The second week of June 1998, Lieder began having a headache he initially thought was "*Föhn*"-related. However, this pain was not like the others. The pain was constant and he felt it over his whole head. During that week, he went on a trip with friends, traveling and playing music, accompanying his friends on his *Diatonische*. Throughout the trip, he felt unwell and tired. He would lie down for several hours but he was still fatigued and had an unrelenting headache.

On the Monday after his trip, Karl returned to work at his bar and liquor store. Although he felt relatively well, his customers noticed something strange about him.

"*Hast du irgendetwas*? (What's wrong?)," asked one of the two customers in the store.

Apparently, this man thought Karl had imbibed too much of his own wine or beer. Thinking nothing of it, Karl continued eating the sausage roll in his hand. The other customer commented on how good the sausage roll looked, and Lieder, always happy to do things for his friends, started to go to the street vendor outside to get another roll. As he went through the door, he suddenly felt dizzy, lost strength on his left side, and fell with a loud crash. Later, recalling the feeling he had at that moment, he remarks that *Schlaganfall* is a good word for stroke since he felt just like he had been hit ("*Schlag*" = hit).

It was at this time that Karl has the distinct memory of lying on his back and watching his left hand fall onto his face. He also noticed that he had difficulty speaking and the tone of his voice was higher than usual. The rest of the events blur into a haze of fear and confusion.

"I thought I was going to die right there."

In a panic, one of the customers called the "*Rettungsleitstelle*" (emergency coordination center) and an ambulance with a doctor was dispatched (*Notarztwagen*). Karl was taken to Grosshadern, a university hospital only a few kilometers away where his wife, Elsa works. Grosshadern has a special stroke unit and the doctors and nurses there immediately began attending to him upon arrival.

"It was like I was on a television show, getting rushed through the hospital halls to the CT scanner and then lysis," Karl remembers. The events were just like a scene from "ER," shown dubbed on German television. Only this time, the events were real and he was the patient.

Because he was a patient with private insurance, either the *"Chefarzt"* (chief of the department) or one of the *"Oberärzte"* (similar to assistant heads of a department) would be his physician. Dr. Lange, an *Oberarzt* at Grosshadern, was on duty on June 15 and thus served as his attending physician.

After medical school, Dr. Lange trained for five years as an *"Assistenzarzt"* or resident, during which time he did four years of clinical neurology and one year of psychiatry. He decided to stay on the academic track rather than work for a municipal non-academic hospital, in a private practice, or as a rehabilitation neurologist, the other options available to him. As an academic physician, Dr. Lange completed a written thesis that is necessary for academic and hospital promotion in Germany. He continues to be involved in research but also shares clinical duties, especially seeing private patients.

At the Hospital

When Karl arrived that day, he seemed to be a possible patient for a protocol on r-TPA lysis in which Dr. Lange was involved. After hurriedly rolling him into the CT scanner, the physicians were encouraged to see that the CT showed no early ischemic changes and no cerebral bleeding. A Doppler ultrasound demonstrated decreased flow in the right middle cerebral artery. His right-sided lesion explained his left-sided weakness and absence of aphasia. Because he was young, not hypertensive, and not suffering from a hemorrhagic stroke, Lieder was an ideal candidate for thrombolysis therapy.

After explaining that Grosshadern was involved in clinical research on lysis therapy in acute stroke, Dr. Lange explained the possible benefits and complications and offered Karl the therapy.

"I had seen a program on television about TPA and how it works, so I thought 'what do I have to lose?' I was afraid but I wanted to try lysis."

The neurology ward is located on floor 8G of the Klinikum Grosshadern, a cold gray building built in the 1970's. Near the middle of the ward are three gray doors labeled "Stroke Unit." The central door leads to the work area for doctors and nurses. The other two doors lead to the intensive care rooms, each with two beds for very sick stroke patients. Near this trio of rooms lie two separate rooms, one with three beds, the other private, both serving as step-down rooms for more stable stroke patients. There are two doctors on-duty during the day, one at night, and several nurses working throughout the day and night.

Karl received the infusion throughout the night in one of the four intensive care beds in the Stroke Unit. All in all, it took one-and-a-half hours from his stroke until the beginning of r-TPA lysis. Fortunately, being a nurse in this hospital, Elsa could stay by his side.

From the top floors of the hospital, a patient can look out the window and see the Alps towering in the distance. But Karl was not thinking of the view as he lay in his bed in the Stroke Unit. Unable to sleep, he watched his left hand, wondering if he would be able to move it again. He thought about the fun with his friends on his recent music trip, troubled by the thought that it may have been his last. He wondered if he would be able to play his beloved *Diatonische* again and teach his grandchildren Austrian songs as he had taught Fabian. His eyes then scanned down to his leg, but the blood pressure cuff interrupted his thoughts, squeezing his arm again, just like it did every half hour before.

With the release of the pressure, his mind began to wander again, accompanied by the rhythmic beeping of the monitors to which he and his neighbor were attached. His neighbor in the Stroke Unit, the man on the other side of the pale blue curtain, seemed to be in worse shape than he. "I'm glad I am not that ill," Karl thought. "But what if I get worse?"

And so it went, idle thoughts in the silence, refusing to give him rest the first night in the hospital; thoughts that he did not want to share with Elsa.

The next morning, the therapists unhooked him from some of the monitors to try to get him to stand up and walk. With several physical and occupational therapists working specifically for the Stroke Unit, rehabilitation efforts are started early. However, Karl could not stand up and fell weakly into their arms. He would try again later, he promised.

Dr. Lange came to see him, disappointed that the lysis therapy had not produced a dramatic improvement. A post-lysis MRI showed an obvious bright white area in the right middle cerebral artery territory. "If the thrombolysis therapy had been successful, we would not expect the MRI to show such a large infarct," explained Dr. Lange.

Despite the discouraging results of thrombolysis, Karl remained cautiously hopeful that his condition would improve. He was moved out of the intensive care room after the first night and found it easier to rest in the quieter step-down room. His stay in the Stroke Unit continued, with the therapists coming every day to work on his leg. Gradually, the strength in his leg improved slightly but he was still unable to walk unaided. During the day, Elsa and Fabian would come to visit, keeping him occupied and keeping his mind off his disabilities. But at night he would often lie awake, not wanting to call the nurse and afraid to go to the bathroom, imagining that he would fall on the way.

As is often the case, the physicians could not determine what caused Karl's stroke. He had no past history or family history of stroke or other cardiovascular disease. His blood pressure was 140/95 on the right and 130/90 on the left. All EKGs were normal, and transesophageal echocardiography (TEE) showed only minimal mitral insufficiency with no vegetations and normal cardiac size and function. Laboratory results were all normal except for elevated cholesterol of 237 mg/dl.

Lieder stayed at Grosshadern for a total of eight days and was finally transferred to a rehabilitation facility on June 22. His medications at the time of transfer were daily simvastatin 10 mg and enteric-coated aspirin 300 mg. He was discharged with diagnoses of left hemiparesis and dysarthria resulting from a right middle cerebral artery territory infarct. Elsa explained that this meant he has muscle weakness on the left side of his body and difficulty with his speech as a result of his stroke on the right side of his brain.

Bad Aibling Rehabilitation

A *Krankentransportwagen* transported Karl to Bad Aibling, a rehabilitation facility about 100 km from Munich. In this new setting, he began intensive physical therapy, exercising his left side five days a week. At first, his left arm only hung limply at his side and he had great difficulty walking. He always had to concentrate, forcing himself to move his arm in order to move his leg. His gait was awkward and his leg would often spring up at the wrong moment, not heeding the signals he wanted his brain to send. The physical therapists made him sit in a wheelchair for a short time, concerned that he was programming the wrong walking pattern in his brain.

After this brief setback, Karl headed out to walk again, doing laps around the garden under the summer sun. Even as he improved, he had to focus exclusively on walking. If he turned his head to see a passing train or attempted to get the keys out of his pocket, he would be unable to continue walking and might even become weak and fall. Unfortunately, the therapists were so concerned about his leg and his walking that they spent relatively little time exercising his hand. By the time he left Bad Aibling, he was able to walk comfortably and was gradually increasing speed but his hand was still very weak. He despaired of ever playing the *Diatonische* again.

Overall though, Karl enjoyed his time at Bad Aibling. He was reassured by his physical improvement and was able to relax in the new environment. Because of the distance from Munich, Elsa and Fabian could only visit on the weekends, but he was working so hard on rehabilitation, he appreciated the time away from home. By the fourth weekend, he was able to return to Munich for the weekends and spend time with his family.

After seven and a half weeks, Karl returned home to stay. At first he paid the bills from Grosshadern and Bad Aibling and then his private insurance company reimbursed him. Halfway through his rehabilitation, the public retirement insurer *Bundesversicherungsanstalt für Angestellte* (BFA) helped DKV with the costs of the extended stay. At that point, Lieder had to move from his private room to a room for publicly insured patients. Karl did not mind the move and noticed very little difference between having DKV and BFA cover the costs.

Once home in Feldmoching, Karl continued to attend outpatient rehabilitation sessions three times a week. He started cycling at an old airstrip and continued to improve the strength in his legs. Beginning in the summer of 1999, physical therapy sessions were cut down to once every month or every two months. Instead, he devised his own training regimen, combining increasing distances of walking and then running. He also joined a nearby sports club to exercise and play ballgames with other people.

"I am part of the housewife class because they are at my level right now, but I hope to move up to the married couples' class soon," he laughs.

Insurance Problems

After returning home, Karl began having problems with his private insurance company. They refused to continue to fund his *"Krankengeld,"* the payments he received to cover the money he was not earning while too ill to work. His options were to either find a job — which he felt unable to do — or go on his retirement pension. The latter choice would be financially difficult since the small amount of pension he would receive would barely cover his insurance premium of DM 780 per month, let alone his living expenses. (Note: On January 1, 2002 the Euro became the official currency of Germany.)

Karl turned to *Verband Deutscher Kriegsversehrter* (VDK), an organization that helps Germans with retirement difficulties and also advises on health insurance problems. They suggested that he apply for unemployment money, a fund he had been making mandatory contributions to while employed in Leipzig. Following their advice, Karl applied and began receiving unemployment benefits from the social insurance system. The *"Arbeitsamt"* (unemployment agency), now in charge of funding his health insurance, took him out of the private insurance system and placed him in public insurance with BARMER. With this change, the *Arbeitsamt* is able to pay much lower premiums. Thus, Karl discovered that unemployment was the only way to transfer from private insurance back into public *Krankenkassen*. Being self-employed for much of his life, he had never wanted to rely on social welfare. But after his unexpected illness, it became his only choice.

A New Development

Although Karl thought the problems from his stroke were over, Christmas 1999 brought a new unpleasant surprise. Several days before the holiday, he began having muscle spasms in his back. He also awoke several nights with a "strange feeling" that something was wrong. One afternoon he suddenly had an episode in which his muscles became tight, he was unable to move his arms, and his face became contorted. "I must be having another stroke," he thought to himself, angry and afraid that this was happening again.

Elsa was at work at the hospital. He tried to call Fabian, who lives downstairs, but was unable to speak on the phone. It was not fear that paralyzed his voice, but a complete inability to move the muscles of his throat. His son called for an ambulance and he was brought to a municipal hospital in Schwabing. There, the doctors determined that he had had a seizure and not another stroke. Karl was hardly relieved by the news, for this diagnosis meant that his battle with the effects of the stroke was far from over. He was discharged that evening from Schwabing, wondering if life would ever return to normal.

Because Dr. Lange maintains a close relationship with his Stroke Unit patients (something that is unusual for hospital-based physicians in Germany), Karl returned to see him for care of this new seizure problem. He could have gone to any outpatient neurologist but chose to come to Dr. Lange at Grosshadern, where there is also an outpatient department. Dr. Lange started him on valproic acid 300 mg three times a day to prevent future seizures.

What Lies Ahead?

By the beginning of 2000, Karl's weakness is mostly gone. He has no problems walking and even running. However, he still has a bit of a facial droop and has problems distinguishing temperature on both his left arm and leg. He still has moments when he feels very tired, his face starts to hurt, and he must lie down to make the pain go away. The most bothersome lingering effects are in his hand and his psyche. He still has difficulty with fine hand movements such as using a fork and most importantly, playing his *Diatonische*. He had played for over ten years and has been trying to play as a way to exercise his fingers. After playing effortlessly for over ten years, the difficulty he now has frustrates and depresses him.

Most disappointing, Karl does not get as much enjoyment out of music as before. This feeling seems to be related to his general mood lability. Ever since his stroke, he cannot concentrate, he is often tired, and he cries whenever he talks with strangers about his stroke. Previously, Karl had never been a man to cry about anything. He feels like he would be unable to return to any kind of worthwhile work because of his lingering hand problems, his seizures, and his emotional instability. In his worst moments, he thinks that nobody cares about his problems or wants to help him in spite of reassurances by Elsa and Fabian. These thoughts haunt his future as he considers what lies ahead.

Dr. Richter, his *Hausarzt*, had prescribed a tricyclic anti-depressant for Karl's depression but Dr. Lange discontinued this medication because he believes the mood lability is caused by the right hemispheric stroke and his job situation. Furthermore, he worries that the anti-depressant may exacerbate his seizure condition.

So, at present, Karl looks like a healthy man on the outside. He is one of the lucky ones to survive an acute stroke and regain virtually all of his previous function. It is difficult to say what role thrombolysis played in his recovery, but the intensive and early rehabilitation efforts certainly helped him improve as remarkably as he did. On the inside, however, Karl is a different man. He is unable to find employment, feels emotionally labile, and lacks confidence in his mental and physical abilities. He is now dependent on the social welfare system, something he has always wanted to avoid. When asked about the future, he replies, "I'm just waiting for my life insurance to start paying at 65 so that I have money to do something again." And surely, he is hoping that the future will include playing music and getting back on the road again with his friends.

Case 12: Frau Baumgartner and Herr Schneider*

Aimee Der-Huey Shu

Frau Baumgartner's Story

Isolde Baumgartner is a 55-year-old retired secretary in Munich, Germany with a history of rheumatoid arthritis (RA) who told me her story in early April 2002 while she received an intravenous infusion of infliximab. It all started in 1986, with intermittent painful wrist swelling and diminished grip strength. Sometimes she could not even grip the doorknob firmly enough to open a door. These symptoms would last for two days and then go away, only to return a few days later. In an attempt to relieve the swelling and pain, she applied cold compresses to her wrists.

When her symptoms returned for a third time, Frau Baumgartner turned to her *Hausarzt* (house doctor, or general practitioner), who referred her to an orthopedic surgeon who had a private practice in the community. For the next five years, the orthopedic surgeon treated her swollen wrists, knees, and ankles by periodically withdrawing fluid from her joints with a needle. However, in 1991 as the fluid continued to

---

*These two cases were written by Aimee Der-Huey Shu in the spring of 2002, when she was a student at Harvard Medical School and participated in the US-EU-MEE student exchange at Ludwig-Maximilians University, Munich, Germany.

re-accumulate, he referred Frau Baumgartner to the rheumatology clinic at Ludwig Maximilian University's (LMU) Innenstadt Hospital.

Tests and Treatment at LMU

LMU is Munich's largest university and medical school. The university's clinical medical faculty is divided between two campuses: Innenstadt Hospital, located in beautiful, historic buildings in the city center; and Grosshadern Hospital, a much larger hospital in the outskirts of Munich.

At LMU-Innenstadt Hospital's *Medizinische Poliklinik* (Medical Ambulatory Clinic), Frau Baumgartner was given a series of tests. Her erythrocyte sedimentation rate (ESR) and C reactive protein (CRP) levels were found to be elevated, sure indicators of inflammation. Other test results, including HLA-B27, anti-nuclear antibodies (ANA), and psoriatic skin findings, were negative. She was given a weak radioactive tracer intravenously and a bone scan was done. It showed enhanced uptake of the radioactive substance in both wrists, right hip, both knees, and bones in her left ankle. The physicians noted "oligoarthritis of unknown origin" in her chart, and treated her with non-steroidal anti-inflammatory drugs (NSAIDs).

Over the next several years, Frau Baumgartner's symptoms continued to wax and wane, and she visited the LMU clinic as necessary. September 1996 was the first time she was told that she has Rheumatoid Arthritis (RA). She had been having symptoms for 10 years by this time, and the pain had been getting worse since 1994. She began to have morning stiffness, but she was thankful that she did not have other symptoms of RA, such as fever, night sweats, skin changes, hair changes, or eye changes. Laboratory tests also showed that she was negative for rheumatoid factor and serum Lyme antibodies.

Frau Baumgartner did not know of anybody else in her family who had RA. Because the pain and stiffness in her joints had lasted so long and was not getting any better, and her lab tests clearly indicated inflammation, her doctor at the LMU clinic prescribed low-dose methotrexate (MTX) 15 milligrams (mg) weekly, folate 5 mg weekly, prednisone 10 mg daily, calcium supplements, and vitamin D supplements. After receiving the RA diagnosis and starting the MTX, Frau Baumgartner was scheduled to visit her rheumatologist every three months.

At first her disease was relatively unchanged, with pain and stiffness but no redness, warmth, or swelling. At one point, her MTX was stopped for four months (August 1997–December 1997) because she had a remission from symptoms. Her first *schub* (flare) was in December 1997, and she started taking MTX again.

From this time on, she continued to take MTX and prednisone. Her flares were related to changes in weather, and they were worst in winter when she would miss one to two days of work per month because of the flares. On occasion she would miss more than three days of work, in which case she required a doctor's note. In December 1999, she enrolled in a clinical study (VIGOR) investigating the effectiveness of rofecoxib [Vioxx] versus naproxen to treat pain. At the study's conclusion in February 2000, she started taking rofecoxib 12 mg daily.

Dr. Anne Marie Schonfeld first met Frau Baumgartner at the LMU clinic in October 2000. Although Frau Baumgartner complained of hair loss, and difficulty walking, she was still working. Full-time work had been a part of Frau Baumgartner's life ever since she took her first office job at age 16. At that time, she was given a choice of *Krankenkassen* (health sickness funds). She decided on *Deutsche Angestellten Krankenkasse* (DAK), a sickness fund for *Angestellte* (salaried employees and civil servants).

I asked Frau Baumgartner why she had chosen this particular *Krankenkassen* but she said it was for no particular reason that she can remember. Under German law, all citizens are entitled to health care

Table 5.1.   Frau Baumgartner's Surgical History.

Frau Baumgartner's Past Surgical History	
1953	Tonsillectomy
1978	Right wrist carpal tunnel release
1988	Bone graft to right wrist
1992	Right total hip replacement
1994	Left total hip replacement
2001	Bilateral surgical debridement of hip spurs

regardless of health or employment status. Each German employee and the employer must contribute a percentage of the employee's income to one of several independent *Krankenkassen*.

I asked Frau Baumgartner, "Are all *Krankenkassen* equal in your eyes?"

"For the most part, yes, but occasionally I hear of 'bad' ones. By this I mean they ask for higher co-pays."

When Frau Baumgartner was 19 years old, she decided to leave her hometown in northern Germany and head for the "big city excitement" of Munich. She immediately liked the Bavarian city in the southern part of Germany, where she met her husband, Wally, and raised her two sons, now ages 32 and 33. She was working as a secretary for a professor in the Department of Astronomical and Physical Geosciences at a technical university in Munich when Dr. Schonfeld became her doctor at the clinic. Dr. Schonfeld is an *Assistenzarzt*. She has graduated from university and is now training under the supervision of the clinic's attending rheumatologists. She manages patients on her own, and consults the attendings when she feels necessary.

Dr. Schonfeld's initial contribution to Mrs. Baumgartner's care was to add leflunomide to her medications. She also attempted to optimize the prednisone dose, and added an opioid for pain. Frau Baumgartner's symptoms improved, but did not completely go away. She kept her clinic

Table 5.2. Frau Baumgartner's Medications.

Frau Baumgartner's Medications February 2001
Prednisone
Leflunomide
Infliximab
Calcium & vitamin D combination
Furosemide
Loperamide
Leflunomide 10/00 — present.
Infliximab 2/01 — present.
Methotrexate 9/96–8/97, 12/97–2/01.
Discontinued because it was ineffective.

appointments every two to four weeks. In January 2001, Frau Baumgartner complained of severe night sweats. She also developed herpes zoster around her eye, and then her lips. She was referred to an ophthalmologist and a dermatologist.

A Medication Change

In February 2001, it seemed that Frau Baumgartner's disease was progressing. Her joints were stiff every morning for about 30 minutes and she continued to have foot pain. Her physicians decided to abandon MTX and try infliximab infusions instead. Frau Baumgartner received her first infliximab infusion on February 23, 2001. She came to the clinic, was hooked up to an intravenous (IV) line for about two hours, had her blood pressure checked every half hour, and returned home when the infusion was finished. Three days later, she enjoyed increased range of motion, and decreased foot pain.

Because Frau Baumgartner has been getting infliximab every six to 10 weeks, Dr. Schonfeld has been especially vigilant about her patient's overall health and possible infliximab side effects. She has investigated Mrs. Baumgartner's complaints of chest pain, diarrhea, headaches, fever, weight loss, and leg edema. She even sees her for unscheduled visits, and has assumed a primary care role. Frau Baumgartner is happy with her care at the university clinic. She often has to wait two hours to see Dr. Schonfeld, but she thinks it is worth the wait.

In addition to her visits to the Innenstadt clinic, Frau Baumgartner has also had a primary care physician for about 25 years. She chose this particular doctor because his office is near her home in Schwabing. She estimates that she sees him about three times a year for check-ups and minor viral illnesses. When she sees him, she takes her notes from the LMU clinic to him. He is not involved in her RA care, and does not write any prescriptions for her RA medications.

Frau Baumgartner had a comprehensive evaluation by the physical therapy department at Grosshadern on November 29, 2001. The purpose of this evaluation was to teach her physical therapy she could do on her own, and to establish a functional status to which future evaluations would be compared. While there, she learned about a support group for

RA patients. She also spent 20 days at a *kur* — a unique German blend of rehabilitation hospital and spa resort — in *Bad Schussenried* from January 8–28, 2002.

I accompanied Frau Baumgartner for her eighth infusion of 200 mg of infliximab, three mg/kg in saline. After a brief meeting with Dr. Schonfeld, she went upstairs to the lab to give a urine sample and have her blood drawn. An IV was placed, and she moved to another room. Dr. Schonfeld was called up to connect the IV. Three other patients were in the room.

RA and Daily Life

While keeping her company during the infusion, I asked Frau Baumgartner how RA has changed her life.

"Well, for one thing, I can't do sports anymore, I can only swim. Up until three years ago, I enjoyed dancing with my husband, Wally, once a week but then I had to stop. I also had to retire prematurely (in April 2001) from my job as a secretary for a prominent professor. As part of my job I had to prepare to welcome the professor's guests. I had to walk to the grocery store to purchase coffee and cookies, but this became increasingly difficult. My feet hurt so much that I even packed my own lunch and brought it from home so I would not have to leave my office."

"How are you managing around the house?"

"Cleaning has become a big effort. After using the vacuum cleaner, for instance, I have to lie down and take a rest because I get so exhausted. Because of the decreased range of motion in my shoulder, I can no longer reach high, so I use a ladder, unless Wally is home. He helps when he can but he still works in automobile manufacturing."

Now that she is retired, Frau Baumgartner collects *Rente* (social security pension), and continues to pay a percentage to her *Krankenkasse*. In the last five years, with German health care reform, she has had to contribute a copay for her prescription medications. This amount is approximately €25 (~$32.50) per month. She paid €81 (~$105) for a series of 20 physical therapy sessions. She considers these fees to be nominal. Frau Baumgartner also points out that because she is considered handicapped, all these copays are tax-deductible. One situation did outrage her, however. For a 20-day *Kur* (rehabilitation spa) visit, her *Krankenkasse* asked her to pay a total of €2234 (~$2904).

By law, patients with chronic illnesses are entitled to *kur* visits for three to four weeks every two years. The sickness funds' rationale for charging steep copays is that there is no evidence to prove efficacy of these *kur* treatments. How much is vacation and how much is medical therapy is controversial.

"What do you think about private insurance?" I asked Frau Baumgartner.

"I think privately insured patients get the same care as I do. Perhaps they do not wait as long. I have seen that privately insured patients often are invited to sit in separate waiting rooms and they are treated by the professors and the heads of departments at the hospital. When they are hospitalized, their rooms have fewer patients in a room."

"What percentage of your pay and your present *Rente* goes to your *Krankenkasse*?"

"I really don't pay much attention to that. I don't know what the percentage is now, but my employer and I each pay the same."

Frau Baumgartner learns about RA from books, television and newspapers. She believes the specialists know what they are doing, and she is happy to let them make the decisions. Other than the RA patients she sees in the waiting room, Frau Baumgartner does not know any RA patients. While at Grosshadern for her physical assessment, she learned of a RA support group. She is awaiting a phone call and plans to attend a meeting next month.

Herr Schneider's Story

Six years ago, Robert Schneider noticed he could not wrap his hands around the barbells he was lifting. His knees also hurt when he bent down. The then-27-year-old avid body builder figured these problems must be related to his intense weight lifting regimen. When the problems did not go away, however, he went directly to see an orthopedic surgeon. He did not need to obtain a referral from his *Hausarzt* because his *Krankenkasse* allowed him direct access to specialist physicians. This doctor had treated him when he was a teenager because puberty had happened so quickly for

Table 5.3. Herr Schneider's Medical History.

Herr Schneider's Past Medical and Surgical History
• 1974 Surgery for undescended left testis
• anosmia, secondary to deviated nasal septum ("the last thing I smelled was butter acid in chemistry class at age 18")
• 1997 Diagnosed with RA, seronegative

him. Between the ages of 15 and 18, he grew 30 cm (almost 12 inches) in height. He finished growing at age 21.

This time, for the hand and knee problems, he was referred to another orthopedic surgeon in Munich who ordered a magnetic resonance imaging (MRI) study of his knee. After reading the MRI, he recommended that Herr Schneider see a rheumatologist. Instead he went to see a third orthopedic surgeon. This physician recommended the rheumatology clinic at Ludwig Maximilians University (LMU).

RA Diagnosis and Treatment

So, in 1997 at age 28, Herr Schneider came to the LMU clinic, where he was diagnosed with Rheumatoid Arthritis (RA). Herr Schneider remembered that his father's sister was diagnosed with RA when she was 32 years old.

Herr Schneider was initially prescribed chloroquine (an anti-malarial drug that reduces inflammation in RA), from 1997–1999; then changed to sulfasalazine from 1999–2002. For pain, he took the NSAID diclofenac. On the day I met him, he was under the care of Dr. Anne Marie Schonfeld. In consultation with the attending physician, she decided to change his medication to Methotrexate (MTX) because his disease was progressing and gave him an information sheet about the drug, including all the side effects.

"Whoa, what am I getting into?" he asked.

Dr. Schonfeld assured him that if he read the side effects of chocolate he might think the same thing.

As I accompanied him to have a chest radiograph as baseline for MTX pneumonitis effects, I asked him more questions.

"How does RA affect your life?"

"Well, I work as a software engineer with a keyboard and mouse, and I can handle them without much complaint," Herr Schneider replied. "I regret that I can't cycle as powerfully as I used to. I used to weight-lift five days a week, but now it's no fun body building when each increase in weight hurts so much that I feel it everywhere."

We walked past the hospital cafeteria and Herr Schneider sniffed ruefully.

"I have to watch my diet now so I don't gain too much weight. Before RA I was so active that I was able to eat anything I wanted."

We sat down to wait outside the X-ray Department.

"Lately I can't bend my knees past 90 degrees." He gets out of his chair to squat and illustrate his point.

"RA changes your way of thinking and living. I have to think twice before placing household items too low or high, because how will I be able to get them later? Things I took for granted all my life now take a lot of thought. Still, I am thankful for my small victories."

"What have you changed in your home to make it 'RA-friendly'?" I asked.

"Really nothing, and so far I am lucky to never have been hospitalized for RA. Now, my knees and hips give me the most trouble. I do physical therapy at a place close to my home. I chose it because it has good facilities, including a cage where I can be suspended and feel like I'm flying while weights are applied to individual joints to stretch them. They teach me exercises I can do at home, and encourage me to keep moving; to be active."

"Where do you live, Herr Schneider?"

"I live by myself in Freising, a suburb north of Munich. I walk three flights of stairs to my apartment instead of taking the elevator so I can get some exercise. I work for a company south of Munich and I have never missed a day of work on account of my RA."

Herr Schneider's Care in the German System

Herr Schneider's *Krankenkasse* is Techniker, which he chose because his field is technology, and because his mother used Techniker as well. He does not recall even considering other *Krankenkassen*.

Herr Schneider's *Hausarzt* is Dr. Bildner in Freising. This is convenient because Dr. Bildner's office is nearby and it is open until 6:00 pm. Although Herr Schneider visits Dr. Bildner every two months to have his RA prescriptions refilled, Dr. Bildner is not otherwise involved in Herr Schneider's RA care. He writes the refills for the prescriptions but never reviews them or prescribes anything different.

When Herr Schneider calls to see Dr. Schonfeld at the university clinic, he usually has to wait three weeks for an appointment. In contrast, to see his *Hausarzt*, he drops by at "speak hour," an open clinic time when patients queue up to see Dr. Bildner; no appointment is necessary. Time devoted to "speak hour" sessions differs by physician, but many do make room for them in their schedules. Thus, Herr Schneider has found it most convenient to go to the "speak hour" sessions to have his prescriptions refilled. He does not pay for any of these sessions.

Since Herr Schneider is generally otherwise healthy, he does not see Dr. Bildner for many other reasons. He did have Dr. Bildner administer a hepatitis immunization a while ago. Herr Schneider was going to travel, and wanted the vaccination. He purchased the vaccine at the pharmacy, and brought it to Dr. Bildner to administer. He explains that his *krankenkasse* did not cover costs for the vaccine because it was for "vacation purposes."

When I asked Herr Schneider his opinion of the German health care system, the first thing he mentions is the difference between private and public health insurance. His income is high enough that he qualifies by law to consider purchasing private insurance. On occasion, he receives soliciting phone calls asking him if he would like to purchase health insurance. After he tells them about his pre-existing condition of RA, however, the agent inevitably says that he will look into this matter and call Herr Schneider back. The answer has always been the same: "Sorry, we cannot take you at this time."

He thinks privately insured patients enjoy benefits like less time spent in the waiting room, wider selection of frames and lenses for glasses, broader dental coverage, wider selection of metals for tooth crowns. He would prefer if private and public patients received the same services. He has noticed that dentists are nicer to private patients because private insurance compensates the dentists better. However, Herr Schneider says he is happy with his RA care, and thinks that a private RA patient would not receive different care for this disease. The two-tiered health care is most apparent to him at the level of eye and dental care.

He has never been concerned about the availability of diagnostic tests; he has gotten them whenever his physicians felt it was necessary. For instance, he had knee MRIs in 1996 to investigate the source of his pain; and a head CT in 1997 to look for causes of his anosmia (loss of sense of smell).

According to Herr Schneider, he does not spend a lot of time thinking about his disease. So far, he has maintained a positive attitude. He does not even think about disability insurance. He does not go out of his way to research the latest treatments because he trusts his doctors will take care of this.

"Anyway, you don't know who to believe. My mother gave me a cookbook that supposedly cures everything," he says with a laugh.

I asked about the cost of his medications.

Herr Schneider paid a total of €15 (~$19.50) for a three-month supply of MTX, folate, and calcium/vitamin D, each costing €5. In the past, he paid €10 (~$13.00) for a three-month supply of sulfasalazine and dicolfenac, also €5 each.

I asked Herr Schneider, "What is your 'wish list' regarding health care?"

"I would like to see the same physician at the rheumatology clinic. Dr. Schonfeld and the other *Assistenzaerzte* (equivalent to US Resident Physician) that I see are technically in training, and they stay at the clinic for only a few years before they move on to other positions. On the other hand, my *Hausarzt,* Dr. Bildner, has known me since I was 15 years old. I also wish the clinic would have better record keeping. They lost my records from a few years ago."

Conclusion

Studying these two very different patients with the same disease, I concluded that the German health care system takes care of patients with chronic illness very well. They were able to get the best health care available at very little personal cost and generally they were satisfied with the treatment offered.

Case 13: For a Breath of Air*

Gregory Sawicki

"In the last four years, I have been through what most people go through in twenty!" This is how Luke Schmidt, a 38-year-old German man with cystic fibrosis (CF), describes his recent medical history. When I met him in April 2001 on the wards of Klinikum Innenstadt, a hospital near the center of Munich, Germany, he had already been an inpatient for almost three months.

Luke was born in a small town 300 km from Munich. In his first three years of life, his parents recall many episodes of coughing and bronchitis, prompting physicians to perform a sweat test, which confirmed the diagnosis of cystic fibrosis. This was a shock to his parents as there was no family history of this genetic disease. His two siblings, Tomas and Horst, also received sweat tests, which were both negative. His parents were informed of the diagnosis in the hospital, but they do not remember having a good explanation of the disease from their local physician.

From the age of two until eight, his parents gave Luke pancreatic enzyme supplementation, but he did not receive any antibiotics, physiotherapy, or inhaled therapy. He was never hospitalized and recalls being able to pursue athletic activities as well as all of his peers. Perhaps because

*This case was written by Gregory Sawicki in the spring of 2001 when he was a student at Harvard Medical School and participated in the US-EU-MEE program at Ludwig Maximilians University, Munich, Germany.

of this, his parents saw no need to seek more information about CF or be concerned about additional treatment. In adolescence, he did not take any medication at all. He did not consider CF an important part of his life.

By the age of 23, Luke was finished with school and moved to Munich to begin a life of his own. He found a job as a computer programmer and enjoyed the attractions the city offered to a young man with a little money in his pocket. After a few years he met Marlena, a programmer for another company, who became his special girlfriend. They got married and Luke envisioned a happy future. Eventually he left his job and started a computer-marketing firm of his own.

In his early twenties, Luke had multiple episodes of bronchitis requiring him to seek medical attention. Since he was living in Munich, he began seeing pulmonary specialists at the Klinikum Innenstadt. At this university hospital, there is an adult CF clinic that cares for approximately 50 patients. The physicians in the group are all trained in adult pulmonary medicine. They are employed by the hospital and are responsible for the inpatient pulmonary ward as well as an outpatient pulmonary clinic. Many of their patients have ambulatory general practitioners who do not follow their patients while in the hospital. The CF doctors prefer that their patients have an outside physician to handle any non-CF related problems. For Luke, however, since his only health problems were related to his disease, he did not see any physicians outside of the pulmonary group in the hospital.

During these visits in his twenties, Luke was prescribed sultanol, a nebulized beta-2 agonist for bronchodilation. These treatments improved his breathing enough so that he rarely sought medical attention, coming for appointments approximately one or two times per year. In addition, he began taking multivitamins and Creon (pancreatic enzyme supplements) to aid his digestion. He had occasional sessions of chest physiotherapy, but they were not a regular part of his treatment routine. For Luke, all of his symptoms were a minor annoyance, but they did not alter the way he lived. He convinced Marlena that they were of no consequence. No one had yet persuaded him of the seriousness of his disease.

When Luke first got a job, his health insurance switched from his parents' sickness fund (*Krankenkasse*) to another fund, Barmer, which was chosen by his employer. A fixed percentage of his salary went to pay his share of health coverage. When he started his own company, he remained with Barmer, but paid a set rate into the fund based on his income level. By 2001, as a self-employed individual, Luke had paid 1100 Deutsche Mark (DM) each month to Barmer for the previous seven years. (Note: On January 1, 2002, the Euro became the official currency of Germany.) With his insurance, he has had a free choice of physicians and has never had to pay for any doctor visits, hospitalizations, home care, or medications. In fact, he never gave much thought to how much his medical care cost.

In June of 1998, Luke's situation began to change. He was admitted for the first time to the hospital for intravenous antibiotic therapy and he could no longer pretend to himself or Marlena that his illness was insignificant. He was an inpatient for one week, and then was taught by a nurse how to administer his IV medicine at home so that he could continue with his treatment for three more weeks. These antibiotics were aimed at curtailing the growth of the various microorganisms, most notably *Pseudomonas aeruginosa*, that had made his airways their home.

Over the next two years, he underwent five courses of inpatient IV therapy. His symptoms were always the same — typical of a pulmonary exacerbation of CF — chronic cough, a large amount of sputum production, fatigue, and inability to take in deep breaths. With each hospitalization, his health improved for a short time, but within a few months, it had worsened again. Over the course of these hospitalizations and home IV therapies, he was given a wide range of medications intended to improve his respiratory status, help his nutrition, and prevent further infection. Luke jokingly compares his situation to the German film "Run Lola Run" in which the main character relives the same day many times over. He feels like every time he makes an improvement, he ends up back in the hospital and has to start all over again.

In 1999, Luke asked his doctors to perform a genetic analysis to look for the exact mutations that were causing his disease. As he recalls, he also wanted the genetic test to re-confirm the CF diagnosis for his own satisfaction. This type of test was now possible because in the years since his initial diagnosis, much progress was made in understanding the genetic basis for CF. In the late 1980's the CFTR gene was identified and by 1999 screening tests for many of the most common mutations of the gene were readily available. Luke's test results revealed one rare mutation (G-T mutation at position 711 of Intron 5) and an intron polymorphism (7T/7T

Intron 8). The test did not detect a second mutation, perhaps because it is likely that it is a rare mutation not routinely screened for in the standard CF mutation analysis.

Luke and Marlena began reading voraciously about CF and tried to learn as much about the disease as they could. They used books, patient magazines, and the Internet as sources of information. Luke began communicating with other CF patients by email to learn about different types of therapies. He found information about "alternative" therapies and decided to give them a try. He made appointments with a Chinese acupuncturist and a German homeopathic physician. The treatments did not seem to help, so he discontinued them. In contrast to his standard medical therapies, which came at no cost to him, he had to pay for these consultations on his own since Barmer did not cover such therapy.

In January 1999, on the advice of his physicians, he spent three weeks at the Dead Sea in Israel, attempting a form of "climate" therapy aimed at increasing the oxygenation in his lungs and decreasing his work of breathing. In Israel, the patients stayed in a hotel with nurses, physical therapists, and physicians on site. The premise of the therapy is that the low elevation of the Dead Sea region would promote increased oxygenation in the lungs. Though there is only scant literature supporting such therapy, Luke's doctors thought he should try it, and Barmer paid for his trip because it was done under a doctor's supervision. Unfortunately, the trip had the opposite effect. Luke felt worse while there, and he returned to Germany disheartened.

His downward progression continued, with several more IV treatments, both at home and in the hospital. He also began to have chest physiotherapy more regularly, arranging for the therapists to visit him at his home. In February 2000, he traveled to the Canary Islands at his own expense to see if the climate there might help, but unfortunately he continued to get worse. By November 2000, he had to stop working and began receiving disability payments of 100 DM per day from his insurance. Marlena took over the day-to-day management of the company. For Luke, his illness had become a full-time job. He required continuous oxygen at home, and at night, he slept with a BiPAP machine, providing extra pressure support for his breathing. During one of his hospitalizations, his physicians first mentioned the possibility of a lung transplant. Luke was hesitant at first, and no further tests were done.

In January 2001, Luke developed a worsening cough and increased sputum production but his main problem was an overwhelming tightness in his chest. He was unable to move air into or out of his lungs, and as a result he was constantly fatigued. Though he had been hospitalized multiple times over the past few years, these symptoms seemed worse then ever before. For the first time he required transport by ambulance to reach the hospital. When he arrived, he was unable to walk a single step.

On arrival, an arterial blood gas was taken showing severe respiratory decompensation. His oxygenation only barely improved after administration of three liters of oxygen. An X-ray showed evidence of his long-standing obstructive pulmonary disease with hyperinflation and diffuse bronchiectasis, which meant that his lungs had lost normal elasticity. No evidence of pneumonia or pneumothorax (air in the pleural cavity) was seen to account for this decompensation. Sputum cultures at the time showed growth of non-mucoid *Pseudomonas aeruginosa*, a common colonizer of the lungs of people with cystic fibrosis, as well as a small amount of *Aspergillus,* a fungal infection.

His cultures had been growing out *Pseudomonas* for over three years, but the presence of the fungus was new. The *Pseudomonas* was resistant to many antibiotics in culture, but was still sensitive to tobramycin and colistin. He was started on IV steroids and IV antibiotics along with his usual regimen of chest physiotherapy and aerosolized bronchodilators. Within a few days, his condition had stabilized enough to perform pulmonary function tests, which showed a marked deterioration from one year ago. His forced expiratory volume (FEV_1) had decreased from 1.6 Liters per second to 0.5 Liters per second.

Upon admission in January 2001, his clinical condition was as bad as it had ever been, prompting discussion of the next possible therapeutic step by his doctors. When Luke and Marlena heard that a double lung transplant might be this next step, they were shocked but they could not deny the seriousness of his condition any longer. In addition to his worsened respiratory status, he had lost approximately 10 kg (more than 22 pounds) over three years.

Within a few days after being admitted, however, Luke slowly began to respond to his intensive medication regimen, which for the first time included IV steroids in addition to antibiotics. Within a few weeks, he was well enough to be discharged to a rehabilitation facility outside of Munich, the Klinikum Berchtesgadener. He stopped taking antibiotics at this facility, and his condition deteriorated once again, prompting readmission to the hospital in the middle of March.

His admission data in March 2001 was as follows:

ABGs	No Oxygen	2L O$_2$	3L O$_2$
PH	7.44	7.43	7.43
PCO$_2$	53.4	55.8	55.3
PO$_2$	45.5	54.3	58.2
O$_2$ Sat	82.9	88.7	90.4

Admission PFTs	Admission Labs
TLC 9.09 L (nl 7.06 L)	WBC 8.3, Hct 43, Plt 316
RV 7.4 L (nl 1.9 L)	Electrolytes WNL
FEV1 0.65 (nl 4.05)	LFTs WNL
FEV1/IVC 39.26 (nl 80.55)	IgE 0, IgG 875 (nl)

At this time, Luke's doctors made the decision to proceed towards transplantation. He had a battery of tests, including Computed Tomography (CT) scans, an echocardiogram, a V-Q scan, and numerous serologic and microbiologic tests. He was evaluated by psychiatry, anesthesia, and ENT. For the first time that he can recall, Luke became frightened by his disease. He was afraid he would collapse and stop breathing while walking to the bathroom in the mornings. He was unable to walk more than 20 meters without gasping for breath, and he coughed incessantly. He realized now that a transplant could buy him more time.

During this hospitalization, he tried several new medications including Pulmozyme, a recombinant form of DNAse, which has been shown to decrease the thickness of secretions in CF patients. Unfortunately, this medication had the opposite effect on Luke and made his cough worse by increasing the amount of secretion. He was also started on anti-fungal therapy because of the growth of *Aspergillus* in his sputum. He was placed on a high calorie diet and gained some weight.

By mid-April, his respiratory status had stabilized, and he was able to walk around the hallways of the hospital on his own. He felt that his condition was improving for the first time in over six months. He and Marlena began to talk hopefully about a summer vacation together on the Baltic Sea. Pulmonary Function Tests when he was discharged, however, showed minimal improvement on spirometry (FEV_1 0.58) and he maintained an O_2 saturation above 95% only when on three liters of oxygen. He was discharged home to continue with IV antibiotics and steroids. Though all of the pre-transplant tests were done, he had still not decided whether to actually put his name on the transplant list.

One week following his discharge, Luke returned to the outpatient CF clinic at the hospital for a follow-up appointment. He was feeling a bit better, and was glad to be back at home for the first time this year. He was grateful for the support and assistance of his parents and Marlena, who basically had put their lives on hold to help him. He continued IV antibiotics at home, and contacted a physiotherapist who would come to his home three times per week.

Now that he had had some time to think further about the transplant, Luke decided that he would proceed if his doctors felt it was the only option. Following this appointment, his physicians went to Grosshadern, a larger University-affiliated hospital on the outskirts of the city, to discuss his case with the transplant team and the following week he had his preliminary appointment with the transplant surgeons. The only thing left for him to do now is to wait, keep up with his treatments, and remain hopeful.

Case 14: A Startling Diagnosis*

Jack Casey

At 40 years of age Leon Weber was extraordinarily active. A longtime resident of a small town near the Bavarian Alps, he was highly involved in sports, participating regularly in running, swimming, bicycling, and skiing. When a swimming instructor told Leon that he had recently observed "unusual positioning" of his arm, he thought little of it. However, shortly thereafter, friends mentioned that they noticed his foot "dragging" as he walked. Although he himself had not noticed any problems and he was feeling well, he decided to make an appointment with his primary care physician (PCP).

Dr. Meyer, his PCP was concerned about his symptoms and recommended that he schedule an office visit with a local neurologist. It was four weeks until his appointment with Dr. Keller but Leon was not particularly worried. He complained to his wife, Grette, that he had been feeling increasingly tired lately, but he thought it was because of the extra time and energy he was spending trying to master a certain elusive swimming stroke. He could not seem to follow through quickly with his right arm, as the instructor wanted him to do.

When the day of his appointment with Dr. Keller finally arrived, Leon had showered and was buttoning a clean shirt when he noticed a slight

---

*This case was written by Jack Casey when he was a student at Harvard Medical School and participated in the US-EU-MEE student exchange at Ludwig Maximilians University in Munich, Germany in the spring of 2004.

tremor in his right hand. At the time he thought little of it, but he mentioned it in the course of the long and thorough medical history Dr. Keller recorded. Leon was surprised when this slight symptom seemed to be of great interest to the neurologist.

In the physical examination that followed, Dr. Keller was able to again elicit the tremor in his right hand. He carefully flexed each of Leon's joints in turn, and found that his right wrist resisted this gentle flexion. Finally, he turned to Leon and said the words that Leon was to remember forever:

"You will need to have more tests, but it appears that you may have Parkinson's disease."

"Parkinson's Disease?" It was an illness Leon had never heard of.

Eager to understand more about this illness, Leon rushed home and together he and Grette read the section of his health encyclopedia regarding Parkinson's disease, yet many of his questions remained unanswered. Unfortunately, he did not have access to the Internet, nor the skill to glean information from it.

With the hope of learning more, Leon purchased several books and borrowed others from his neurologist. He felt terrified as he read about the potentially devastating course of the disease and the possible outcomes. He read that Parkinson's was a chronic, progressive, degenerative disease that occurs when cells in a certain part of the brain die, resulting in reduced production of a substance called dopamine. He was appalled to learn that 80% of these cells usually die before symptoms are noticed.

Leon's concerns centered mostly on the welfare of his family in the event that he become too ill to provide for them. He owned a driving school and realized that his deteriorating motor skills might soon make it impossible for him to continue to drive and teach his students. His fears were at times overwhelming, but this did not deter him from seeking treatment. He continued to see his neurologist and was promptly started on a drug regimen for Parkinson's disease.

Disease Progression

Even with progressively increasing doses of these medications, Leon's symptoms gradually became more prominent over the next several years.

He considered his worsening tremor and difficulty moving his right arm particularly worrisome and he feared that if his clients noted these changes he might not be able to continue his livelihood as a driving instructor.

In 1996, he met with Dr. Meyer, his primary care doctor, to discuss his disease progression. Together, they decided that he would attend a specialized rehabilitation program in picturesque *Schwarzwald* (the Black Forest). For four weeks, he participated in daily activities including exercise, massage, and psychiatric treatment at Parkinson-Klinik Wolfach. Aside from paying a small supplement for the cost of his meals, his stay at the Parkinson's Klinik was fully covered by the German social insurance system. When he finally departed, he felt much better and his symptoms had regressed to the level they were a year or two before. He was now more knowledgeable about Parkinson's disease and felt increasingly confident upon returning to work. However, over the next several months his health began to worsen again.

A New Hope

In 1999, Grette saw a television special featuring a relatively new treatment for Parkinson's disease, called *tiefenhirn* stimulation or deep brain stimulation. She taped the program and when Leon came home, he and Grette eagerly watched it several times. Although he was still working full-time, he was very concerned about his symptoms, and although this procedure sounded risky and frightening, he thought it might hold some hope for him. He scheduled an appointment to discuss the procedure with Dr. Keller, the neurologist who had been guiding his treatment for almost a decade. To Leon's dismay, after a few minutes discussion, Dr. Keller stated that he thought that undergoing the treatment at this time was "nonsense." He argued that Leon's disease had not progressed sufficiently to warrant this risky operation for which there was little supporting data.

Although he was disappointed at this reaction, Leon decided to seek a second opinion. He traveled two hours to Munich, where he met with Dr. Lehmann, a neurologist at the Klinikum Grosshadern, a leading academic medical center. During an hour-long *poliklinik* (outpatient clinic) visit, the neurologist evaluated Leon and concluded that, in his opinion, he would be a good candidate for *tiefenhirn* stimulation. He then carefully explained the operation in detail, including the potential risks and benefits.

One to two weeks before the surgery, Leon would stop taking his medications for 12 hours and undergo tests to determine the severity of his Parkinsonism when he is off medication. He would also be given psychological tests to establish a baseline of his present cognitive and psychological functioning and whether he can withstand the psychological stress of the operation, which requires that he be conscious and lie perfectly still for many hours. Wire probes would be inserted deep into the subthalamic nucleus of his brain and Leon would need to be able to answer questions by the surgeons to determine the best placement of the probes during the operation. There was no guarantee that Leon's symptoms would improve, although the operation had been having substantial success. On the other hand, his memory and thinking could become somewhat worse.

Leon felt that adequate time was taken to answer all of his questions during this initial visit and he and Grette discussed everything the doctors told them. Before moving forward with the procedure, Leon returned to the neurology *poliklinik* for two more visits. He also met once with Dr. Becker, the neurosurgeon who would perform the procedure. Finally, under the guidance of the specialists in Munich, Leon agreed to undergo the operation in December 2000, ten years after he was first diagnosed with Parkinson's disease.

Dr. Meyer, Leon's PCP, however, was not aware of this decision, and in fact did not even know that Leon was considering the procedure until he scheduled an office visit to obtain pre-operative health information requested by the doctors at Klinikum Grosshadern. This was not particularly unusual because in Germany the world of outpatient, or primary care medicine and that of specialists and hospital-based medicine is clearly separated. When Leon informed Dr. Meyer that he was scheduled for surgery in Munich, the doctor was surprised but supported Leon in his decision and agreed that it would be prudent to undergo the procedure.

In the weeks prior to surgery, Leon continued to worry about the welfare of his family, but was comforted by his faith in the doctors. When asked, he said that he had no financial concerns regarding payment for this costly procedure and had no idea how much his care would cost, as it was fully covered by his insurance plan. (In the US, this operation cost between $50,000 and $75,000 in 2004). Leon has been a member of *Barmer*, a national *Krankenkasse* since he began working at age fifteen. He states, "They cover everything."

Indeed, his insurance so far has covered almost all of the cost of his extensive medical care, including his office visits to his PCP, visits to the specialists at the Klinikum Grosshadern, medications, transportation to and from medical care (with limits), and his pre-operative work-up. It also paid for his four-week rehabilitation program in the *Schwarzwald* and it will pay for the expensive *tiefenhirn* stimulation surgery.

While his *Krankenkasse* has provided broad coverage, there are a few small costs not covered by the sickness fund. All *Krankenkasse* members are required to pay a small co-payment, or "day-fare," of about €10 (~$11.40) for each day of hospital admission. Fortunately, since age fifteen, Leon has participated in a supplemental "day-fare" insurance fund through Continentale, a private German insurance company, for which he pays €8.90 (~$10.15) per month. All "day-fare" payments are covered for members of this plan.

As the date for his surgery approaches, Leon can see that the tremor and other motor symptoms of his disease are getting worse and his medications seem to be having less effect. Although he knows that it is not a cure for his Parkinson's disease, he is satisfied that he has made the right choice to go ahead with the surgery.

Leon reports to the hospital early the next morning, ready for the long day of surgery. The plan is to implant electrodes in each side of his brain, but if the surgeons encounter difficulties, or the patient is too tired, they may defer the second side until tomorrow. Leon hopes that it will all be completed in one day. His head is first placed in a frame that is bolted to his skull with special screws to ensure that his head does not move during the delicate surgery. Two coin-sized holes are drilled in his skull and a huge arched contraption is moved over his head. It will help to drive the electrodes millimeter by millimeter into his brain while the physicians work to guide them to the best location. They will need Leon's active participation to move an arm or a leg and answer questions when asked. Local anesthetics are used for the preliminary procedures, but the brain does not have pain receptors, so needs no anesthetic.

The hardest part of the surgery for Leon is lying with his head so absolutely still for so long and with very little movement of the rest of his body. He can see how this is the most trying part of the operation for the patient. A kindly nurse who gently rubs his feet is his greatest comfort.

Leon and his family are happy when the operation is finally completed without complications. One week later, under general anesthesia, two pulse generators are implanted under the skin below his collarbone on either side of his chest and wires threaded under the skin of his scalp and neck to connect to the electrodes in his brain. He is discharged home the next day.

During the following year, Leon felt better than he had in years and his symptoms were less prominent. But by 2001, his situation began to worsen. Since then, he has continued to be hospitalized at least once per year for adjustment of medications and stimulation parameters and replacement of the pulse generator batteries every two to four years. However, there is little that doctors have been able to do to arrest the progression of his illness. Over the past three years, Leon has been forced to reduce his work hours from a weekly average of fifty to about seven. For the past three months, he has been unable to work directly with clients, although he does continue to perform managerial office work. Leon has had to hire employees to do tasks he once completed on his own, so his business has become less profitable. Grette has started working to cover the family's expenses, and he hopes to sell his business sometime this year.

Moving Forward

Leon continues to see the neurologist in Munich every three months. He does not always get to see the same doctor but during these visits the neurologist reviews the history of his disease and treatment and performs a brief physical examination. He modifies his medication regimen if needed and checks that the batteries of his pulse generators are working well. Leon mentions that attending these quarterly office visits is now mandated by his *Krankenkasse* (sickness fund) as a condition for their continued coverage of the cost of his medications.

Through all of his struggles, funding for his health care has never been a concern. Since January 2004, Leon, like all Germans, has had to submit a co-payment of €10 during any quarter in which he attends one or more appointments with his PCP or a specialist. However, he is awaiting legislation that may exempt chronically ill patients from this expenditure.

While Leon is upset that his worsening health will necessitate the sale of his driving instruction business, he remains optimistic about the future. He plans to return to Parkinson-Klinik Wolfach later this year, soon after the sale of his business is completed although he has not yet informed Dr. Meyer of these plans. He will likely stay for about three weeks, completing a course of physical therapy, psychotherapy and speech therapy similar to his experience at the center in 1996. He hopes that this visit will be as beneficial as the prior one. Although his health condition has significantly worsened since 1996, he remains as active as possible. He continues to jog and swim, and while he has had to give up downhill skiing he is able to continue cross-country skiing. He knows the worst is yet to come, but he is confident that the nation's health care system will meet his needs.

Case 15: A Ray of Hope*

S. Elissa Altin

Herr von Walther sits pleasantly on a couch in the day room where we chat. His hair is thinning but not so much that he cannot coax it into a sort of genteel mohawk. He is wearing slacks and loafers and a pastel rugby shirt with the collar impishly upturned. He is a 41-year-old man currently in the fourth month of his seventh hospitalization for schizophrenia. His English is far better than my German; he learned it in school over twenty-five years ago. When I ask him to tell me about his experiences with his disease and in the hospital, he offers this assessment, "It's terrible."

Things were not always terrible for Herr von Walther. As a child, he reports a happy youth when he played soccer, visited his grandparents, and enjoyed a loving family with his parents, brother, and sister. His father worked as a lawyer for the German equivalent of the CIA, called the *Bundesnachrichtendienst* or BND, while his mother was an anesthesiologist in a local hospital. He comes from a well-off, well-respected family, which has been infinitely supportive of him throughout his illness.

I asked Herr von Walther when things started to go awry for him.

---

*This case was written by S. Elissa Altin when she was a student at Harvard Medical School and participated in the US-EU-MEE student exchange at Ludwig Maximilians University in Munich, Germany in the spring of 2005.

"It was at the start of puberty, when I was about 14," he replied. "I began to have problems with girls. I couldn't even get on a bus when there were girls around without getting red in the face."

"Was that your only problem at that time?" I asked.

"No. It was around this time that I started using marijuana and having problems in school. I smoked at least once each week and sometimes several times a week. Eventually I failed out of the *Gymnasium* track at grade 11. My problems with girls had not improved either and I began to withdraw socially."

"Did your education end at that time?"

"No. After I left the *Gymnasium* I enrolled in a three-year agricultural trade program where I studied farming. I graduated at age 22. All this time I continued using marijuana regularly and my social problems continued to get worse."

"What did you do then?"

"With my agriculture degree in hand, I found only odd jobs or was unemployed for the next two years. In 1986 I left for a three-month trip to Goa, India, mostly to smoke pot. During this time I also tried LSD for the third time."

"How was that?"

"It was a horrible, frightening experience. I vowed never to do it again, and I haven't. But after I came back home I found it harder and harder to function. I began to experience strange thoughts and hear strange sounds. It was terrible and scary. I don't even like to think about it."

This marked the beginning of Herr von Walther's long experience within the German mental health care system. Because he is from a well-to-do family, his care was covered under private insurance so his story was somewhat different from many others.

First Hospitalization

After returning from his trip to India, he began to see a psychotherapist for these paranoid and hallucinatory symptoms and was treated with Orap (pimozide), a typical antipsychotic used at that time in Germany and the US mostly for suppression of motor and phonic tics in patients with Tourette's syndrome but with off-label usage for psychosis. Despite this treatment, the symptoms worsened, and all Herr von Walther can remember is a haze of time when days ran together in the fog of his cloudy mind.

From March to June 1987, he was hospitalized at the Max-Planck Institute in Munich with delusions, hallucinations, disorganization, and paranoia. He was diagnosed with schizophrenia, paranoid type. The DSM-IV criteria for this diagnosis includes many of the symptoms and social dysfunction that Herr von Walther exhibited. During this hospitalization, his psychosis improved without further auditory hallucinations or delusional thoughts, and he was discharged on Haldol (haloperidol), an antipsychotic, Tegretol (carbamazepine), an anticonvulsant that can be used for refractory schizophrenia, and Fluanxol Depot (flupentixol), and long-acting antipsychotic.

In and Out of the Hospital

Over the next few years, Herr von Walther was maintained on these medications as an outpatient, although more psychiatric symptoms became evident. Clozapine, 150 mg per day, was added to his medications, but he continued to decompensate and from January 1991 to September 1994, he spent a staggering 41 months as an inpatient. He was first hospitalized from January to April of 1991 because he became psychotically hostile to his father. His medications were increased and he was stabilized and cautiously managed as an outpatient for four months at a nearby day clinic. But then he became so overwhelmed and psychotic that he was hospitalized again, this time in the *Ludwig-Maximilians Universität* (LMU) psychiatric inpatient ward from July to November 1991.

At LMU, several of Herr von Walther's medications were titrated up to the maximum and several more were added. Despite these hefty doses, his symptoms remained refractory to treatment. Eventually his medications were changed to clozapine 550 mg and Haldol 30 mg, at which point he was discharged to a day clinic. This lasted only three months and he returned to the Ludwig-Maximilians ward from February to September of 1992. During this seven-month hospitalization, many medication combinations were tried, even a Haldol dose up to 70 mg daily, which either did not help the psychosis or induced akathesia, an inability to sit still.

Finally, because of the lack of success with medical treatment, Herr von Walther's doctors decided to try electroconvulsive therapy (ECT). He eventually received 12 unipolar ECT treatments, which resulted in slight improvement that unfortunately did not last. This was not too surprising since there is no evidence that ECT is a viable long-term treatment for schizophrenia although some patients, especially those like Herr von Walther whose disease is not helped by standard treatment, do find short-term improvement. In addition to ECT, more medication combinations were tried, with higher doses of Haldol and clozapine, as well as clomipramine, a tricyclic antidepressant.

I asked Herr von Walther how he felt at this point.

"This hospitalization was particularly disheartening and difficult for me, and I think for my doctors, too," he recalls. "I don't remember many details, but I only thought I would never get better."

On his chart I noticed a half-hearted suicide attempt where Herr von Walther drank a bottle of shampoo and opened the window without attempting to jump out. Since he did not mention it, I didn't want to ask him about it. Clearly, his long illness and psychosis were taking a toll on him at that time but after this there was a small ray of hope. His medication was switched to an altogether different drug to which he showed some improvement. He was eventually discharged in September of 1992 to the Ludwig-Maximilians day clinic.

This improvement was brief, and within one month at the day clinic Herr von Walther became overwhelmed and acted aggressively, gaining re-admission to the Ludwig-Maximilian psychiatric ward for another seven months from October 1992 to April 1993. He responded again to a change in medications and was discharged to *Herzogsägmühle*, a therapeutic community of nearly 1700 people organized by the Protestant church. Residents here are varied, including the homeless, drug addicts, elderly, people in debt, and the mentally handicapped, in addition to psychiatric patients. This was intended to be a transitional placement for Herr von Walther until he could function in normal society. Within less than a month, though, he decompensated and became psychotic and aggressive again. For the sixth time, he was hospitalized at the Ludwig-Maximilians hospital from May to September 1993. During this hospitalization, a variety of medication regimes were tried and eventually one was found that helped him.

Transfer

At discharge, he was transferred to a nearby psychiatric hospital serving the western greater Munich area. This hospital, built in the early 1900s, is a large municipal psychiatric, psychotherapeutic, and neurology hospital complex with over 1200 beds on a large campus. Its wards are organized into about 130 individual house-like buildings. Unlike the university hospital of LMU, which can pick and choose patients because of its status as a teaching hospital, this is a public hospital that almost necessarily has to admit patients refused by other local psychiatric units. The admitting office accepts anywhere from 10–60 patients each day, and on average they remain about 4–6 weeks in the hospital.

What is immediately striking about the wards at this large hospital as compared to the LMU hospital is how many patients are in each room — up to six or seven, depending on how crowded the hospital is at the time. Also, the ward seems somehow slightly more dilapidated than the well-kept, newly designed university hospital. Despite these problems, this hospital provides amazing service to the Munich community. Any person who needs acute psychiatric hospitalization can get it. They do not need to be actively suicidal or psychotic to be admitted. A day in this hospital costs a private patient around €250, similar in price to LMU. Herr von Walther remained there for a year on the vocational rehabilitation ward, moving from a locked ward to an open ward once the neuroleptics began to help him.

"How was your experience at the large public hospital?" I asked.

"This was my worst hospital experience so far. The hospital was overcrowded and full of "crazy" patients. My own delusions were not under good control. I think some of the nurses physically abused patients."

"Did this ever happen to you?"

"No, but I heard screaming in the ward at night. I did get sick there once, though, and was sent to the neurologic intensive care unit."

"What happened?"

"I'm not sure, but I became very thirsty and drank a lot of water and had a convulsion."

According to Herr von Walther's medical records, he "presented with polydipsia leading to hyponatremic status epilepticus and was treated in the neurologic intensive care unit." After his return to the ward, he made slow improvement and was discharged in September 1994 on daily doses of lorazepam 6 mg, Risperdal 6mg, pipamperone (an antipsychotic) 30 mg, and clomipramine 125 mg. By December of that year, he was readmitted for a brief period because he was not taking his medications regularly, but for the next 10 years, he showed steady improvement with only outpatient management.

Payment for Herr von Walther's Care

Because Herr von Walther's parents are among those who earn more than €3,900 a month ($5,185) or €46,800 a year ($62,220) they are eligible to opt out of the German public health insurance system and purchase private insurance. (These are the figures for 2005. This income level is set anew every year). This makes sense for people earning a higher income because the amount they are required to pay into the public insurance system (approximately 14% of income) becomes quite expensive at higher income levels. Fully 10% of Germans are privately insured.

With private insurance Herr von Walther's parents have free choice of physician and hospital, the guarantee of a one- or two-bed room in the hospital, and treatment by the most senior attending physicians on service. Some disadvantages include paying premiums based on existing medical conditions rather than by flat rate, having to pay premiums even after retirement, having to insure each member of the family separately with additional premiums, and difficulty, if not impossibility of opting back into the public health insurance later.

Herr von Walther has not had a job since his diagnosis with schizophrenia. Because of this, his father can continue to carry him on his insurance plan. They are insured with *Allianz Versicherung*, one of about 50 private insurance companies in Germany, which costs Herr von Walther's father €1000 a month, or €330 each for himself, his wife, and his son. This covers all inpatient and outpatient care, all of his son's lengthy hospitalizations, all medications (which add up to €500 per month), ambulance or taxi rides to the hospital, and all except a small portion of the cost of dental care and eyeglasses.

At discharge from the hospital, the patient with private insurance receives a bill from the hospital itemizing all costs and services.

The patient then pays out-of-pocket to the hospital and files to *Allianz* for reimbursement of the entire amount. A similar process occurs for prescription payments and outpatient treatments. First the patient pays the health care providers directly, and then submits the bill for full insurance reimbursement. Physicians and hospitals like to have privately insured patients because they can bill up to two or three times the amount they bill the public insurance companies, owing to special services like private hospital rooms and treatment by the senior physician.

For psychiatric care, *Allianz* offers nearly full coverage for in- and outpatient treatment. For the acute hospital admission, the hospital does not need prior authorization to admit a patient, and only after a reasonable length of stay (usually around one month, depending on the admitting diagnosis) does the insurance company require a physician's report justifying the length of stay and treatment, which is then reviewed by an independent physician review board. Usually, the insurance company will approve further treatments when medically necessary, as some psychiatric patients can spend months as inpatients. In Herr von Walther's case, he has been hospitalized up to one year at a time, which his insurance paid for in full.

The second level of psychiatric care is for placement of sub-acute patients in day clinics, group home rehabilitation settings, psychotherapeutic rehabilitation clinics, and other similar settings. In this case, insurance pre-authorization is necessary, and usually granted given the referring physician's judgment of medical necessity. Often, insurance companies gladly pay for these treatments because they are significantly cheaper than a hospital stay (€150–200 per day versus more than €500 per day for privately insured inpatient treatment). Herr von Walther was frequently cared for in such day clinic settings when he was discharged from the hospital, which his insurance always approved.

There is a third level of rehabilitation clinic that is distinctly German offering a mix of allopathic and homeopathic therapies. Called the *Kur*, these treatments combine therapeutic bathing and environmental stimuli with allopathic treatments and represent the more pluralistic approach to medicine in Germany than in the United States. In many cases, the private insurance companies will not pay for these treatments because their medical necessity is questionable.

Finally, outpatient psychiatric appointments for psychopharmacology as well as psychotherapy are completely covered by *Allianz* if they are medically necessary. For a patient with schizophrenia like Herr von Walther, it is not difficult to prove this need and he has virtually unlimited access to outpatient treatment without paying for it himself. There exists a grey area for approval of long-term life crisis. In this case, health care providers must obtain pre-approval from the insurance company, which they may or may not grant based on the presumed medical necessity.

For private patients, reimbursement is more generous, and often it is these patients who subsidize the treatment of the public patients in a practice. The psychiatrist can charge up to double the public insurance rate to the private patients and restrictions about number of sessions are significantly more lenient, as we have seen in the case of Herr von Walther. In either case it is relatively easy to obtain initial treatment authorization, but continuation beyond a certain point is harder with public than private patients. With public insurance patients, most *Krankenkassen* will endorse 30 hour-long psychotherapy treatment sessions. Greater than 30 sessions are harder to obtain, unless the patient continues to be acutely in need of services. Authorization for psychoanalysis is also very hard to obtain. Only a small minority of patients pay out of pocket for psychotherapy, as compared to practices in the United States.

Back to Herr von Walther

After his discharge from the large municipal hospital, and after struggling for seven years with his disease, Herr von Walther was finally able to live at home with outpatient follow-up. The length of his hospitalizations during those seven years is astounding by American standards, but with such refractory disease, it seems that he had few other options. Once settled at home, he lived in a small garden house on his parents' property where he enjoyed taking walks and making pottery. He is such a prolific potter that his small house overflows with vases, bowls, and plates that he created at his potter's wheel and painted in his studio.

Herr von Walther was treated during this time by a psychiatrist, Dr. Zander, whom he has seen for one hour a week for the past 11 years. They have an intense and trusting relationship with one another. Herr von

Walther feels comfortable and safe telling his doctor what he is feeling and as a result his physician knows him extremely well. As for the costs of Herr von Walther's weekly sessions, Dr. Zander charges *Allianz* up to a maximum of €200 per hour-long session. With both private and public patients, he must obtain pre-approval before starting psychotherapy treatments. Dr. Zander admits that he has been surprised over the past eleven years how freely *Allianz* has paid for these weekly treatments but hypothesizes that the money was well spent because it kept Herr von Walther out of the hospital for so many years.

During this time his schizophrenia remained relatively well controlled with improved, newer generation medications, but anxiety and obsessive-compulsiveness became his major issues. He was managed for a time on Zyprexa (olanzapine) a newer antipsychotic, which worked very well until he unfortunately developed diabetes mellitus from it and he was switched to metformin. He was also switched to various other agents including quietapine, benperidol, clozapine in combination with Fluanxol (flupenthixol), and others but none worked well to stabilize his anxiety. This led to two short hospitalizations in August 2004 in a local Munich area hospital in Gauting. This was the first time he began to complain of visual hallucination of colors. He describes these colors as on his body and all around him, that they torture him, even with his eyes closed, and they make him occasionally feel physical pain.

Hospitalization February 2005–June 2005

"How has life been for you this year?" I asked when we met in early June 2005.

"It was really pretty good for awhile," he replies. "I was happy to be at home and to have my pottery to keep me occupied. My father and I enjoyed long walks. But here I am, hospitalized again."

"What happened?"

"Starting in February, I noticed more and more psychotic thoughts. The colors were torturing me and I was becoming more and more anxious. Thoughts were put into my mind that I was the devil and the lowest human being on earth."

"Were these voices that you heard?"

"No, they were just thoughts that I couldn't get rid of. I never heard actual voices but I can tell the difference between 'normal' and 'psychotic' thoughts. Besides, I became intensely afraid of corners. Because of this, I couldn't take walks alone because when I came to a corner, I was struck with such incredible paralyzing fear that I couldn't go on."

I read in Herr von Walther's chart that in the weeks preceding his latest hospitalization, he would not leave his house unless his father was with him. When he walked with his father, his fears were less, but still present. The combination of the delusions, color hallucinations, and inability to function because of his anxiety compelled his psychiatrist to refer him to Ludwig-Maximilians hospital for electroconvulsive therapy (ECT) in February 2005. Interestingly, Herr von Walther is the first schizophrenic patient in 15 years to be referred by his psychiatrist for ECT because the newer medications are generally so much more effective than before.

For four months, Herr von Walther again remained refractory to many drug treatments but finally was tapered off his admission meds and maintained on a simpler regimen of clozapine and Fluanxol. Despite his psychiatrist's preference that he be treated with ECT, it was three months into his hospitalization before these were started. The explanation for this delay is that German physicians are hesitant to use ECT as there is a negative perception of the treatment as violent. Herr von Walther's psychiatrist explains that this has to do with the history of how the mentally ill were abused during the Nazi regime. Both lay people and physicians have a poor impression of these therapies and they conjure up memories of the violent handling of many patients during those war years. Of the many psychiatric hospitals in the greater Munich area, only the clinic at the LMU actually performs ECT.

Finally, in May Herr von Walther started treatment with 12 rounds of bipolar ECT, to which he showed reasonable improvement. His psychosis decreased and he became less anxious and was able to function in an outpatient setting. According to Herr von Walther, his experiences at the LMU hospital have been the easiest for him as a patient. He finds the care good, enjoys its central location to town, and appreciates the relatively small-sized wards with fewer patients. He believes that by getting treatment from the most senior attending (*Chefartzt*), whom he sees weekly for about 20 minutes, that he is receiving excellent care and is generally pleased with his experience in the German health care system. He notes that it is much easier to sleep in a private room than in a conventional patient suite, where five or six patients may stay, indicating this as a real advantage of private insurance.

Herr von Walther represents at once the best and worst case patient scenarios. He is lucky to come from a family with the means and desire to support him fully. His father has visited him each day during his numerous long hospitalizations; his mother, an anesthesiologist, is savvy about navigating the healthcare system, helps him fill his prescriptions, and reminds him to take his medications. Their health insurance is generous and makes it easy to access necessary care, plus they are able to provide their son with housing of his own on their property. He can live independently there while being close to his family for regular daily support. Additionally, with his own pottery studio, he has access to productive daily activities. The worst part of Herr von Walther's story is that his disease has been so difficult to manage and resistant to treatment.

Despite all his setbacks, Herr von Walther retains his faith in the medical system and believes that ultimately treatments will help him. Interestingly, he maintains a "doctor-knows-best" attitude, which is apparently more common in Germany than in the United States. To a certain extent, patients in the US have become consumers of health care, partially motivated by increased access to medical information via the Internet, partially because of increased direct marketing of pharmaceuticals to consumers, and also because patients have to act as their own advocates in the sometimes difficult-to-navigate health and insurance system.

For private patients in Germany there is great availability of quality care with special treatment by senior attendings and small patient rooms. For public patients, though, there is similar access to high quality care. Although some private patients stay in separate wards, essentially all patients, private and public, are treated in the same hospitals, by the same medical, nursing, and support staff. It must be stated that although treatment between public and private psychiatric patients is generally equivalent in teaching hospitals such as the LMU, in large municipal hospitals there are some discrepancies. Notably, public patients in these hospitals generally only see a physician once every few weeks, and the majority of their interactions are with the nursing staff. In contrast, private patients in municipal hospitals have greater access to physicians and see the senior attending more frequently.

Home Again

After the successful ECT treatment at LMU, Herr von Walther was discharged on June 10 and returned to his little house on his parents' property. He will have regular follow-up at the LMU day clinic. Inpatient stays in Germany are often lengthened by the limited communication between their inpatient and outpatient physicians. Upon discharge the hospital sends a letter describing treatment and progress, but sometimes this letter takes a few weeks to reach the psychiatrist and outpatient appointments may already be scheduled before the information reaches the doctor. In this case, the outpatient provider has to rely on patient accounts until information from the hospital arrives. This is not a problem for Herr von Walther. Because Dr. Zander completed his psychatric training at LMU he knows many of the hospital physicians and maintains good communication with them about his patients' hospital treatment.

At our last meeting, Herr von Walther said, "I told you my illness was 'terrible,' but I want you to know that it has not kept me from having joy and meaning in life during times when my disease has been under control. It is the hope of getting better that keeps me going."

Case 16: Herr Oscher and German Social Solidarity*

Alden Vincent Chiu

Before I went to see Rudolph Oscher in the Klinikum Innenstadt (central city hospital) in Munich on a fine April morning, I had been given a little information about him. He had a remarkable past that included at least three careers, three marriages, and severe pulmonary disease. He was admitted to the hospital from St. Joseph's nursing home where he had been a resident since February. It was a story not unlike those commonly heard in US emergency departments.

A quick look at Herr Oscher's chart told me that his primary diagnosis was chronic obstructive pulmonary disease (COPD) but he was in the hospital recuperating from deep vein thrombosis (DVT) and pulmonary embolism. Obviously, he had recently been a very sick man. His most recent pulmonary function test revealed a forced expiratory volume in one second (FEV_1) of 0.45L, only 16% of expected. This, I knew, indicated a poor prognosis with studies showing the five-year survival rate to be around 11%.

When I met Herr Oscher, however, I was surprised to find him smiling and cheerful in spite of a nasal cannula delivering a steady two liters of

*The story of this patient is based on a case written by Alden Vincent Chiu when he was a student at Harvard Medical School and participated in the US-EU-MEE student exchange at Ludwig-Maximilians University in Munich, Germany in April and May 2005.

oxygen. He motioned me to a chair beside his bed. "So you are the medical student from the United States who has come to learn about the German health care system?" he said, his inflection indicating more of a question than a statement.

I was thankful that I had made several local German friends and could understand his Bavarian accent. In my best medical student manner I said, "Tell me what brings you to the hospital."

"Perhaps I should start at the beginning," he replied. "I was born in 1939, so that makes me 66 years old. After the war, I was able to get training as a *Schweißen*, or welder. I worked at that occupation for 18 years, until I was 36 years old. During that time I was married and we had a son. When he was about ten years old, we divorced and I moved to Obrigheim and started a new career working in a nuclear power plant, specializing in heating systems and pipelines."

"How was your health during that time?" I asked.

"Oh, I was young and it was fairly good. I started to smoke at age 13, so of course I did have some coughing and caught colds easily. Eventually I smoked one and a half packs a day, and only quit three years ago. While I worked at the nuclear power plant, I began to complain of night sweats and my supervisor sent me for an X-ray. In 1980 I was diagnosed with tuberculosis and took the recommended antibiotics for about two years."

"How were your medical expenses taken care of?"

"I have been a member of Bavaria's regional sickness fund, *Allgemeine Ortskrankenkassen* (AOK) my whole life. It has covered the expenses for all my inpatient and outpatient medical care. Throughout my working life I have paid about 14% of my income to AOK to provide this care. In addition, I pay €100 per year (about $130 in 2005) to purchase supplemental insurance from AOK that covers all my medications without co-payment. I have been very fortunate to have this insurance because after I was diagnosed with tuberculosis, I continued to have pneumonia frequently. Each time I was prescribed antibiotics and I recovered without any serious complications."

Herr Oscher paused to catch his breath. I could tell that talking was tiring him but he seemed eager to continue.

"Did I tell you I was married again in 1975 and I have a daughter, Christina, who is now 26 years old? She works here in Munich as a hairdresser, but unfortunately, I do not see her very often. She is very busy and I don't want to trouble her. Her mother and I divorced in 1984."

I wanted to ask Herr Oscher more about his experience with Germany's social welfare system but he had more medical and social history to tell me.

"I married once again in 1985–for the last time," he laughed, "and my son, Matthias, was born in 1986. I worked at the nuclear power plant until 1993 and then decided to take an entirely different direction in my life. By this time I was coughing a lot and I was often very tired. I thought the work in the nuclear power plant was too strenuous and I went to work in a nursing home. Around this time my *Hausartz* suggested that I see a pulmonary specialist. He ordered a lot of tests and diagnosed me with COPD."

"Were you able to see a pulmonologist of your own choosing?" I asked.

"Oh yes. I have always had the freedom to choose my own doctors and I have always had excellent care. I don't have any complaints about the German health care system. I am sure my smoking has caused a lot of my respiratory problems. By the time I quit, I had a 75-pack-year smoking history."

Remembering to ask about family history, I asked Herr Oscher if he had any brothers and sisters.

"You may be surprised to know that I have a twin brother. I also have an older sister and brother, and of course, my son who is now 40 years old. I really don't have much to say about them. I have drifted away from all of them, including my three wives. Matthias's mother and I were divorced when he was 10 years old and I rarely see or hear from her. I am lucky to still have contact with Christina and Matthias. He is now 19 years old and is an apprentice in training to be *Gebäudereiniger,* a house cleaner. Neither he nor Christina makes much money, so I am fortunate that I have not had to depend on them for help."

"Was the job in the nursing home your last job?"

"No. I worked there for five years, but I was always interested in cooking, and finally got a job as a cook in a small bistro and worked there from 1998 until 2000. Unfortunately, by 2000 my COPD had gotten so bad that it was difficult to keep on working. I was on many medicines, including heavy corticosteroids, all of it completely paid for, thanks to my supplemental insurance with AOK."

"I understand you have recently been living at St. Joseph's nursing home."

"Yes. Probably because of the steroids, I now have osteoporosis and I had a painful fracture of a vertebra in my back. I finally had to listen to Christina and Matthias who had been urging me to retire. I have been on constant home oxygen for five years now. With the oxygen, while I still lived in my own apartment, I was able to walk outside and sit in the sunlight. Without oxygen, I can walk only three or four meters until I have to stop and rest."

"How do you like living at St. Joseph's?"

"After living independently for so many years, it was hard to admit that I could no longer take care of myself. Christina and Matthias urged me to go to St. Joseph's and I really like it very much. At St. Joseph's I have time to enjoy painting, something I have not done since I was a child. And I enjoy visiting with my fellow St. Joseph's residents, most of whom are female."

"How does the German social welfare system cover your expenses?"

"Of course AOK continues to pay for my health care. My illness and physical limitations qualify me for the highest level of coverage under *Soziale Pflegeversicherung,* the statutory long-term care insurance program. This enables me to live at St. Joseph's with no out-of-pocket expenses. In addition, my retirement pension from the government provides a little spending money each month. It is fortunate that Germany has such a comprehensive social welfare system because I have few other options. It is just bad luck that I had to get this DVT and pulmonary embolism. As soon as they have my anticoagulation medicine adjusted, I'll be out of here and back at St. Joseph's. I have every expectation of living out the rest of my life with adequate health care services and personal support."

I thought of how Herr Oscher's story, with his history of broken relationships and serious disease, might have been different if he did not have the strong social welfare support network Germany has built up to help people in his situation. The challenge will be to maintain the system in the face of increasing costs, an aging population, a smaller workforce, and a slower economy. The continuation of Germany's health care system and social welfare state will depend on the willingness and determination of the people to solve these problems.

Case 17: The Amalgam Question*

Anna Ratiner

Michael Benz is a 38-year-old unmarried West German man who currently lives in Munich. He was born in the small city of Straubing in south-central Bavaria, and came to live in Munich in 1991, when he was 26 years old. Currently he works as a professor in photo-design at the University of Applied Sciences in Munich.

One Saturday morning in 1998 he was leisurely reading the morning paper, *Deutsche Welle,* when a small advertisement caught his eye:

> Research subjects wanted for study of amalgam dental fillings. Will receive free dental care at Ludwig Maximilians University School of Dental Medicine. Call +49 89 1234 4321.

It was the mention of amalgam fillings that drew Michael's attention. Off and on he had read in the paper that amalgam fillings were bad for one's health. Some of his friends at the University of Applied Sciences showed him articles in a newspaper about amalgam fillings. The articles stated that

---

*The story of this patient is based on a case written by Anna Ratiner in March 2003 when she was a student at the Harvard School of Dental Medicine and took part in the US-EU-MEE exchange at the Ludwig Maximilians School of Dental Medicine.

amalgam fillings were toxic to the body and were causing unspecific ill-nesses in many people. Michael was curious and concerned about this because, of course, he was one of millions of people with amalgam fillings in his mouth. They had been placed there after his permanent teeth erupted and he began to have dental caries at about the age of six or seven.

Michael had always been a believer in alternative medicine. When he came to Munich in 1991 he found a physician who practiced mostly homeopathic treatments along with allopathic medicine. This Dr. Grauerstein has been his primary physician or *"Hausartz"* for the past seven years. Michael once asked him what he thought about the theory that amalgam dental fillings could be harmful.

"It does make some sense," Dr. Grauerstein replied. "There is a high percentage of mercury, especially in older fillings. The ratio was 8:5 until 1959 when Dr. Wilmer Eames recommended a 1:1 ratio and this new for-mulation was adopted. Mercury has been known to be a biological toxin, particularly damaging to renal and neurological tissues. Look at how much publicity there is about avoiding mercury in fish! Chronic mercury poisoning by exposure to its vapor in a higher amount than is considered safe can indeed cause a multi-symptom disorder that presents as depres-sion, anxiety, tiredness, memory loss, tremor and a host of other non-specific symptoms."

"Do you think I should have my amalgam fillings removed?" Michael asked.

"You have had persistent feelings of weakness and fatigue as well as a low leukocyte count," Dr. Graustein replied. "It might be something you want to consider."

Michael thought this over and started to pay more attention to the media on the topic of amalgam fillings as well as to other articles in news-papers, books on homeopathic medicine, and magazines. All of these stated the same thing: that amalgam fillings are "bad for the body" and need to be removed. It seemed there was a worldwide debate on the matter.

Michael's Medical History

When Michael was a child, he and his parents noticed that he was prone to frequent infections, particularly tonsillitis. When he was about eight or nine years of age, his parents brought him to the town doctor to find the reason for these frequent infections and possibly a cure. The doctor did a number of blood tests, which revealed that Michael had a low white blood cell count. In fact, the number of leukocytes was found to be only one-third to one-quarter of the normal level. Other white blood cell levels were within normal limits, as Michael recalls. The physician told his parents at the time that such a low level of leukocytes was not too much of a concern and that nothing needed to be done. Therefore, Michael had received no treatment of any kind.

During his entire life as far back as he can remember in childhood, Michael has felt tired, weak and fatigued on a daily basis. These symptoms were not severe enough to interfere too much with his daily activities as he grew up, graduated from the *Gymnasium* and went to college. This problem was never addressed or treated by a physician but he discussed it several times with Dr. Grauerstein as he was treated for less serious illnesses, such as allergies, flu, and colds, usually with homeopathic medicines. The homeopathic remedies always seemed to work for him and he was satisfied to let it go at that. Otherwise he has no other health issues, or illnesses. At the moment he is not taking any medications or any recreational drugs. He also has no history of smoking or heavy alcohol consumption.

The Dental Connection

Seeing the newspaper advertisement for the amalgam filling study at Ludwig Maximilians University brought the matter to the forefront of Michael's mind again. At first he did not think about enrolling in the study mentioned in the advertisement, but decided that he would broach the subject with his own dentist. He called on Monday morning and made an appointment.

Michael has been seeing Dr. Schwartz, a private dentist who works in a group practice with two other general dentists and a pediatric dentist. When it comes to payment for dental or medical procedures, Michael has no problems because he has private insurance (DKV), which he acquired since he moved to Munich in 1991. His insurance is such that for dental treatments any fillings are covered completely; more complicated procedures such as crowns are covered 85%. For any medical problems or illnesses, most of the treatments and procedures as well as medications are covered nearly 100%. The only reason he has chosen to have private insurance is because it covers the alternative medicine physicians and treatments that he favors. Even if it should cost some out-of-pocket expenditure, he decided to ask Dr. Schwartz to replace his amalgam fillings with composite fillings.

When the day of his appointment came, Michael told Dr. Schwartz about his decision.

"Oh, I don't think you want to do that," said Dr. Schwartz. "Don't be persuaded by what you read in the newspapers and hear in the media about amalgam fillings. Amalgam has been successfully used as a restoration material for tooth decay for more than a century. It has been estimated that currently every year five hundred million amalgam restorations are done worldwide. This debate over the issue of toxicity of amalgams has triggered numerous studies done by dental schools or other dental organizations to answer the question of whether amalgam indeed poses a danger to people's health. In Germany and many other countries research about this topic still continues in search of answers. However, because of the difficulty in establishing parameters of measurements and cause and effect relationship, as well as the subjectivity of the results due to the patient personal beliefs, a clear-cut answer is very difficult to find."

"If you really want to have your amalgam fillings replaced," Dr. Schwartz continued, "you should have them replaced with gold. That is the best and most durable choice of material and is much superior to composite."

Michael told Dr. Schwartz that he would think it over, but privately he thought Dr. Schwartz was seeing "*geld*" dancing before his eyes in the form of higher payments. He was not sure his insurance would pay for gold fillings, and he thought that he might consider finding a new dentist.

The Ludwig Maximilians Study

When Michael arrived at work at the University of Applied Sciences his friend, Robert, came into his office waving the copy of *Deutsche Welle* that Michael had read over the weekend.

"Look! Here is a study going on about amalgam fillings at the Ludwig Maximilians University School of Dental Medicine. I know somebody who has enrolled as a subject and all of his amalgam fillings have been replaced free," Robert said excitedly. "Why don't you call this number and enroll?"

Michael had never considered taking part in a scientific study and was a little hesitant. "Did they replace the amalgam with composite?" he asked.

"Yes, they did." answered Robert. "Here's the phone. Give them a call."

"Hey, is somebody paying you money to recruit subjects for this study?" Michael asked.

"No, no! I just know you have been interested in having your amalgam fillings replaced. What did your dentist, Dr. Schwartz say about it?"

"He recommended that I have him replace them with gold."

"It figures. If you're not sure what to do, why don't you read some of the scientific articles that have been published by universities or medical or dental schools? I have read studies conducted in Germany, US, and other countries, most of which have shown that amalgam is not a source of toxicity to people. In a study published in 1995, for example, a German group of researchers developed a new technique to measure the amount of mercury vapors in the oral cavity and in the saliva, and they showed that the amount of mercury released from a tooth filling is far below toxic levels. Similar conclusions were reached in 1997 by researchers from the University of Göteborg. There are numerous other studies conducted all over the world that showed that amalgam does not seem to produce toxic effects in humans. Then there is the other side, particularly in the media and in people's personal beliefs and experiences that seem to indicate that amalgam fillings are harmful. You can look at both sides."

"I know, but I don't always trust the scientists. They will say that something is true or is not true but actually it is just because they have not done the right studies to prove it one way or the other. For example, most scientists reject homeopathic medicine completely and discount the positive experiences people have had with it for years. The absence of proof is not disproof. Most scientists do not believe that alternative medicine treatments have any value, yet many people have been helped by them."

"What do you say to the argument that removal of amalgam can cause even higher levels of mercury vapor to be released and greater toxicity than if the amalgam fillings had stayed in the mouth an entire lifetime?" asked Robert.

"I think it's not that harmful to temporarily have a higher level of mercury vapor released because then the cause of the toxicity will be permanently removed."

"Have you heard how the Ludwig Maximilians study got started?" Robert asked, and continued before Michael had a chance to respond. "About six years ago, 1100 people — patients from all over Germany filed a lawsuit claiming that amalgam fillings caused them numerous health problems. A public prosecutor became a representative of these people and has filed a lawsuit against the amalgam producing company, Degussa. The company, of course, claimed that these allegations were false. The prosecutor has ordered this company to contribute money to various institutions in Germany to conduct a study and answer some of the questions raised in the lawsuit. One of the studies is the one at *Poliklinik für Zahnerhaltung und Parodontologie* at LMU."

After Robert went back to his own office, Michael again pondered the idea of becoming a subject in the LMU study. After all, he did want his amalgam fillings removed, and he had great confidence in the quality of the work at the University because of their expertise and experience. And as a subject he would be aiding science. He picked up the phone and dialed the number for the study.

Aiding Science

Michael was accepted into the study and was promptly given an appointment to have his amalgam fillings removed. They were replaced with white composite, which he had to admit also improved his appearance. Over a period of a few weeks he has noticed that his feelings of fatigue and weakness have significantly decreased, however they have not gone away completely. He also believes that he is getting fewer colds and other minor infections than he did before. He knows there can be a strong placebo effect but he believes his leukocyte count has increased, even though he has not yet had a blood test. If this proves to be true, that will be concrete evidence and proof enough for him.

Case 18: A Life with DM*

Charles R. Wira III

In 1951, the year J.D. Salinger published *The Catcher in the Rye* and Charles Schultz's Peanuts comic strip was first published in US newspapers, a young West German boy in the town of Cham, Bavaria was diagnosed with Juvenile-Onset Diabetes Mellitus at the age of six. His name was Martin Fehling and he was the hoped-for son in a family with three older sisters. In this time period, the German and worldwide understanding of diabetes was developing, and management was experimental. There was no family history of Type I diabetes among young Martin's relatives prior to his diagnosis, although his maternal grandmother had Type II diabetes.

Cham is a small town of 10,000 people just 16 kilometers south of the Czech Republic border. In this rural region there was little knowledge about diabetes by local physicians in the 1950s, but the Fehling's family physician (*Hausartz*) recognized that the child was seriously ill. He arranged for Martin's parents to take him to Children's Hospital in Frankfurt for one month. There he was placed on an insulin regimen and his parents were taught how to administer the medication.

The family physician caring for Martin upon his return home from Frankfurt was typical of other generalist physicians in Germany at this time

---

*This case was written by Charles R. Wira III in 2000 when he was a student at Dartmouth Medical School and participated in the US-EU-MEE exchange program at Ludwig Maximilians University in Munich, Germany.

who had little knowledge about the management of diabetes. Consequently there was poor control of glucose levels and as a child, Martin experienced many periods of frequent urination and extreme thirst, which correlated with poor hyperglycemic management. His parents did the best they could to care for him but were constantly worried at these recurrent bouts of illness.

During this time period Germany was still recovering from shortages and deprivations following the end of World War II. The management of Martin's diabetes was hindered by a shortage in the national supply of oxen insulin in the entire country. Consequently, there were many occasions when the insulin was delivered late to pharmacies or delivered in deficient amounts. As a result, Martin never took more than four units of insulin per day as a child, nor did most other diabetic children in Germany at this time. This was still true when he suffered his first hyperglycemic coma at the age of nine.

Summer Camp

Martin's health continued to be precarious until the age of 14 when his family physician discovered a summer diabetes camp near the Swiss border established by the German Diabetes Association. It was founded by Dr. Herzig, the first physician in Germany to formally organize pediatric patient education about diabetes. Martin's parents were persuaded to allow him to attend the camp. There were three dozen other children participating in this program and for the first time, Martin did not feel like a freak among his peers. Afterwards, his insulin dose was increased to four units twice a day and he did not have so many episodes of illness.

Martin did well in school and received excellent marks. He had no restrictions other than exemption from his physical education class. At age 16, however, he began to have increasing symptoms of dizziness and drowsiness and couldn't follow his lessons. To the disappointment of his parents, he dropped out of school. He undertook a bank-teller apprenticeship and began formal work in a bank in less than a year.

Within four months of dropping out of school, monitoring of urine sugar levels became available. Martin attended another summer camp where he was taught to self-administer two units of insulin between doses if his urine glucose strip was positive. His self-management improved his health remarkably, however, his physician was skeptical about the additional insulin and stated explicitly to Martin's family that he could not be responsible for the administration of insulin between doses. He did concede to write the prescriptions, nevertheless and this was his only role in the management of Martin's illness. Later Martin said he believed his physician "had no understanding of the disease."

Career and Marriage

At the age of 22, Martin, now a successful assistant bank manager married Katrina, a girl he met at the summer diabetes camp when he was 16. Because of the diabetes mellitus in both of their histories, they thought they would probably not plan to have children. Still, they enjoyed their quiet life in Cham and recreation in the nearby Bavarian Alps.

I met Martin Fehling many years later, in 2000, when he became "my patient" to follow in the US-EU-MEE medical student exchange. He was 55 years old and was a regular patient in the Endocrine Department at Grosshadern Hospital in Munich. He spent a generous amount of time with me sharing the ups and downs of his medical history. It was apparent that both he and his wife had become quite educated over the years on the subject of diabetes mellitus.

Complications

"When did you first notice any complications of diabetes affecting your health?" I asked.

"It was in December 1979 when I was 34 years old," he replied. "I was working in the bank in Cham when I had a sudden onset of blurry vision in my right eye. I immediately saw a physician at the local hospital where they also discovered that I had extremely high blood pressure. They sent me to an ophthalmologist in Cham, but my vision became progressively worse and began to involve both eyes. They called Katrina and an ambulance took us to Munich two hours away. In Munich I had four laser therapy treatments and things quieted down for awhile."

"I went back to work at the bank but my eyes still gave me trouble," he continued," I developed a vitreal bleed in my right eye and in 1981 I had to have a vitrectomy to remove the vitreous gel in that eye because it had become clouded with blood. Glaucoma developed as a secondary complication and subsequently that eye had to be removed (enucleated). Over the next year there was progressive vision loss in my left eye to the point where I could only distinguish between light and darkness. So in 1982 at 37 years of age, I was declared legally blind and I would never be able to work again."

"That certainly was hard for you and Katrina," I sympathized.

"Katrina has been my mainstay through everything. Fortunately I was immediately put on disability and we were able to manage on the 80% of my salary the government pays. My primary insurance is Hamberg Manheimer, the same insurance that covered my family when I was a child. It covers everything imaginable. Since I am unemployed the payments to my sickness fund are split 50–50 between myself and my social security insurance."

"Are there any special support services because of your visual impairment?" I asked.

"Yes, services for the visually impaired are organized by the Federal government but provided by the states. Several states have had to drop these services because they ran out of money but that has not yet happened in the State of Bavaria. For example, they provided 60 hours of instruction in skills of day-to-day living and how to get around by myself by a teacher who commuted 200 km to Cham. They would have taught me to use a Seeing Eye dog, but I couldn't meet the qualification of being able to walk 5–10 km per day because of my peripheral vascular disease."

"During the hospitalizations for my eyes in the Ophthalmologic Hospital they mismanaged my diabetes. My blood glucose levels were out of control because the doctors there had no idea how to manage diabetes. My serum glucose ranged between 0 and 1000. During one admission I developed hyperglycemic coma and was transferred to the Intensive Care Unit for one week. During another admission I developed acute renal failure for the first time."

Specialist Care

"I see from your medical records that you began to be cared for at the University of Munich Endocrine Clinic around this time."

"Yes. An endocrinologist in Munich started to closely manage my diabetes. I was the first patient to get intensified insulin therapy in the University of Munich Endocrine Clinic in 1982. At this time blood glucose levels became measurable by using a glucometer so there was better control of the blood glucose. However, my serum creatinine levels progressively increased even after I was started on diuretics and my endocrinologist informed me that there was a high likelihood that I was having further kidney deterioration. At this time the endocrinologist gave me three options: watch and wait, start hemodialysis, or undergo a preventative renal/pancreas transplant."

"Those were tough choices."

"They certainly were, but in this discussion with my physician I felt that I was informed of all the possible options. I felt that it was my decision to make, rather than to have my physician choose the direction of management of my disease. I chose to wait."

"How did that turn out?"

"Things were all right for awhile, but three months later, the renal insufficiency progressed to a level where I had to have dialysis. Even then I had a choice of the type of dialysis — in the hospital three days a week or at home. I opted for peritoneal dialysis at home and to be placed on the waiting list for a double simultaneous renal/pancreas transplant."

"There was a nurse at the Munich hospital specially trained to educate patients about dialysis. Both Katrina and I participated in this session and were trained to operate the equipment. To perform the peritoneal dialysis at home with proper sterile precautions, a special catheter attachment machine had to be ordered from the United States. It automatically attached my catheter to the dialysis bags."

"So you and Katrina became peritoneal dialysis experts."

"Well, not exactly, but we did well. I had only one episode of peritonitis and that happened when I was in the hospital for carpal tunnel repair."

Transplantation

Over several subsequent conversations, and by reading his medical records, I learned more about Mr. Fehling's experiences with his disease.

One evening in the fall of 1983, six weeks after he had been placed on the simultaneous double transplant list for a kidney and pancreas, he was called by a representative at the Grosshadern Hospital in Munich who notified him that a 23-year-old man had tragically died in a motorcycle accident and that his organs matched Mr. Fehling's blood and HLA profile. (Currently in Germany information about donors is strictly confidential). An ambulance fully paid for by his insurance, arrived at Mr. Fehling's home and brought both him and his wife, Katrina, to Munich for the operation. The cost of the renal operation was covered by Mr. Fehling's insurance, while the cost of the pancreatic transplant was paid for by research funds at the University of Munich.

Mr. Fehling's operation was only the sixth double simultaneous renal/pancreatic transplant performed in Germany. Post-operatively he remained in the hospital for three months and required close monitoring of his immunosuppresive medications. Upon discharge he was eligible for home assistance services but did not need this help because Katrina took very good care of him. He also was not sent to a rehabilitation center because his rehabilitation was included in his three-month post-operative hospital stay.

There was initial success with the simultaneous graft placement. His creatinine normalized and his glucose levels improved dramatically. He could eat whatever he wanted and exogenous insulin was not required. However, this happy state was not to last long. In 1985 at subsequent follow-up appointments his serial creatinine measurements were found to be elevated, he developed recurrent symptoms of early uremia and ultimately the renal graft was rejected.

A fistula was created in his left arm for hemodialysis. His physicians thought peritoneal dialysis was not a good choice this time because they believed the peritoneal inflammation and scar tissue formed from the operation would limit its effectiveness. He was placed on the waiting list for another renal transplant and again underwent the typical pre-testing of tissue typing, blood tests, and a heart catheterization.

Mr. Fehling's hemodialysis was performed at a hospital in Roding, Germany, a small town 15 kilometers from his home. This was the closest of four hospitals in Bavaria that provided hemodialysis. A taxi, paid for by his insurance, picked him up and transported him to the hospital for his six-hour treatments three times a week. The same taxi transported four or five other hemodialysis patients from the region and they became a friendly little group sharing a common experience.

I asked Mr. Fehling how he felt about his situation at that time.

"Of course it was a great disappointment when the renal graft failed. I knew from the beginning that this might happen, but those few good years gave me hope that it wouldn't."

"How did you feel about going back on dialysis?"

"I was not happy about it at all and I had more difficulty tolerating the hemodialysis than the prior peritoneal dialysis. I had frequent episodes of seriously low blood pressure following the treatments. The dialysis staff also didn't know how to manage diabetes so this had to be closely monitored by the staff physician in the dialysis department."

In late 1985 Mr. Fehlman's glucose levels became elevated. A biopsy of the pancreatic graft revealed a cellular rejection pattern and interstitial fibrosis. Exogenous insulin injections were re-started and he was now placed on the transplantation waiting list for a repeat double simultaneous renal/pancreatic transplantation.

The waiting time for the second transplant was two years. Towards the end of this time his endocrinologist placed him on high urgency since he was tolerating the hemodialysis poorly. Once again he went through the battery of now familiar pre-op tests and procedures. His surgeon went over the standard informed consent protocol with him and he signed the appropriate forms certifying his understanding of the risks and benefits of the procedure. His second transplantation was performed in February 1988.

Within two weeks of discharge, coincidentally after he had the flu, the pancreatic graft started failing and his serum glucose levels rose. He underwent six subsequent operations to try to augment the blood supply to the graft but they were not successful. Four weeks later the surgeons had to take out the pancreatic graft to preserve the kidney graft.

Post-Transplant Diabetes

"This was certainly a low point for me," Mr. Fehlman said. "After removal of the rejected pancreas my endocrinologist tried other methods for managing my diabetes. At first we tried an external insulin pump.

The cost was covered completely by my insurance plan. An internal insulin pump was not considered because these were not widely used in Germany at the time. However, the external pump caused skin irritation and was difficult for me to operate alone without vision so it was discontinued after just a brief trial. Then we tried insulin pens, which were very successful. I still use them today."

There were further complications caused by Mr. Fehlman's diabetes. In 1993 he developed numbness and paresthesias consistent with peripheral neuropathy. He also had two falls related to the "stocking distribution neuropathy," as the loss of sensation progressed from his feet up his legs. Fortunately he did not lose consciousness during the falls and escaped without hip fracture or other serious injury.

The doctors discovered at this time that Mr. Fehlman also has diffuse atherosclerotic disease that has caused peripheral non-occlusive vascular disease. In August of 1999 he developed intermittent claudication in his right lower leg after walking five or six blocks. A duplex scan revealed partial occlusion of the right external iliac artery. A stent was placed in the artery instead of a bypass graft for fear of damaging his functional renal graft. His symptoms improved greatly after the stent placement, but he still experiences leg pain if he walks long distances, usually more than three to four miles.

Mr. Fehlman's hypertension has remained under control with antihypertensive medications. He has not had any symptoms of ischemic heart disease. A heart catheterization in 1998 revealed a left ventricular ejection fraction of 82% and moderate left anterior descending (LAD) artery occlusion (30–50%). A scan, with the vasodilator Persantine, in the same year demonstrated mild ischemia in the LAD distribution. Mr. Fehlman does not have any scheduled follow-ups with a cardiologist, but his endocrinologist, whom he sees every six weeks, keeps an eye on these cardiac issues.

Since the second transplant, Mr. Fehlman's glucose levels have been controlled well with exogenous insulin. He has not had any episodes of hyperglycemic coma, and has only had two episodes eight or nine years ago of syncope related to hypoglycemia. He also has never had diabetic foot ulcers for which he credits Katrina's routine checking and care of his feet. His peripheral neuropathy has not progressed in the past seven years.

Current Diabetes Management

I ask Mr. Fehlman how he presently manages his diabetes.

"First of all, Katrina keeps me on this complicated regimen of medications," he says, indicating a neatly typed list. "She knows what all the 'qs' and 'qds' mean and sees that I get the right medicine at the right time."

Mr. Fehlman's Medications

Cortisone 2 mg qd

Lasix 40 mg qd

Cyclosporin 100 mg bid

Metoprolol 1–1.5 tab q

Azathioprine 50 mg bid

Norvasc 5 mg bid

Entero-coated aspirin 100 mg qd

Enalapril 10 mg bid

Actrapid 1 tab with meals

Corvaton 1.5 mg tid

Protophan 4U 3 am, 2U 7 am, 5U 11 am, 12U 11 pm

Lispro 2 U prn (prior to sugar intake, glucose > 300)

"Who pays for all this medication?" I ask.

"It depends on the amount prescribed and whether there is a generic form or not. There is a cap on what I must pay and after that amount is reached each year, I do not pay any more."

"What about the other expenses related to your illness?"

"I have no idea what the charges are for outpatient visits, labs, tests, or studies ordered by my doctors. These bills go directly to my sickness fund and I never see them. On the other hand, I am notified of all the amounts of the hospital bills, but the sickness fund pays them also. Years ago I purchased private disability insurance that helps me to buy equipment to assist with activities of daily living. For instance I have a scale, wristwatch, and calculator, all of which announce their respective readings aloud. I also have a special device called "Reading Edge" made by Xerox that scans printed material and reads it aloud. Some of this equipment I have had to pay for up front but most of the cost has been reimbursed by my sickness fund or my private insurance."

"How do you keep track of your glucose?" I ask.

"I measure my blood glucose six times a day. I have been using a glucometer since 1982 when they became widely available in Germany and replaced the blood indicator sticks. Just recently my insurance paid for an $800 glucometer that reads my glucose level out loud so now I can completely monitor my own glucose levels, even without Katrina's help."

"Oh yes," says Katrina, joining our conversation. "He is becoming very independent. He also measures his own blood pressure, temperature, and weight. He neatly records all these values in a logbook at the request of his endocrinologist."

I sense that Katrina has had a lot to do with bringing him to this point of independence. "Do you get any exercise?" I ask.

"Exercise is not a problem," Mr. Fehlman replies. "I get exercise every day. Sometimes Katrina and I take walks, but I can walk alone to the center of Cham to visit friends in various shops. I use a walking stick to identify objects in front of me and I can determine the terrain of the road whether it may be dirt, cobblestone, or pavement depending on which section of the city I am in."

"He is remarkable," says Katrina. "He has a very keen memory of the town's geography and knows his exact location by the smells and sounds of different shops, like the perfume of the flower shop and the delicious aroma of the bakery and butcher's shop. He always knows exactly where he is and has never been lost. He usually walks one or two miles a day."

There are also organizations for people with diabetes in which Mr. Fehlman participates. On a monthly basis a diabetic support group coordinated by a local generalist physician meets in Cham. They have educational workshops on topics such as nutrition and medications. Occasionally there are health maintenance exams performed by visiting specialists such as ophthalmologic exams, neurological exams, and blood pressure measurements. All of these services are provided by the state and are free. The majority of Mr. Fehlman's and his wife's education about diabetes comes from these groups and from his endocrinologist. I am impressed by how much they have learned without having access to the Internet. The Bavarian Blindness Association sends books on tape and another organization in Berlin sends monthly magazines on tape.

Mr. Fehlman does not have other health care providers such as a social worker or dietician primarily because Katrina fills these needs.

"Is she strict about your diet?" I ask.

"Oh yes, but I'm really lucky that I don't have too many dietary restrictions," he replies with a chuckle. "I watch my carbohydrate intake, and usually don't eat concentrated sweets. If I want to indulge in ice cream or a piece of cake occasionally, I take two units of short acting insulin. I don't smoke and I only drink alcohol occasionally."

Mr. Fehlman has appointments with his endocrinologist in Munich every six weeks. A taxicab paid for by his insurance plan picks him up in Cham, drives him the four-hour round trip to Munich for the appointment, and the driver waits for him while he is in the clinic. He could travel by other means if he wished. As a visually impaired person he and one escort have free access to public transportation by bus, train, and subway within a 50 km radius of their home. If he had a car he could park in reserved handicapped spaces or park free at any meter.

At Mr. Fehlman's appointments with his endocrinologist the physician reviews his medications, tests his serum glucose and hgbAlC, and performs a physical exam. Typical appointments range from 15 minutes to one hour depending upon issues that arise or exams that are needed. Mr. Fehlman routinely gets a neurological exam, blood pressure check, eye exam, examination for foot ulcers, cardiovascular examination and other appropriate studies and basic lab work performed at these clinics. His most recent hgbAlC was 6.5 indicating exceptional control of his blood glucose levels.

Mr. Fehlman does not see any other physician regularly. He only sees his primary care physician in Cham when he needs prescription refills, basic lab tests, or care for illnesses not related to his diabetes such as colds or flu, or more recently, a bout of pneumonia that was slightly more severe and required antibiotics. If Mr. Fehlman is seriously ill, his primary care physician comes to the house. He is not entirely satisfied with this physician.

"Appointments only last for ten minutes," he complains. "He is so busy and has so many patients to see in one day that he doesn't even look at my feet. It is Katrina who makes sure I never get blisters or diabetic ulcers on my feet. I always have to take the initiative to ask for lab results or the results of other tests or I would never get the information. If I have several questions, he always interrupts after five minutes and says, 'let's talk about this at the next appointment.'"

"Is there anything you like about this physician?" I ask.

"Well, yes. If I am really ill he will come to pay a house visit, and he spends more time with me on those occasions so I do respect him for that. I am grateful for the medical care I have received throughout my life from all of my doctors and realize that I wouldn't be here without all they have done to help me."

I thank Mr. Fehlman for his time and marvel at how he and Katrina and his physicians have managed his complicated illness over the years.

6

Cases Written by German Students in the US

Case 19: One More Cruise*

Marion Bohatschek

"You know my dear, next month I'm going on a cruise to the Caribbean and I'm so looking forward to it," Mrs. Stein says, turning to her daughter, Deborah, with a big smile.

Every time Mrs. Stein thinks of the forthcoming trip her eyes gleam with anticipation. The expression in Deborah's eyes, when thinking of her 89-year-old mother's pending journey, however, is one of worry instead of joy.

Since the death of her husband 12 years ago, Mrs. Stein has been living on her own in a spacious apartment on Manhattan's Upper East Side. Both of her adult daughters live only a few blocks away, but she has never considered moving in with either of them. On the contrary, she very much appreciates the situation as it is, having a place of her own and being independent, yet at the same time seeing her family frequently. "During the last months even too frequently," she thinks. She is a little uneasy about some new facets of the relationship with her daughters that began to evolve after an incident in May 1998.

---

*This case was written by Marion Bohatschek in 1999 while she was a medical student at Ludwig Maximilians University, Munich, Germany and participated in the US-EU-MEE student exchange at Weill Medical College of Cornell University, New York City, New York.

A Trip to the Hospital

On that day, Deborah and her sister Linda stopped by their mother's apartment for what was to be a casual afternoon visit. Instead, they found her lying next to her bed in a physically and mentally disturbing state. Mrs. Stein had a severe cough, difficulty breathing, and fever. What worried them even more was the fact that their mother was completely helpless and not oriented to time and place.

This was a new and frightening experience for the sisters who prior to this time had seen their mother only as a strong, self-determined and organized person. Realizing the situation was too much to handle alone at home, they called Dr. Smith, Mrs. Stein's primary care physician. Unfortunately, they found that he was on vacation. The doctor covering for him told them to bring their mother to the emergency room at the New York Presbyterian Hospital.

Dr. Smith has been Mrs. Stein's primary care physician for almost four years, and she and her family are very happy with him. After the doctor she went to for almost all her life died, Mrs. Stein did not have a primary care physician for a while. This was not a decision made on financial grounds. She has traditional Medicare A and B and a Blue Cross/Blue Shield medigap plan and therefore is able to chose any doctor she wants, but apart from severe osteoarthritis, which especially affects the joints in her legs and which eventually led to a knee replacement operation in 1994, she feels very healthy. Mrs. Stein only started seeing a doctor on a regular basis again when borderline hypertension was discovered in the pre-operation check for her knee replacement. The physician treating her suggested she should see Dr. Smith, a general internist, for regular follow-ups. Dr. Smith is a member of the Cornell Internal Medicine Associates (CIMA) and sees patients once a week at the outpatient clinic of the New York Presbyterian Hospital.

But now, with Dr. Smith away, the sisters called an ambulance and had their mother transported to New York Presbyterian Hospital. In the Emergency Room Mrs. Stein was diagnosed with pneumonia and admitted based on her poor general condition. When Dr. Smith returned he would continue to see her in the hospital on a daily basis. The concept that a Primary Care Physician continues to take care of his patients when they need inpatient care is different from the German system. There, hospital and primary care services are usually completely separated. The continuity of care is certainly an advantage of the American system. Mrs. Stein knows and trusts Dr. Smith and he is familiar with her situation. This is likely to facilitate her treatment and there should also be fewer problems caused by insufficient communication concerning her past medical history and lab tests that have already been performed. On the other hand, this system is very time consuming and financially unattractive for the doctor who must commute between his office and the hospital.

Admission to the hospital, however, had no immediate benefit for Mrs. Stein. In this new and foreign environment her mental status deteriorated even further, especially during the first night when she became very agitated. She pulled out her IV lines repeatedly, fell out of the bed and kept striking out at the nurses. To guard Mrs. Stein from seriously injuring herself, the nurses decided to put her in physical restraints.

In the United States, the decision to mechanically restrain a person lies within the purview of the nurses. The purpose of restraints is to protect both the patient and the caregivers from harm. In Germany the use of restraints is limited to emergency situations and has otherwise to be approved by a judge. No such outside control to protect the patient seemed to exist in the United States in 1998.

Naturally, Deborah and Linda were not happy to see their mother being tied to the bed the next day, but they realized she needed more supervision than could be expected from the nurses on an ordinary ward. Both of the daughters had jobs that demanded a lot of time and energy so they could not provide consistent care for their mother. For the next two nights they hired a nurse's aide to care for Mrs. Stein. They paid $10 per hour (in 1998) out of pocket for this service, a luxury they could well afford. On the second day of Mrs. Stein's hospitalization, the daughters met with one of the social workers employed by the hospital to make plans for the time after hospital discharge.

Patients who are likely to need prolonged care after the hospital treatment are usually referred to a social worker who assesses the social and financial situation and then provides the patient or the family with information on the available options. If the patient is not capable of giving information on her background, it is also the job of social workers to track down relatives and find out more about her general living conditions. The social worker is usually the one who initiates the paperwork necessary to apply for further professional care or financial support and helps with other administrative matters.

Mrs. Stein was a comparatively easy case. She had great support from her family and was financially secure. The main thing the social worker should have done in her case was to discuss the different options after hospital discharge with Deborah and Linda. Both of the daughters, however, thought this did not happen in a comprehensive way. With little knowledge of Mrs. Stein's history, the social worker was convinced that the only adequate option for her would be a nursing home.

The complete loss of independence, the one thing Mrs. Stein cherished so much, would have meant a major change in her life. Deborah and Linda both knew their mother would have fought the decision. Still, seeing her mother in this disoriented state, Deborah more readily agreed with the social worker and one of the doctors, who told her that a nursing home would be a reasonable choice. Thus she started looking into admission procedures for several nursing facilities.

Linda, on the contrary, did not approve at all. She was convinced that it was too early to take such a drastic step and wanted to see how her mother recovered. She opposed the idea of a nursing home especially having had the experience of seeing her mother-in-law's rapid decline after being admitted to one. She was realistic enough, though, to see that at least in the days immediately after hospital discharge, some sort of care would be necessary for her mother. She began discussing the alternative options of home health care with a friend of hers, a trained social worker experienced in this field.

Within the next three days, Mrs. Stein's physical state improved steadily. Her fevers and chills ceased and her breathing became much better. Her mental state recovered somewhat as well. Despite the history of a fall, no diagnostic tests to clarify the etiology of the disorientation had been done during Mrs. Stein's hospital stay. As her cognitive functions slowly improved and she recognized her family members again, further steps to determine the cause of the confusion were scheduled by her primary care physician in an outpatient setting. Her discharge from New York Presbyterian Hospital was planned for day five after admission.

Now that Mrs. Stein was more responsive, Deborah and Linda carefully began to approach the topic of how to arrange her living conditions after the hospital discharge. As expected, Mrs. Stein insisted that she was perfectly able to continue living on her own as she had done before, but after long discussions she reluctantly agreed to hire a 24-hour Home Health Aide (HHA).

HHAs receive only very basic nursing training and their main duty is custodial care. This involves assistance with the activities of daily living such as bathing, cooking, and shopping but not the actual treatment of disease. This seemed perfect for Mrs. Stein, who did not need medical care and required only a little assistance with the activities of daily living. The main reason for employing a Home Health Aide was to have someone around in case of an emergency throughout the day and especially at night. The sisters turned to an agency recommended by one of Linda's friends. After a first assessment of Mrs. Stein's needs by a registered nurse, two HHAs were assigned for her care. The agency charged Mrs. Stein $13.60 an hour for this service. The costs quickly add up to considerable sums: $326.40 a day, $2284.80 a week and so the question of who pays for this care is of great concern to many American families.

Medicare does not cover custodial services, either at home or in nursing homes, so the total costs have to be paid out of pocket by Mrs. Stein. If she had to rely on the Social Security she receives this would quickly become unaffordable. Fortunately she has other sources of income and thus money is not a limiting factor in her case.

Diagnosis

In the week after the hospital discharge Mrs. Stein had a follow-up appointment with Dr. Smith and it was only then that Mrs. Stein and her family were given a name for the cognitive problems she had experienced in the past. This name was Alzheimer's disease, a dreaded diagnosis. Dr. Smith based this diagnosis mainly on Mrs. Stein's history and clinical appearance. The only lab tests he performed were blood electrolyte checks and a thyroid function test to rule out a metabolic cause. Dr. Smith said the symptoms Mrs. Stein showed are so classic for early stage Alzheimer's disease that he even refrained from doing any cranial imaging. And indeed, looking back at the past years, the family could identify a number of signs of Mrs. Stein's slow deterioration that are really typical for this type of dementia.

Mrs. Stein had been a very active and self-determined woman all her life. As a girl, she convinced her parents to send her to college. After receiving a BA, she started working as a social worker, despite her whole family's disapproval. After marrying an engineer, who also successfully ran a men's clothing company and real estate business, she reluctantly quit her job and stayed at home with her two daughters. But she kept up one of her passions: traveling. For most of her life, she and her family spent at least one month a year on vacation in Europe and another two months driving through America. Even after her husband died, she continued traveling on her own. Her last longer vacation, a trip to Mexico, was only six months prior the hospital admission. Socially she has been very engaged in various groups and she frequently visited Jewish women's clubs. For many years she also participated in the Senior Program of Hunter College, where she attended mainly art and literature classes.

In retrospect, her daughters say there were some slight but noticeable changes in their mother's behavior and a slow gradual decline in her cognitive functions during the last two or three years. She started forgetting names and dates and sometimes she could not remember meetings or recall telephone conversations. Two years ago, she also stopped taking college classes and only rarely attended theater performances and concerts. Deborah and Linda noticed all of those things, but they considered them as normal signs of aging — nothing to worry about. Mrs. Stein herself still thinks this way. She acknowledges that she has become more forgetful throughout the years but says, "At my age you are allowed to forget some things."

In the spring of 1998 Deborah became more aware of the problem when she realized that her mother had difficulty keeping track of her finances. Up to then, Mrs. Stein had been meticulous about paying bills and doing her taxes, but now Deborah realized that a number of bills had not been paid in months. Mrs. Stein is still responsible for her finances and has her own checkbook, but now the daughters double-check.

The actual diagnosis of early stage Alzheimer's dementia in May 1998 did not have a big impact on the plans the family had made. They agreed on hiring the 24-hour home attendants and they saw no immediate need for other action. In practice, however, the Home Health Aides turned out to cause more tension and stress than relief. Instead of supervising Mrs. Stein constantly, they let her go for walks on her own. In addition, they did not prepare meals and the daily journal they were supposed to keep was only rudimentary. And, what was even more important, Mrs. Stein did not get along with them. Thus after only four days, Deborah asked to replace the two women with different ones.

The new HHAs were more reliable, but Mrs. Stein was still very unhappy about the whole situation. By the end of the second week, her cognitive functions were not back to the old level, yet she felt secure enough to be on her own again. Mrs. Stein is a very friendly person and being in the early stages of the disease, her skills of basic social interaction are still fully intact. In conversations she is charming and funny and only after talking for a while one realizes that she has difficulty following more complex thoughts and a tendency to repeat herself.

But despite all this, she again had major quarrels with the HHAs. Having someone around for 24 hours a day was very disruptive for her. She could not stand the idea of being watched constantly and having a stranger living in her apartment. In her opinion this was just a waste of money and a needless cutback of her independence. Linda agreed with her mother on this issue. She did not see the absolute necessity of constant supervision, especially as her mother's psychological wellbeing obviously suffered under it. Deborah on the contrary, was convinced that Mrs. Stein still required persistent surveillance. However, after five weeks of what she considered imprisonment and over $11,000 in costs, Mrs. Stein seized the moment and fired the HHAs while Deborah was on vacation. Linda took no steps to repeal her mother's move and when Deborah came back, she had no other choice but to accept the situation.

Long-term Adjustments

On their next meeting with Dr. Smith, Mrs. Stein, Linda and Deborah again discussed the problems of her living alone in her apartment. In general, the doctor had no major concerns about Mrs. Stein being unsupervised throughout the day and only suggested some precautionary modifications to the apartment to make it safer. This especially included removing rugs and unstable furniture to prevent falls. Linda and Deborah also started to check on their mother more often. Now usually both of them call her in the morning. Deborah visits her mother every day in the early afternoon and helps with the grocery shopping. Linda generally stops by after work and takes care of the laundry. They both invest a lot of time in taking care of their mother and this is often an exhausting job.

Apart from a few disconcerting incidents like a burnt brisket when Mrs. Stein forgot that she had put the roast in the oven, and the time she forgot to take her medication, every thing went more or less smoothly during the next months; only the decline of memory became more and more obvious. Thus, in October 1998, when Dr. Smith suggested a trial of Aricept, Mrs. Stein and her daughters agreed. They were aware that this drug could not bring back the old cognitive abilities but might slow down the progression of the disease. Dr. Smith started with an initial dose of 5 mg daily and provided Mrs. Stein with sample tablets for the first four weeks.

In the follow-up visit one month later, Mrs. Stein reported no side effects and Linda said there even might have been a slight improvement in her memory. Because of that, Dr. Smith decided to continue the treatment and prescribed a supply for another month. Aricept is a rather expensive medication so he was starting it cautiously. In pharmacies, the patients have to pay up to $150 for 28 pills (1998 price), but there is also the possibility of obtaining the drug at a discount through different organizations, such as the American Association of Retired People (AARP). Dr. Smith told Deborah they could buy a four-week supply for only $104 through AARP. As medication is covered by neither Medicare nor by Mrs. Stein's gap-insurance (this is pre-Medicare Part D instituted in 2006), she has to pay the total costs out-of-pocket. Because of that she was grateful that Dr. Smith informed her of the AARP discount.

At the same visit, Deborah mentioned that recently her mother often seemed depressed. Linda disagreed, but Dr. Smith decided to refer Mrs. Stein to Dr. Davids, a geriatric psychiatrist for consultation. Dr. Davids found Mrs. Stein to have broad, but relatively mild deficits in memory, language, abstraction and visual spatial function. On the Mini-Mental Status Exam (MMSE) she scored 24 out of 30 possible points. She could

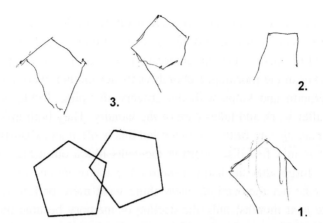

Figure 6.1.   Mrs. Stein's Attempts to Copy Intersecting Pentagons for the MMSE in April 1999.

not perform the serial sevens or spell "world" backwards, had severe problems recalling the three objects she had learned earlier and completely failed in copying two intersecting pentagons (see Figure 6.1).

Mrs. Stein was fully oriented to her person, time and place, but was not able to recall recent news items or produce the names of the US president, her doctor or her granddaughter. Overall, Dr. Davids could not see any signs of depression or psychosis. Thus he suggested she continue taking Aricept and made an appointment for a follow-up visit four weeks later. Like Dr. Smith, he discussed the possible risks of Mrs. Stein living on her own, but seeing how adamant she was about keeping her independence, he agreed with the daughters to respect her wishes as long as this was feasible.

The one thing he was seriously concerned about, though, was the trip Mrs. Stein was planning for the following spring. From late October on she had expressed her plan to go on a cruise, and she insisted on going on her own. Her daughters, especially Deborah, were very worried about it as well. Even though Mrs. Stein never got lost in her immediate environment they feared that she could not cope with completely new surroundings anymore.

On various short trips they had taken to family gatherings she had repeatedly become slightly disoriented. On these occasions not only her sense of orientation, but also her general cognitive performance and well-being seemed to suffer. Yet, Mrs. Stein firmly held to her plan of going on this cruise. In a joint effort, her doctors and her family finally convinced her to take someone along. So now both of her daughters and her son-in-law will accompany her on this journey.

Since then, four months have passed and Mrs. Stein's status has not changed much during this time. She still scores 23/30 on the Mini-Mental Status Exam and has no problems coping with basic everyday life. What is troublesome though and might be the beginning of a later stage of the dementia are two episodes of wandering at night that occurred at the beginning of this year. Mrs. Stein was about to leave her apartment building dressed only in a nightgown and could not explain where she intended to go. Both times she was stopped by the doorman who then called one of the daughters.

Even though this suggested further progression of the dementia, the daughters still see no need to take precautionary legal steps to anticipate the time when Mrs. Stein might not be able to give valid consent anymore. They have not set up a power of attorney or a will. As Mrs. Stein does not acknowledge her disease and tries to keep her independence, her daughters say she would never agree to such a document. She has signed only a health care proxy and a Do Not Resuscitate (DNR) order.

Mrs. Stein's case clearly illustrates two of the main issues caregivers of people suffering from dementia disorders have to face at some point. First, it demonstrates that Alzheimer's dementia cannot be seen as an isolated problem of the person diagnosed with it. This disease also affects all the people around the patient as well, and it is often hard for them to witness the steady decline of a loved one when they can do nothing to stop it. The other point which it illustrates is the difficulty of finding the right balance between leaving the patient as much autonomy, independence, and quality of living, as possible but at the same time making sure she is safe.

Finally the Trip

In a few weeks, Mrs. Stein and her daughters will be on a cruise ship in the Caribbean. Was it a good decision to make this trip or was Deborah, the more concerned of the daughters, right to oppose it? As each case is unique, no one can answer this question confidently. No one can say what will be the right thing to do for Mrs. Stein after they come back, either. There is no universal solution, but together, Linda, Deborah and their mother seem to have found a reasonable middle ground to balance risks and benefits. Knowing this may be her last vacation trip, the sparkle of anticipation in Mrs. Stein's eyes tells them they are right.

Case 20: The Obesity Battle*

Benedikt Aulinger

For a number of reasons I have decided to use two patient stories in this case report. Both will undergo surgical treatment at the New York-Presbyterian Hospital/Columbia Center for Obesity Surgery in New York City, which cooperates with the Weill Cornell Medical Center, but the two patients have a totally different history and their ways of coming to the point of considering surgery couldn't be more diverse.

Meeting Frank

I met my first patient, Mr. Frank Burns, at the entrance hall of the Weill Medical College. Although I had never seen him before and there were other people around, I stepped towards him and greeted him by name. He was not surprised. If my disease of special interest was for example, diabetes, arthritis or any other of those common chronic diseases, it would have been difficult to distinguish Mr. Burns from the other people nearby. That's the condition obese patients have to live with. Their disease is immediately obvious and carries with it an undeniable stigmatization.

---

*This case report is based on cases written by Benedikt Aulinger in 2003 when he was a medical student at Ludwig Maximilians University in Munich, Germany, and took part in the US-EU-MEE student exchange at Weill Medical College of Cornell University in New York City.

But as opposed to those who are obviously disabled — sitting in a wheelchair for example — society doesn't regard them as patients with a severe illness.

Mr. Burns and I exchanged greetings and settled down in a comfortable conference room for our conversation. I knew from his medical records, which he had previously given me permission to examine, that he was 38 years old and had several other medical problems that were aggravated by his obesity.

"Please call me Frank," he said, when I addressed him in my formal, European way. In the presence of this well groomed, but enormous young man, I was suddenly at a loss to know where to begin. He made it easy for me, saying, "Go ahead. Ask me anything you'd like to know."

Given this permission I asked, "What do you think is the reason that you have gained so much weight?"

He paused a moment and replied thoughtfully, "I think it is because I have always eaten too much and too fast."

"Have you always been heavy?" I asked.

"I was somewhat heavy as a child. Then I got heavier during my high school years and in my mid-twenties. As a child I always got what I wanted if I insisted on it. I think this was a learned misbehavior that contributed to my weight problem."

"Do your parents have a problem with their weight?"

"My father doesn't, but my mother was moderately overweight at one time. My brother and two sisters are all obese or even severely obese, so I think there might be a genetic problem."

"Do you think the kind of food you eat has contributed to your weight gain?"

"No, I think I had good nutrition during my childhood and adolescence, and I don't think I eat the wrong kinds of food now — just that I eat too much of it."

"What has been your highest weight and what do you weigh now?"

"I probably hit a peak somewhere around 400 pounds. I don't know exactly because the scales in doctors' offices stop somewhere around 350. I think I weigh about 370 now."

At his height of six feet two inches, Frank's Body Mass Index (BMI) is approximately 48 kg/m². That means he belonged to the group of patients with severe or so-called morbid obesity, which is related to several serious health problems. Ironically, it is the obviousness of this disease that leads to stigmatization and psychological problems and is the reason insurance companies often deny treatment. Body weight is regarded as a matter of personal vanity and not of health status and therefore treatment is considered a cosmetic intervention. Fortunately, this attitude on the part of some insurance companies is changing with the realization that it is wise from a medical and economic point of view to treat obesity.

"Have you tried to lose weight?" I asked, feeling a little foolish to ask such a question.

"Oh, yes! I've tried just about everything. My first try was between the age of 25 and 26. That was the only time in my life when I found the willpower to eat significantly less. For one year I cut down my food intake so drastically that I lost approximately 150 pounds. My weight was down to around 250 pounds."

"Did you do this under the supervision of a doctor or a nutritionist?"

"No, I did it completely on my own. I didn't follow any particular diet but just ate a lot less."

"Did you follow a regular exercise program during that time?"

"No, I've never been fond of exercise or sports of any kind. I did it all by reducing my food intake. Unfortunately, during the next five years I couldn't keep up my motivation and by the time I was in my early thirties, my weight was back to the mid to upper three hundreds."

Frank's history of obesity is similar to so many others I have heard. Along with some temporary success in losing weight, there is a continuous weight gain in nearly every obese patient's history. When you ask them what kind of diets they have tried you will always hear one answer: Everything! Of course no patient has tried every existing diet but many have tried at least a respectable number of them and therefore many obese patients are discouraged by repeated unsuccessful attempts. The long-term result of these diets is usually a temporary triumph over eating habits but no sustained weight reduction. Although frequently there is some weight loss in the beginning, almost no one can maintain the lower level of body weight and in most cases will even put on more pounds.

"You said you were not under the care of a physician for losing weight," I continued. "Did you see your Primary Care Physician (PCP) at all during the time you lost and gained back weight?"

"Oh yes. During this time I had a lot of health problems. I developed high blood pressure, sleep apnea and osteoarthritis in the joints of my ankles and feet. My PCP treated me for all of these medical problems, which were very obviously related to my body weight, and gave me the usual advice on diet and exercise."

I guess most obese patients get that "usual advice" although it doesn't promise any positive result for either the patient or his body weight. Those patients are expected to lose their extra pounds if they really want to and so we leave them to struggle with the problem alone. Some insurance companies have also historically taken this attitude.

Frank's list of health-related problems and diagnosed diseases includes nearly all of the common co-morbidities persons with severe obesity are likely to have, but also some really severe and life threatening diseases. He was hospitalized in December 2001 because of breathing problems and diagnosed with cardiomyopathy and congestive heart failure (CHF). Furthermore he has two aortic aneurysms: one 4.8 cm at the aortic valve and another one 4.3 cm at the ascending aorta. These were surely triggered by his elevated blood pressure.

To complete the list, Frank was diagnosed with sarcoidosis and colitis ulcerosa in 1997 and 1993, respectively. As I could see by the list of medications in his medical records there were some psychological problems worth mentioning. It's likely that those were related in some way to his obesity. All of those drugs were prescribed by his PCP or later by the obesity specialist, Dr. Blake, and he never received psychosomatic or behavioral therapy.

Insurance Coverage

Frank was working for a large global security company and therefore he received insurance coverage from his employer. He was participating in the employer's group health plan at BlueCross/BlueShield, one of the largest insurance networks in the USA. They operated with local insurance providers to offer many kinds of managed care plans like Health Management and Preferred Provider or indemnity plans. Frank's monthly insurance fee was $282 of which approximately $50 to $60 was taken from Frank's paycheck to cover the employee part of the premium. This was paid from pre-tax income, so you could say the US government supports this kind of insurance enrollment.

In addition to that, Frank paid a $20 out-of-pocket co-pay every time he saw one of his physicians, no matter if it is his PCP or a specialist and no matter how much the visit might cost. Because of his many health problems Frank visits the doctors' offices quite frequently. Based on the number of single appointments with some of his specialists, I estimate a total of approximately 20 visits per year and therefore an amount of $400 as out-of-pocket expenses only for the appointments with his physicians. This doesn't include expenditures for hospital stays or medication.

Frank's out-of-pocket co-payments for the above-mentioned medications were about $150 a month (in 2003). His PCP or one of his specialists prescribed all of these drugs. The co-payments of the single drugs range between $10 and $15, depending on whether it is a generic or brand name drug.

I asked Frank if these costs held him back from seeing a doctor when he feels he needs one. He replied, "Costs don't make me hesitate to go to

Medication	Substance	Purpose
Wellbutrin	Tri-cyclic anti-depressant	Possible weight reduction
Glucophage	Oral anti-diabetic	Possible weight reduction
Norvasc	Calcium channel blocker	Blood pressure, CHF
Coreg	Alpha + Beta-blocker	Blood pressure, CHF
Altace	ACE inhibitor	Blood pressure, CHF
Lasix	Diuretic	Blood pressure, CHF
Spironolactone	Diuretic	Blood pressure, CHF
Protonix	Proton pump inhibitor	Acid reflux
Ambien	Sedative/Hypnotic	Insomnia

the doctor. I don't cut back on medical care but instead I reduce my spending for personal entertainment like movies, books and so on."

Because of structural changes in his company, Frank was likely to lose his job at his current employer in the near future and therefore medical coverage was an important issue for him. Fortunately, he could continue his group insurance under a government-approved plan called COBRA for a maximum of 18 months, but this was very expensive. Because of some lucky circumstances, namely severance pay from his employer, a certain amount of unemployment support by the government and the fact that he lived in his uncle's house with a very low rent, he could afford the monthly premium for awhile until he found a new job.

"The best thing my PCP did," Frank continued, "was to refer me to Dr. Blake about three years ago. He is an obesity specialist at Cornell. I have developed a good relationship with Dr. Blake and have a lot of confidence in him."

"What treatments did he recommend?"

"At first they were all 'natural' treatments. He prescribed, and I tried different medications from herbal substances to psychiatric drugs. Dr. Blake closely supervised all of these treatments and monitored my general health. For example, he watched my blood pressure closely as the side effects of some medications include elevated blood pressure. I had some degree of success, but it was not enough and did not last long-term."

"Finally Dr. Blake and I came to the decision that surgery might be a new option for me in my struggle against excess body weight. He referred me to the New York-Presbyterian/Columbia Center for Obesity Surgery, which cooperates with the Weill Cornell Medical Center."

Considering Surgery

The first time Frank considered surgery was about two and a half years ago when Dr. Blake mentioned it matter-of-factly during one of their appointments. Frank's next step was to collect information on the Internet and to get in touch with previous gastric surgery patients through the help of various support groups. He also talked about his idea of having an operation to his sister-in-law, a nurse in an intensive care unit (ICU) for cardiothoracic patients.

"She told me this horror-story of a patient, who had surgery and then came to the ICU because he had all of these organ failures. I was too afraid of suffering the same complications and couldn't take any further steps toward surgery at that time."

There followed a long period of time in which Frank weighed the pros and cons of a surgical intervention nearly every day. Although he still was afraid of possible complications, he finally agreed to gastric bypass surgery and the operation was scheduled for July 10, 2002. He came to his decision because he realized that conservative treatment had failed so far and a significant weight loss was urgently needed to improve his health and elevate his quality of life. At this point he finally gave up the hope of achieving sufficient weight loss by any non-surgical means.

This should have been the turning point in his obese life but one week prior to the operation, Frank had a consultation with the anesthesiologist, who would perform the narcosis during the operation. She regarded his risk profile as very high and asked Frank if he was totally informed about this fact. In her opinion the surgeon who did the pre-operative consultation with Frank did not consider his high risk adequately. Therefore she wanted him to be aware of the fact that he might not survive this operation. This obviously met with some success because Frank was "frightened to death" and immediately canceled his appointment with the surgeon.

"Today I wish I had done it at that time," he said.

Instead, approximately nine months later, Frank was starting another attempt. He was waiting for a new appointment for the operation at the same hospital and he was considering his personal situation differently. As mentioned before, Frank would have to look for a new job and that would bring certain new challenges into his life. Although COBRA would cover him until he found another employer he couldn't afford this kind of insurance for an unlimited time.

Frank said about his current situation, "Now that I have these different events taking place at the same time, I know I have no choice but to do the surgery now, because when I start a new job I really can't afford to go out on medical leave right away. So I am going to schedule my surgery and hope for the best."

Frank did a lot of research about the center where he will be operated on. For example he talked to some people who were having this operation and he searched in different media for information about the hospital and the surgeons. He was referred to a Dr. Pierce and has come to have a lot of confidence in him.

"My understanding is that Dr. Pierce is one of the best surgeons for performing weight loss surgery so I do feel comfortable with him," he explained. "They perform a lot of this type of surgery at this center and have a mortality rate that is below the national average. They have an extensive program of preparation and support afterwards. It's not just taking someone in, performing surgery on him and then telling him, Good luck!"

To qualify for bariatric surgery, and to meet insurance company criteria, the patient must have:

- Clinically severe obesity (BMI > 40 or BMI > 35 with co-morbid conditions).
- A history of obesity for at least five years.
- Failure of other methods of weight loss verified by a physician.
- Psychological screening confirming a mental attitude needed for successful treatment.

At the New York-Presbyterian Hospital Center for Weight Loss Surgery the patient is required to attend a series of seminars and meetings with a nurse practitioner who explains the different types of surgery and the nursing follow-up program. All risks are explained, including the possibility of death and the permanent lifestyle changes that will be necessary in regard to eating and nutritional supplements afterwards.

There is a thorough pre-op work-up of history, physical exam, blood tests, x-rays, and upper GI exams in preparation for the surgery. Any special exams are scheduled if needed. Then the patient meets with the surgeon who goes over all the details of the operation again. One week before the scheduled surgery, final tests are done and the patient decides on the type of operation to be done (if there is a choice) and schedules the operation appointment. One week prior to that appointment the last exams and preparations are done.

After surgery the patient might go to an intensive care unit (ICU) for a short term and will be discharged normally after 2–3 days. After a gastric banding operation the patient might be discharged the same day of the operation because this procedure is not as stressful and there are fewer complications than with other types of bariatric surgery. Gastric bypass patients get an upper GI exam on the second day to detect leaks and thereby avoid severe complications.

When patients hear that the recovery time is about four to six weeks, some become nervous, but they are relieved when they are told that they usually can return to work after two weeks. Regular medical check-ups take place two weeks after the operation, then every six months during the first two years and finally once a year.

Difficult to Determine Costs

Frank's insurance is a Preferred Provider Organization (PPO) plan that allows out-of-network benefits. This made it possible for him to have surgery at the New York-Presbyterian Hospital Center for Obesity Surgery with Dr. Pierce, his preferred surgeon. As Frank fulfilled all the requirements for the surgery, his insurance company had already given its pre-approval for the operation as a medical necessity and would pay 80% of what they regard as reasonable and customary (R&C) costs.

If Frank had gone ahead with his surgery last year, Dr. Pierce was a member of his insurance network and the cost would have been covered. This year Dr. Pierce has changed networks and Frank has had to subscribe to the PPO to be able to go to the surgeon he has come to know and trust. Frank thinks it will be worth it, even though he will have to bear more of the expense.

Actually Frank didn't really know how much the insurance would cover and how much Dr. Pierce was going to charge him. He didn't know how much "reasonable and customary" cost was for this operation and he also didn't know if the hospital stay and the follow up examinations were completely covered by his insurance plan. He felt a bit uncomfortable about this lack of knowledge. He told me, "Well, there is a good chance that this whole procedure may only cost me $200 but on the other hand, it may cost me around $3100 and I am prepared for that. Until I get out of the hospital and start getting the bills, it's tough to know in advance."

Frank hopes that most of his out-of-pocket costs will be covered by his "flexible spending account." This is an amount of money he is allowed to set aside through his employer each year to pay for deductibles, co-payments and other medical or dental expenses that are not covered by his insurance. Because this is pre-tax money, it is advantageous for Frank to calculate carefully the amount he is likely to need for these expenses throughout the year, as he will at least save the taxes on this amount of income. It is also a way of governmental support for health care expenditures for people who have a regular income and foreseeable health care costs, for example because of chronic disease. If Frank doesn't use all the money put in the account each year, he will forfeit it at the end of the year because it cannot be carried over into the next year.

Following his operation, Frank will have extra ongoing costs for the nutritional supplements he will need to take, but he might also save money because of less prescribed medication and fewer co-payments for physician visits.

Frank's Expectations

"At first I wanted gastric banding because I thought it is less intrusive and has a lower risk, but at the time it was considered experimental and not proven, and I was not sure my insurance company would pay for it. After more discussion with Dr. Blake I decided to have the gastric bypass operation, also called the Roux-en-Y gastric bypass. I am waiting now for an appointment for my operation."

When I finished this case report, Frank was still waiting for his operation to be performed. I don't know if everything went perfectly and if the results would bring the hoped and expected results for his body weight and his general condition. Still I think this is a good chance for him to start living a new life without the obesity he experienced for almost 30 years.

"As everything has developed so far and I am having these severe health conditions," he said, "I don't believe this can give me a new life with the chance of being totally healthy again, but I do think that it can improve my situation significantly and my quality of life is going to reach a satisfactory level."

A Second Case

The second patient I will include in this report is Jennifer Diaz, a 31-year-old Hispanic woman who had problems with her body weight as well. With her weight of 202 pounds and a height of five feet two inches, she had a BMI of approximately 37, which means she was in the classification group of Obesity Grade II. When we met, she asked me to call her Jennifer, or Jenny.

Although she had been steadily gaining weight since about the age of 19, she only recently had the feeling of being definitely too heavy. I asked her why she suddenly felt that her weight is a problem.

"My son, Ricardo, was born a little more than two years ago," she replied. "After his birth I never lost the weight I gained during pregnancy and then I put on even more weight. Over 200 pounds at five feet two inches tall is definitely too much! This last year really was unbearable."

"Why do you think you suddenly gained so much weight?"

"One important factor is the lack of physical activity caused by the office job I have had since I went back to work."

"Have you tried any medical or non-medical weight-loss programs on your own," I asked, again feeling foolish at asking a question with a predictable answer.

"I never tried any weight-loss medicines or supplements," she replied. "I don't take any medicine regularly except contraceptives. Of course I have tried many diets on my own and I joined Weight Watchers™ without long-term success. I even tried a diet professionally supervised by a nutritionist for a while but I couldn't achieve or maintain any weight reduction. These countless attempts to lose the extra pounds have worn me out with trying any more conservative measures. I have decided that bariatric surgery is the only answer for me."

At this stage of her illness Jennifer had not had very many side effects of obesity, which is the opposite of Frank's situation. Not being able to wear high heels because of joint problems in her feet and a recurrent carpal tunnel syndrome are the most severe problems she has had to deal with until then. But coming from a high-risk family, this could change quickly especially if she gained more weight in future.

"Living in a Hispanic family," she said, "I certainly grew up in an environment that enhances calorie intake of the wrong kind and quantity of food. Along with all the delicious high-calorie Hispanic food, we drank all sorts of sodas and 'sweet stuff.' There is a high incidence of obesity and type 2 diabetes in my family. Nearly my whole family is suffering from obesity and metabolic syndrome. All of my sisters are obese and there are several cases of diabetes among my closest relatives."

"What made you think of gastric surgery as your best chance for weight loss?" I asked.

"Mostly it was the positive experience of my sister, Juliana, who had weight loss surgery last November. Now I am trying to get approval from my insurance company."

Jennifer's Insurance

Jennifer had employer-sponsored health insurance in a Health Maintenance Organization (HMO) with the Aetna Insurance Company. She only had access to the doctors having contracts with the insurer, so her choices of physicians and treatment locations were limited. Fortunately her insurance company had contracts with another weight loss surgeon at the New York-Presbyterian Hospital/Columbia Center for Obesity Surgery where her sister had her surgery. If she got the longed-for approval from her insurer, she would see no bill at all for the operation. Her costs would only be the usual deductibles for hospitalization and physician co-payments. Besides, she needed a referral from her PCP to this obesity center to be allowed to get treatment there.

Even though Jennifer was obviously restricted very much in the choice and number of physicians and specialists she could see, she was happy with her health care. She was enrolled in another HMO plan offered by her employer for the first two years of her employment but it did not please her. Now she regarded the care she and her son received as adequate and extensive. Jenny liked the low premiums, the predictability of her medical costs, and the uncomplicated system of direct payment by her insurer to the physician so she never saw bills.

Waiting for Approval

Jennifer will have to fulfill the same criteria as Frank if she is to be approved for one of the types of bariatric surgery performed at New York-Presbyterian. Whereas Frank had no problems fulfilling those criteria, Jennifer is still struggling to get approval from her insurance company. With a BMI of 37 and her relatively short history of obesity, and without further risk factors she is not considered to have an adequately high risk profile. The surgery itself and the possible complications don't worry her too much, which is another big difference from Frank.

Ironically, Jennifer told me in confidence that she is currently trying to eat more than she would like so she can gain enough weight to improve her chances of getting approval for the surgery.

"I hope my insurance company will see that I need to break out of the pattern of obesity-caused health problems in my family and I think bariatric surgery is the only way. I think I will gain enormous benefits from it."

I asked Frank and Jennifer how satisfied they are with their health care and what they think about the American health care system. Both told me they feel privileged to have their health insurance and the high tech medical care they receive and therefore are very happy with the system. But Frank adds, "Medical choices are significantly limited for anyone who is uninsured because of having a job without insurance, or is poor and has only Medicaid, or is elderly and has only the default Medicare benefits without any coinsurance, which is quite expensive."

Case 21: The Poetry of Life and Breath*

Oliver Fuchs

Hands

Out there
We are alone in the world
Our clubbing fingers stand out
Like sore thumbs.
Here
We come together.
Hands bind
Like sunshine.
Our rays embrace
The universe
Our love binds us.
Loneliness
Disperses in the darkness
Behind us.
I am
Whole
Here.

Ana Stenzel — CF Adult Retreat, Summer 1998

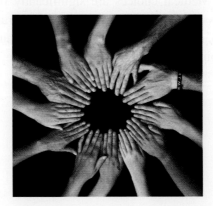

---

*This case report was written by Oliver Fuchs in 2001 when he was a student at Ludwig Maximilians University and participated in the US-EU-MEE program at Children's Hospital, Harvard Medical School in Boston. Poems and photographs used by permission of the authors and The Breathing Room Organization.

Two People with CF

In the not-too-distant, past Cystic Fibrosis (CF) was a disease of young people. Up until 1957 most patients did not survive past age three. Through diligent research and medical advances, people with CF are surviving into adulthood, with the average life expectancy now at age 32 (in 2001). The following case report is based on two patients who are cared for at Children's Hospital in Boston. The first story details the experiences of Jennie Robertson (names have been changed of course) as she moves in and out of care at Children's Hospital over a period of years, simultaneously dealing with issues of family, insurance, and disability status.

The second is a snapshot of 25-year-old Thomas O'Connor who is admitted for a typical short-term "clean-out." It serves as an example of what admission to IV antibiotic therapy and routine care looks like at Children's Hospital in 2001.

Jennie Robertson

Jennie had always been a thin child. The difference compared to her peers was apparent and sometimes made her feel uncomfortable, especially when she was a teenager and the boys called her "Skinny." By the age of 13 she suffered from chronic coughing and recurrent sinus infections. When she was 15 she began to see little streaks of blood in the mucus she coughed up. This went on for several years, but when she turned 19, she began to cough up bright red blood and the hemoptysis became impossible to ignore. In her senior year in high school she was barely able to do simple exercises in gym class without becoming seriously short of breath.

Living just outside of Boston, her parents naturally turned to Children's Hospital for help. They arranged for an appointment with Dr. Baker, a pulmonologist, and thus began a long series of treks to the hospital on Longwood Avenue. After her first battery of tests, which included x-rays and two bronchoscopies that were not a pleasant experience for Jennie, Dr. Baker sat down with her and her parents and explained the damage that had already occurred. In medical terms, this included bronchiectasis, a stiffening and loss of elasticity in her lungs, mainly in the upper lobes, and nodular densities in the right lower lobe.

The bronchoscopies both confirmed the presence of a non-tuberculous mycobacterium (NTM) identified as *Mycobacterium fortuitum* complex.

This was all medical mumbo-jumbo to Jennie and her parents, but they understood that she was seriously ill. She was admitted to Children's and had an open lung biopsy. Dr. Baker wrote in her chart, "granulomatous inflammation with focal necrosis principally involving terminal bronchioles, occasionally of the tubercoid type with Langhans' giant cells and a rare acid-fast bacillus in the cytoplasm of histiocytes and no caseous necrosis indicating infection with mycobacteria other than NTM, supported by lung culture. Anaerobic culture showed isolation of *Actinomyces meyeri*."

More mumbo-jumbo!

Dr. Baker ordered a sweat test, which was positive (sweat chloride, 99 mEq/l) and confirmed the diagnosis by genetic testing. Her illness now had a name: cystic fibrosis (CF). Dr. Baker prescribed high dose penicillin, Oxacillin and Tobramycin. Because she improved, he decided not to start therapy for mycobacterial disease at that stage. Her baseline pulmonary function tests (PFTs) on discharge were: forced vital capacity (FVC), 96% and forced expiratory volume (FEV_1, the amount of air Jennie could exhale in one second after a full breath), 87% of the expected value. These were numbers that Dr. Baker thought were pretty good. They were numbers Jennie would hear many times in the future as she and her doctors struggled to get back to that magic baseline.

A Nursing Career

After high school graduation Jennie was accepted into the four-year nursing degree program at Boston University and managed to stay out of Children's for those four years. Her parents' insurance covered her regular visits to Dr. Baker until she graduated and began to work as a nurse. She realized that good health insurance coverage was going to be important for her entire life and enrolled in the Bluecross/Blueshield Value Plus HMO through the Massachusetts Nurses Association (MNA). She would have had the opportunity to be insured through her job, but the cost through MNA was much less as her employer didn't contribute any money toward the insurance.

For five more years Jennie continued to do well. Her symptoms did not impair her in her daily activity as they had some years ago. Dr. Baker kept a close watch on her medications, which included oral trimethoprim (Bactrim), hrDNAse (Dornase alpha, from July 1993 on) and the necessary vitamin supplements (vitamins A, D, E, K). Her weight was stable and she required only three in-patient courses of intravenous antibiotics during that time.

Marriage and Motherhood

Jennie married her college sweetheart, Jake Robertson in 1993 at age 25, and two years later their son Charles was born. As a nurse, she knew she was walking a fine line between sickness and health but she was determined to make the most of the important experiences of marriage and motherhood in her life. On the medical side, repeated sputum cultures inconsistently showed *Pseudomonas aeruginosa*, *Staphylococcus aureus*, *Candida*, and *Aspergillus* and persistently yielded her old nemesis, NTM, finally classified as *M. abscessus*, because of its susceptibility to the cephalosporin antibiotic cefoxitin.

Her pulmonary function tests (PFTs), however, showed a slow decline of approximately 2% of the expected value per year, together with minimally changing chest x-ray appearance. Dr. Baker and her other physicians at Children's decided to begin a high dose of ibuprofen (NSAID) in February 1996 to slow the progression of her lung disease.

In May 1996 increased cough, low grade fevers, decreased energy, right upper lobe infiltrates and now a 15% decrease in her PFTs (FVC, 82% and FEV_1, 56%), and sputum positive for NTM, got her admitted to Children's again. Despite several courses of antipseudomonal and antistaphylococcal antibiotics, her PFTs stayed stubbornly below baseline, but she was allowed to return home.

In November 1996 Jennie was back at Children's for a high-resolution computerized tomography (HRCT) scan because of the concern that she had active mycobacterial infection. Surprisingly, bronchoscopy and bronchoalveolar lavage (BAL) showed no signs of that, but the presence of NTM was revealed again. Another course of dicloxacillin and itraconazole failed to completely normalize her clinical condition, although she became well enough to leave the hospital.

Jennie continued to have shortness of breath and periodic fevers. But now she had a one-and-a-half year old son to be concerned about, and she continued to work periodically as a private duty nurse, hoping that she and Jake could soon afford their dream — a home of their own. However, her symptoms progressed to the point where in February 1997 she took a six-month leave of absence from work, and in March she applied to the state of Massachusetts for disability status. When her leave ended in August 1997 she decided not to return to work and officially resigned her position as a part-time nurse. She would surely miss it, but her fevers and coughs helped neither her nor her patients. This same month she was approved for disability and began to receive disability income.

Back in the Hospital

In September Jennie was admitted to Children's again. She was spiking high fevers and this time active mycobacterial infection was shown by chest x-ray and CT scan. Smear-positive culture after bronchoscopy showed presence of acid-fast bacilli (*M. abscessus*). On the basis of these findings and her escalating clinical condition she was begun on intravenous cefoxitin (2nd generation cephalosporin), amikacin (aminoglycoside), and oral clarithromycin (macrolide). Levels of amikacin were kept as low as possible because she developed tinnitus (ringing in the ears) and was at risk for progressive hearing loss.

Jennie remained hospitalized on this regimen for five months. Jake visited regularly but she missed her son Charlie dreadfully and often felt totally frustrated by her inability to take care of her family. Dr. Baker and the other physicians at Children's considered surgical removal of the upper left lobe of her lung, but abandoned the idea, much to her relief, because her NTM disease was not located in the left upper lobe alone and the loss would have outweighed the potential benefit.

After five months at Children's, Jennie was able to come home although she needed help to care for Charlie and she could not do heavy housework. Luckily, a follow-up high-resolution CT ten months after her therapy in the hospital showed complete resolution of the former visible abscess cavity, however her sputums remained smear negative but culture positive.

Jennie actually felt pretty good again. She was asymptomatic with stable PFTs (FVC, 90% and FEV_1 63%) for the next three months, but then her clinical symptoms recurred with evidence of a further abscess shown on chest CT. Because of this finding she was re-treated for another five- month course at Children's with intravenous cefoxitin, amikacin, and clarithro-mycin in addition to nebulized amikacin. This course of medication was discontinued because of a drop in her creatinine clearance. Dr. Baker surmised that the amikacin was toxic to her kidneys and was causing interstitial nephritis. After therapy she was symptom free again, with stable pulmonary function tests and chest x-rays but still her sputum cultures were positive.

Unforeseen Problem

Throughout her years of treatment for CF at Children's Hospital, Jennie was also under the care of a Primary Care Physician (PCP) affiliated with her Blue Cross/Blue Shield HMO for routine matters such as flu shots and annual gynecological exams. After her second five-month course of IV antibiotics at Children's, this physician who had cared for Jennie for many years called and told her during the telephone call that she could no longer be her primary care physician. She offered to look for another primary care practitioner for her.

Jennie was shocked. She asked, "Why?"

At first the physician said her office was too far away from Jennie's home, which was not a reason that rang true, especially after Jennie had kept appointments there with no difficulty for many years. Finally the physician added that as her primary care physician she felt uncomfortable that she was not included very much in the decision-making process regarding Jennie's CF therapy at Children's, the follow-ups, and the in-patient periods.

Having had experience with medical politics as a nurse, especially involving HMOs, Jennie surmised that the actual reason was that she was too expensive for the practice and her physician's colleagues had asked her to drop this cost-intensive patient. The last thing Jennie needed at this point was any insecurity in her medical care. She felt she had no choice but to accept her physician's offer to find her another practice willing to take over her basic care.

However, time went by and her physician did not find anyone. Jennie was obliged to stay with this practice two more years. The only contact with her PCP was to get necessary referrals to satisfy her HMO's requirements and when she needed her primary care physician's signature for therapy reasons. She felt the patient-doctor-relationship had been badly impaired with that telephone call and she was very uncomfortable when she had to call the practice.

In August 1999 Jennie was finally notified that she was eligible for Medicare coverage. Medicare is available for all individuals over 65 years of age, those with diagnosed end stage renal disease and the permanently disabled. According to the rules, 24 months had to elapse after being approved as disabled before she could enroll. After thinking it over, Jennie chose not to exercise this option because her coverage at Bluecross/Blueshield Value Plus HMO was excellent and it was not mandatory for her to go onto Medicare at this time.

Another Insurance Problem

Much to her surprise, in December 1999 Bluecross/Blueshield discontinued the Value Plus HMO for all subscribers. Jennie attempted to buy a policy from another insurance carrier but was denied because she was eligible for Medicare. She considered going on her husband, Jake's insurance, but that would exclude her from coverage for a year after enrolling because of her "pre-existing condition." So she finally went onto Medicare coverage in January 2000, as she was unable to insure herself any other way. There is a monthly premium that is deducted directly from her disability payments. In addition to Medicare, Jennie purchased supplementary Medex insurance for $350.00 per month to cover Medicare deductibles and co-pays.

If not for the "pre-existing condition" exclusion, Jennie would have preferred joining Jake's insurance plan. It would cover another possible six-month course of IV antibiotic therapy at home instead of in the hospital, which Medicare and Medex will not cover except for IV chemotherapy.

Medex would cover 80% of the antibiotics, but none of the supplies or equipment such as pumps, or nursing care to reaccess her portacath.

Outlook for the Future

Despite eight hospitalizations at Children's since her diagnosis of CF, Jennie feels well at the moment. She sees her pulmonologist, Dr. Baker every third month for a follow-up when her PFTs are measured and her ongoing therapy is determined for the near future. She has found a new Primary Care Physician and considers the information flow between this new doctor and Dr. Baker to be very good.

Besides the follow-ups every three months, Jennie goes to Children's every month to get her portacath flushed with heparin to prevent blood clots. At these visits she also has the opportunity to talk to social workers who are a part of her interdisciplinary care team. Five days a week a physical therapist comes to see her at home for chest percussion and vibration to help her breathe easier and to loosen the thick mucus from her airways. Like most CF patients, Jennie dislikes this necessary therapy and when she is busy with other things she is inclined to skip the visits. This means that she does not receive all of the physical therapy for which she is eligible. Eighty percent of the cost is covered by Medicare and 20% by Medex. Jake and Jennie's mother try to see that she does not skimp on this important care.

Jennie has been very satisfied with her care at Children's Hospital. There has been an easy flow of information between physicians and patient and she has been able to enter into decisions about her therapy. On her part, she expects compliance and honesty from herself. Her goals are to come back to her baseline functional status as measured by PFTs and appearance of her chest x-rays. Most of all, Jennie wants to be able to live, see her son grow up, and to enjoy a high quality of life. Actually, the term "quantity of life" has become even more important to her. To extend the "quantity of life" and keep the quality as tolerable as possible, she would use oxygen or agree to a lung transplant if necessary. Jennie hopes she won't have to deal with another five or six-month inpatient stay at Children's, but nothing is guaranteed and she thinks it is better to plan for the worst, hope for the best, and then deal as well as she can with whatever comes along.

Therapy

An endless rhythmic beat
A sort of faint knocking in the distance.
The hands of a mutual therapist
Pounding hard on the delicate chest
Beating delicately on the hard chest.
A cruel and merciless treatment
Squenching our precious time on this earth.
Depleting such valuable energy from our souls
As the timer ticks away - anyway.

Faster! Faster!

Harder! Harder!
Day in, day out
A mindless routine sets in.

The anxiety of every breath grows stronger
With each cupped pound.
The aching back, sore muscles.
The bleeding hands gloved for protection
The cup overflows.
What meaning gives this bizarre and undignified practice
To the core of our existence?

"I love you!" says the beating rhythm.
With each beat a reminder that you are no burden
A cherished moment of togetherness
Of deep connection between you and me.
A synchronicity of beating arms
Is a synchronicity of love and affection.

Isabel Stenzel Byrnes

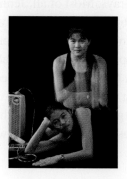

A Second Case: Thomas O'Connor

Thomas O'Connor is a 25-year-old student at Boston College whose Cystic Fibrosis (CF) was diagnosed soon after birth. As a newborn he had a meconium ileus, (a blocked lower intestinal tract) that was the first tip-off and the diagnosis was confirmed by sweat test. There was no family history of CF. He has lived near Boston his whole life and his CF treatment has been at Children's Hospital since the beginning.

Besides his studies, Thomas works at his father's waterproofing business where he answers phones in the office or helps to deliver supplies. He was admitted to Children's on March 3, 2001 for an elective "clean out." This means that he has been referred by his primary care physician (PCP) and will be hospitalized for about two weeks. He will have Pulmonary Function Tests (PFTs), IV antibiotic therapy, and a routine physical exam. The goal will be for him to get back to his baseline level of functioning as measured by his PFTs, and new x-rays will monitor the condition of his lungs.

Thomas is accustomed to these periodic stays at Children's. Although he doesn't welcome the interruption in his regular life with friends and school, he understands they are necessary and feels comfortable here. He definitely trusts his doctors and knows Children's is the best place for him to get treated. There is a good flow of information between his primary care practitioner and the doctors at Children's but if he has any acute problems his primary doctor is always the first one he turns to.

Thomas's Insurance

Thomas is insured through an HMO called Tufts Health Plan. He has never had any problems regarding his insurance or payments for therapy. Luckily he has no out-of-pocket costs for hospitalization but he has co-pays for medications, doctor's office visits, and any Emergency Room visits. He depends on regular care to keep him out of the ER.

As a child, Thomas did not have many questions related to his therapy, but since he turned 18 years of age seven years ago he has become more involved in the decision-making process. He always has the choice to say "yes" or "no" whenever a certain treatment is being considered and he can always ask for a second opinion. Sometimes too many opinions are overwhelming when the attending physicians and the residents in the hospital each seem to have a different slant on things. When his level of frustration rises, he has to remind himself to keep an open mind and listen to what his doctors are saying. Of course he realizes that it is in his best interest to be as compliant as possible with their recommendations. He also learns a lot about how to live with CF from the other patients.

A Clean-out at Beanpot Time

This is not Thomas's favorite week to be hospitalized. The annual Beanpot hockey tournament among Boston college teams gets underway this week and he will miss going out with his friends and having a few drinks and attending the games. He will watch them on TV though, that is for sure.

At admission Thomas presents with progressive cough and has had greenish sputum production over the previous two weeks. This signals an acute infection and precipitated his PCP's recommendation for a clean out at this time. Generally he feels quite healthy. This was the reason he deactivated himself from the lung transplant list. He thought it was too early to think about such an issue. What really bothers him at the moment is his dyspnea (shortness of breath) at rest and with a very low level of exertion. This leaves him feeling uncomfortable around his friends a lot of times and makes any conversation a torture.

During the past two or three years Thomas has been hospitalized three times for a clean out. The last one was in November 2000 when he spent three weeks in the hospital. That was more than his average length of time and more than the average for most CF patients at children's for this routine antibiotic therapy. The length of hospitalization is normally about 14 days. During these weeks he is treated with Imipramin, Tobramycin, and Clindamycin. He sees Dr. Davis, his pulmonologist, as an outpatient regularly every two months.

Thomas has had other stays at Children's beyond the clean outs. In 1982 a chronic infection turned into advanced bronchiectasis and in the end he had a left upper lobe lobectomy. In 1998 he had a G-tube placed to increase his nutritional status. The success of this is obvious as he now presents as a reasonably well-nourished young man. In February 2000 he had a bout of severe hemoptysis that required embolization and a stay in the hospital.

Today Dr. Crane, one of the residents greets him familiarly with, "Hi, Tom."

After the admission examination Dr. Crane will show him to his room where he will spend the next two weeks, and not more, if things go as planned. At the beginning Tom will have to share the room with another patient but he hopes he will soon have a room to himself, just in case his roommate doesn't like hockey.

Besides scattered bibasilar crackling due to the lung infection and the visible digital clubbing, Dr. Crane finds the rest of the physical examination normal including heart and lung sounds. Tom has no signs of wheezing, of chest pain or hemoptysis. On examination, no sinus tenderness is detectable. That is good because sinusitis is quite common among CF patients and Tom has suffered from the resulting headaches and lingering reservoir of infection in the past.

Clinical Practice Guidelines

Everything that will happen in the following days is determined by the Clinical Practice Guidelines (CPG) for CF patients. This is a document that has been designed by a committee at Children's Hospital to provide clinicians with an analytical framework for evaluation and treatment of CF, nevertheless, the clinicians' adherence to these guidelines is voluntary. According to the CPG, orders on admission include IV access, a physical therapy consult and the all-important pulmonary function tests (PFTs). Today Tom's PFTs are: FVC, 53% and FEV_1 29%.

"Those values will definitely have to improve," Dr. Crane observed.

Tom thought to himself that he would be happy to maintain his current PFTs and his weight, but he did not say so out loud. Of course, one had to balance the goals with what could be reached.

Dr. Crane also determines the actual regimen used for the IV therapy this time. According to the latest sensitivity study this would be Aztreonam, Clindamycin and Tobramycin. They will avoid Piperacillin, as Tom previously had signs of serum sickness after being treated with it.

The new sputum, that was sent for culture will give more information about current sensitivities and microbes. The rest of his medication will include Pancrease Tabs (lipase), Serevent (salmeterol), Flovent (fluticasone), Albuterol inhaler, ADEK as vitamin supplement, Prilosec (omeprazol) and Nutren 2.0, a nutrient.

Dr. Crane ordered a chest x-ray, bid Tom a pleasant "good day," and went on his way. The specialized nurse responsible for placing a peripherally inserted central venous catheter (PICC) came to insert the line. This is a familiar but not welcome procedure to Tom. This nurse is skillful and the line is placed quickly and successfully.

By the next morning the residents and the attendings have online access to the results of all the studies on Tom's pre-admission orders and the monitoring of his IV therapy, which had been started yesterday. According to the reports his electrolytes were normal, chemistries showed slightly elevated blood urea nitrogen (BUN) and alkaline phosphatase, (probably side effects of his IV antibiotic therapy) and Tobramycin levels were in the expected range. The rest of ordered studies include monitoring of the vitamin supplement therapy, and protein analysis with special attention to the IgE levels as a sign of aspergillus infection and hematology/coagulation. All of these results were normal.

In addition to the goal of his therapy to reestablish his PFT baseline, his nutritional status also has to be monitored. A GI consult might be called because of recent reflux symptoms. Perhaps he or she might order a pH probe or recommend increasing his Prilosec (omeprazol) dose if the symptoms persist. Because of possible nephrotoxicity of Tobramycin his renal function will be watched especially carefully.

A physical therapist comes to see Tom to determine this aspect of his treatment during the next two weeks. The goal is, as usual, to improve his pulmonary status by increasing aeration and to mobilize the sticky secretions in his lungs. After that a dietitian visits him to plan this important part of the therapy. He and his doctors definitely want to maintain his weight or even have him gain a few pounds. The rounding doctors came in an amorphous blob to inquire if Thomas had any other current problems besides the dyspnea, increased cough, and reflux. Having none, they shuffled off to the next patient and left him to turn on the TV and check on the schedule for the Beanpot hockey games.

Case 22: A Contrast in Care*

Corinna Jenderek

Arthur Taylor

Arthur Taylor's experience with COPD is fairly typical. He was born on July 13, 1923 in Brooklyn, New York. When he was still a very young boy his mother became seriously ill with tuberculosis and eventually died from it. After the death of his beloved mother he lived with his sister and his father. Immediately after high school, at the age of 18, he was drafted into the US Army and eventually sent to Italy to fight in World War II. During his time in the army he came down with pneumonia twice, but recovered quickly.

After the war was over, Arthur left the military service and attended college in New York. In college he was an excellent athlete. He loved to play tennis and did cross country running. He became interested in law and afterwards went to law school and graduated with a law degree from Brooklyn Law School in 1954. For many years he owned a small law firm in Manhattan where he employed six people. He enjoyed his work as a trial lawyer. When he was 71 years old, his physician diagnosed him with COPD and emphysema. This surprised him because at this time he did not

*These cases were written by Corinna Jenderek when she was a medical student at Ludwig Maximilians University and participated in the US-EU-MEE Student Exchange at Weill Medical College, Cornell University, New York in the spring of 2005.

have any trouble breathing. Even though almost everybody in the army smoked, he did not smoke until age 25 when he was in college. He smoked one and one-half packs a day until age 35 when he quit smoking because he started to wheeze. Since that time he has only smoked an occasional cigar. The ten years of smoking one and one-half packs a day added up to 15 pack years.

Arthur Taylor's Insurance

Arthur Taylor continued to work as a lawyer after his diagnosis of COPD, but about a year later he started to feel slightly short of breath when exercising and his cough in the mornings got worse. He decided to go to the outpatient clinic at Mount Sinai Hospital in New York City for treatment. He did not need to worry about the cost because like everybody else in the United States who is 65 years or older, he was covered by Medicare Parts A and B. Medicare Part A is hospitalization insurance and is taken care of by the US government through payroll taxes paid by employers and employees. Part B is medical insurance and covers most doctors' services and other medically necessary laboratory tests and medical services, except routine physical exams. Mr. Taylor pays a monthly premium for Medicare Part B, which was $66.60 per month in 2004, and a yearly deductible ($100 in 2004).

In addition, he purchased a good private health care plan for himself and his employees from a company called Transamerica Life Insurance. This supplemental plan covers the Medicare hospital deductible each time he stays in the hospital, the 20% co-payment for medical visits and the yearly Part B deductible. He has to pay for his prescription drugs out-of-pocket because the private insurance does not have a prescription drug benefit, and Medicare did not cover drugs until the institution of Medicare Part D in January 2006.

This private insurance provided good coverage for most treatments beyond what was paid for by Medicare. Mr. Taylor and his employees could freely choose the doctor or hospital where they wanted to be treated. As the employer, this insurance was very expensive and every year the high premium continued to rise. He considered it as part of the price of doing business, and felt it was worth the money because it not only provided for his own medical needs, and those of his wife, but kept his six employees happy and saved him the expense of high employee turnover.

Treatment at Mount Sinai Hospital

Mr. Taylor was very familiar with the Mount Sinai outpatient clinic because he went there regularly for follow-up care and basic preventive medicine, such as a yearly flu shot. After his diagnosis with COPD the doctors added a chest x-ray and Pulmonary Function Tests (PFTs) to his routine examinations. The PFTs, also called "spirometry," measure the volume of air inhaled or exhaled by the lung and how efficiently the lungs transfer oxygen from the air into the bloodstream. In spite of his slight shortness of breath, Mr. Taylor continued to work at his law practice.

When he was 75 years old, Arthur Taylor experienced another medical crisis. He suddenly awoke one morning with poor vision. He went to an ophthalmologist and was diagnosed with retinopathy pigmentosa, a disease of the retina that causes night blindness and a reduction of the visual field. Soon afterwards he retired as an active lawyer because he could not see properly in the courtroom and felt that he could not represent his clients adequately. He continued to follow up on his old cases though, and loved to keep in touch with what was going on in court.

As his COPD gradually became worse over the years, Mr. Taylor was able to do less and less of the physical activities he previously enjoyed. He fondly remembered skiing at the Matterhorn in Switzerland and regularly running in Central Park in Manhattan. He enjoyed playing tennis and other outdoor activities. About five years after his diagnosis, his breathing started to get a lot worse, and now, after five more years he has trouble keeping up with his same-aged friends and can walk only two or three blocks until he has to stop to catch his breath. He can climb two or three flights of stairs at a slow pace and then has to stop and rest. He and his wife, Samantha, live on the Upper East Side in Manhattan and lead a happy life together but his COPD and his shortness of breath bothers him a lot.

Luckily, Arthur Taylor has never been admitted to the hospital because of a COPD exacerbation. His cough and dyspnea has been worsening but has remained on a stable level over the past few years. Only once when he was feeling a lot worse than usual, his pulmonologist gave him prednisone, which he took for four days and felt better. At age 79 he decided to go into a private pulmonary rehabilitation program to try to increase his lung function. Medicare covered the costs but his health did not improve significantly. On the MMRC Dyspnea scale (a scale that measures breathlessness after certain defined physical activities) he scored 2 on a scale of 0–4. His cough produced yellow-tinged sputum about two or three times a week.

Treatment at New York Presbyterian

When he read in an article in the New York Times Magazine about the treatment of different diseases at various hospitals in New York that ranked New York Presbyterian Hospital first for research and treatment of emphysema and COPD, he decided to go to their outpatient clinic, hoping for more successful treatment. At New York Presbyterian spirometry was done again showing FVC (forced vital capacity) 62% of predicted, FEV_1 (forced expiratory volume in 1 second) 33% of predicted and Diffusion Capacity (DCLO, how efficiently the lungs transport air into the bloodstream) 40%. After Mr. Taylor was given a puff of bronchodialator medication, his FEV_1/FVC was 0.41. This indicates severe COPD according to the definition of the Global Initiative for Chronic Obstructive Lung Disease (GOLD III). He is prescribed appropriate medication and scheduled for follow-up appointments.

Because he has the means to pay for private health insurance in addition to Medicare, Mr. Taylor is not at all worried about the cost of his tests and treatment. In addition to his primary care physician, who is an internist, he regularly sees a cardiologist, a pulmonologist, and an ophthalmologist. His wife receives all the medical care she needs as well. They are both very satisfied with their medical care.

Richard Coleman

Richard Coleman was born on June 20, 1954 in the Bronx in one of the poorest areas in that borough of New York City. His father, William, worked as a carpenter after serving in World War II and his mother,

Amanda, cared for Richard and his two older sisters, Lydia and Cathy. Richard went to public high school in his neighborhood and there he soon got his first taste of nicotine when he started to smoke cigarettes at age 13. "Everybody smoked at my high school and I wanted to be part of the gang," he said.

It was never very hard for Richard to get cigarettes because both of his parents were heavy smokers. Often Richard's two uncles would stop by for a drink and leave their half-full cigarette packs with the 13-year-old boy. Thus cigarettes became a part of the daily life for the adolescent Richard, and by the age of 14 he was smoking one and one-half packs a day.

After finishing high school, Richard decided to go into the army. This was a good opportunity for him to get out of the Bronx. He spent four years in Europe in active military service and another four years in the Army Reserve in the United States. After returning to New York he worked in many different jobs. First he worked as a carpenter for a few years, then he worked in a jail, and later he worked as a security guard at court. Although he always had a job, his salaries were low and living in New York is very expensive.

Illness Strikes

A few years ago, when Richard was working as a security guard, he noticed that he was not able to go from the subway station to his work without resting to catch his breath after a few blocks. Prior to this he also had bouts of chronic sinusitis and bronchitis. He often coughed in the mornings after getting up and his nose dripped constantly. Now he coughed every morning and his shortness of breath had slowly worsened over the last two or three years. His cough produced about a cupful of white, clear sputum every morning. Richard did not pay much attention to these symptoms at first because he had been a healthy man all his life. Apart from the usual childhood diseases he had only undergone surgery for a hernia in 1975. He did not consider going to a doctor to receive treatment for his breathing symptoms.

But one morning in March 2002, Richard Coleman could hardly stop coughing. He remembers that the sputum he was coughing up was not clear anymore, but had a yellowish color. He wanted to get ready to go to work, but getting dressed was too much exertion for him and he quickly became short of breath. His roommate finally called an ambulance and he was taken to the emergency room at North Central Bronx Hospital where he instantly received oxygen to relieve his severe dyspnea. He was earning a relatively small salary as a security guard, but still too much to be entitled to Medicaid. At that time in New York State he had to earn less than $7908 a year as a single adult to qualify for Medicaid.

Richard had always gone to the VA Medical Center in the Bronx when he needed to see a doctor and for his medication. As a veteran he qualified for care there and did not have any other health insurance. This time the ambulance brought him to North Central Bronx Hospital because it was closer to his house. He could receive treatment for his acute shortness of breath there because it is one of the few public hospitals in New York City that serves as a provider of choice for the more vulnerable populations; the medically underinsured, uninsured, and recipients of Medicaid. He could have been treated at other hospitals as well because of a US law called EMTALA (Emergency Medical Treatment and Active Labor Act). According to this law, Emergency Departments in US hospitals have to accept all patients but they are only required to examine and stabilize them and arrange for appropriate transfer. He would not have been admitted as an in-patient.

Since Mr. Coleman had a productive cough for more than three consecutive months in two consecutive years, his illness met the definition of chronic bronchitis. He also had a history of dyspnea and exposure to risk factors such as cigarette smoking; therefore COPD was a highly suspected diagnosis. To confirm this diagnosis spirometry was performed. His post-bronchodilator FEV_1/FVC of less than 0.7 confirmed the presence of airflow limitation that is not fully reversible, thus the diagnosis of COPD was confirmed. After being treated for a week with appropriate medication and antibiotics at the North Central Bronx Hospital he was discharged.

Now Mr. Coleman's treatment could be continued on an outpatient basis at the VA hospital. He was advised to quit smoking to improve his symptoms. He did try nicotine patches for a while and stopped smoking for a few days, but then his cravings for cigarettes became overwhelming and he lit his first cigarette again.

Homeless

Two years ago, something happened that changed the direction of Richard's life. He was staying in a small apartment in the Bronx and he got into a fight with his roommate, who kicked him out. From that day on, he did not have a place to stay, and he suddenly found himself living on the streets. He did not have any close friends that he could live with and his parents had both died from lung cancer; his father in 1976 and his mother in 2001. His two uncles living in New York City had also died of lung cancer. After he left home to join the army in 1972, Richard did not have any more contact with his two older sisters, Lydia and Cathy.

Shortly after Richard became homeless, he lost his job as a security guard and so was forced to "retire" at the age of 48. Since he served in the army for a total of eight years, he was entitled to receive a small pension from the Veterans Administration (VA). After living on the streets for a few weeks, Richard Coleman decided to turn to a Neighborhood Center to ask for help. They gave him a referral to the U.S. Department of Veteran's Affairs and their domicile program. This is a place where he and other homeless people can stay during the day. They get hot food, they can change and wash their clothes, and hang out during the day. If they leave the domicile during the day they have to be back at 5:30 p.m. At night a van takes them to different churches around the city where beds are available for them and they can stay overnight. In the morning a van takes them back to the domicile.

The VA Domicile Program and Relapse

To actually get accepted into the domicile as a full-service client, Richard needed to stay in a VA hospital for 28 days in July 2003. This was required to stop smoking and get "clean" before he could be allowed to stay at the domicile. During his stay in the VA hospital Richard was not allowed to smoke at all. He received nicotine patches to lessen his craving for cigarettes. He also got acupuncture treatments twice to help him quit smoking, although he did not think it worked. After his 28-day stay at the VA hospital, he was allowed to go to the Veterans Affairs domicile.

Unfortunately, as soon as he left the VA hospital, Richard started to smoke again. At the beginning he smoked eight to ten cigarettes a day while being on nicotine patches, which was potentially dangerous to his health. Soon he was back to smoking one and one-half packs a day.

Three years later, his coughing has gotten worse. He coughs every morning, when he exercises, and after smoking cigarettes. His cough produces a lot of sputum and he is only able to walk up two flights of stairs or two blocks until he has to stop and catch his breath. His disease is now diagnosed as GOLD stage III according to the Global Initiative for Chronic Obstructive Lung Disease. On the Medical Research Council dyspnea scale (0–4) he is rated as a 2. Another spirometry was done that showed severe obstruction. He continues to be treated and receive his medication at the VA hospital and does not have a primary care doctor. Because he is homeless and only receives a small pension from the VA, his medical care is covered completely and he does not have to make a co-payment for his treatment or pay for his prescription medications.

After smoking an average of one and one-half packs a day for 37 years, Richard has a history of 57 pack years. He does not intend to quit smoking because he has half-heartedly tried several times without success and he feels that he needs the nicotine and the cigarettes to stand the stress of being homeless and sleeping in churches at night. Continuing to smoke will not only make his COPD worse, but it also puts him at great risk for other smoking-related diseases such as lung cancer. He also has a strong family history of this disease because his mother, father, and two uncles died of it.

Every homeless person at the VA domicile is assigned to a social worker. Richard Coleman's social worker is working on getting him a housing voucher and finding him a place to stay so he can take better care of his health and his future can look a little brighter.

Case 23: Bluegrass Music and Back Pain*

Malte Rieken

Adam Manson's Story

In early June 2001, Adam Manson is referred to the Freedom Trail Clinic by a social worker in his subsidized housing complex in central Boston. A few weeks later he signs his treatment contract at this psychiatric outpatient clinic and is registered as a new patient with the diagnosis of paranoid schizophrenia. MassHealth, the Massachusetts Medicaid program for low-income people, or those with disabilities or who have been out of work for a long time will pay for his treatment.

That same day he is seen by Dr. Miller, his new psychiatrist. Dr. Miller remembers Mr. Manson as a friendly 52-year-old man, who has been living alone for a long time in an apartment not far from Boston's public garden and the Charles River. Mr. Manson worked for more than 25 years as a civilian employee of the army, but had to leave his job following a hospitalization in March and April 2001 and is now awaiting a pension. His diagnosis and treatment for mental illness concerned the supervisor at his place of employment and he suggested that Mr. Manson should retire.

---

*This case study was written by Malte Rieken when he was a medical student at Ludwig Maximilians University, Munich, Germany and participated in the US-EU-MEE student exchange at Harvard Medical School in 2005.

Dr. Miller notes that the appearance of his new patient is unkempt and he is reluctant to converse about his mental illness; instead he complains about his back pain and insomnia.

"Doc, I have had this terrible pain ever since my back went out on me in 1982, and I haven't had a good night's sleep in three or four years."

"How have you been mentally? Is your schizophrenia causing problems?" Dr. Miller asked.

"Oh no, no. I'm not schizophrenic!"

Dr. Miller notices in his chart that Mr. Manson takes antipsychotic medication. He also notes that he shows signs of a tardive dyskinesia, especially of the jaw. Tardive dyskinesias are involuntary movements of the tongue, lips, face, trunk, and extremities that occur in patients treated with long-term dopaminergic antagonist medications but Mr. Manson states emphatically that he never took such a medication.

In general Mr. Manson seems to have little insight into his illness and it is hard for Dr. Miller to get more information from him because his concentration is impaired and he cannot remember details about his life. Moreover, Mr. Manson gets more and more anxious during the conversation and several times spontaneously starts playing Bluegrass music on his harmonica.

To get more information about his new patient, Dr. Miller calls Mr. Manson's social worker at the housing complex where he lives and Mr. Manson's former employer as well. He finds out that Mr. Manson has been on medication for several years, which led to partial remission of his illness. He had always been capable of gainful employment and although he was hospitalized a few times, he worked for the army for more than 25 years. But since early 2001, Mr. Manson began to decompensate gradually and his condition deteriorated. He became more and more disorganized and the easiest things seemed to become too complicated for him. Finally, he could not even log-on to his computer and it became apparent that he was no longer able to do his job. His employer had no other option than to admit him to a hospital. With this information things became clearer to Dr. Miller and he thought about what he should do next.

Mr. Manson's History

Mr. Manson was born in 1948 and spent his youth in a small town near Boston, Massachusetts. After he finished high school he went to junior college for two years. From 1968 to 1972 he worked in a post office, sorting letters, packing parcels and doing documentation work. He typically worked the night shift, from 6 pm to 6 am. When he came home from work, he was often not able to sleep, although he tried to.

"So I was watching TV the whole day, trying to get some sleep. But I couldn't sleep for more than two hours. In the evening I went back to work, often without having slept one minute," he told Dr. Miller when they met again.

The hard work at the post office often led to back pain, but at first he did not take this pain seriously. Finally he left the job because he was not able to stand the pain any longer.

By now Mr. Manson had developed a level of confidence in Dr. Miller and talked more freely about his past life.

"In 1975 I got a feeling I never had before. I began to have the feeling that cars were following me. When I walked down the street, I often turned around to look for suspicious things happening behind me. I thought that someone put a tracer on my parent's telephone and I feared that there was a plot against me. When I was 27 years old, I joined the army, because I hoped the army would protect me from my persecutors. Feeling that someone is following you by car, it is like fight or flight. So I fled. I joined the army."

Mr. Manson's army experience lasted only a few months, but he was given a civil service discharge and his persecution mania disappeared.

"I don't know if it was imagination or it was real. But the feeling went away," he said.

Since 1976 Mr. Manson worked as a civilian employee of the army. He worked at the same place doing paper work until he retired in 2001. In 1980 his back pain increased and the doctors told him he had a herniated disc. They never suggested surgery, but they did prescribe analgesic medication, which he continues to take. Around the same time, his primary care physician (PCP) referred him to a psychiatrist. For Mr. Manson it has never been clear why his PCP took that action and he denies the existence of any symptoms at that time.

"Why the hell did my PCP refer me to a psychiatrist? I needed an orthopedic doctor, not a psychiatrist," he declares vehemently.

New treatment efforts

Dr. Miller thought carefully about the information he had about Mr. Manson. Although Mr. Manson's medical records indicated a diagnosis of schizophrenia, for Dr. Miller the diagnosis was far from certain. Mr. Manson's withdrawn behavior, his memory and concentration impairment, the flat mood and the anxious affect can all be symptoms of schizophrenia, but can occur in many other mental illnesses as well. According to the DSM-IV-Diagnostic Criteria for Schizophrenia two or more of the following characteristic symptoms must exist, each for a significant period of time during a one-month period, to diagnose schizophrenia:

- delusions
- hallucinations
- disorganized speech
- grossly disorganized or catatonic behavior
- negative symptoms, like affective flattening, alogia or avolition

Only one of the symptoms listed is required if delusions are bizarre or hallucinations consist of a voice keeping up a running commentary on the person's behavior or thoughts, or two or more voices conversing with each other. Furthermore, in many patients, major areas of functioning, such as work, interpersonal relations, or self-care are markedly below the person's usual level.

Thinking about these criteria and applying them to Mr. Manson, Dr. Miller decided to try prescribing the anti-psychotic medication, olanzapine. Although Mr. Manson did not show psychotic symptoms, his behavior was disorganized and in conversation he revealed thought disorders, especially incoherent thoughts.

In the following weeks, Mr. Manson's condition improves. His mood stabilizes, he is less anxious and as he is getting used to his new therapeutic environment. He begins to share his greatest passion with the people there: the passion for music, especially Bluegrass music. He often arrives earlier for his appointments at the Freedom Trail Clinic so he can play his harmonica for the other patients.

"I just want to entertain these people a little bit."

At the beginning of December 2001 Mr. Manson accepts the opportunity to enroll in a medication trial, the CATIE-study. The CATIE-study is a randomized, double blind trial, comparing the efficiency of different antipsychotic medications. Neither Mr. Manson, nor Dr. Miller knows which medication Mr. Manson's is receiving.

Because clozapine is included in the study, which can lead to serious side effects in one to two percent of patients, Mr. Manson now has to have blood tests every week. During the first weeks of the study his condition deteriorates continuously. He is getting more disorganized, restless and anxious. He is suspicious about things happening around his apartment, but has no further explanation. The social worker at his housing complex reports episodes of delusion of persecution happening at home, but Mr. Manson denies this. He sees his medical problems as caused by his back pain, which influences his mind, but in his view, there is no connection between schizophrenia and his complaints.

Hospitalization

Finally, Mr. Manson becomes clearly psychotic. On January 9, 2002 he goes to the Emergency Department of Arbour Hospital, a psychiatric hospital in Boston. He is anxious, disorganized and paranoid. He is convinced that someone put a drug into his Diet Coke and he is worried about the effects the drug might have on his body. He is very frightened and has no understanding of the things happening around him.

"I don't know what happened," he says. "Someone slipped me a Mickey. I think I need a new therapist and psychiatrist because I heard that Lindeman went down last night and they are going to have to rebuild it all over again." (Lindeman is the Lindeman Mental Health Center where the Freedom Trail Clinic is located.)

When he is admitted to the hospital, Mr. Manson is frightened but cooperative. He denies hallucinations but appears to be deluded. Despite his disorganized and psychotic state, Mr. Manson asks the clinicians to get in touch with his therapists and arrange follow-up.

The clinicians immediately take Mr. Manson off the CATIE study drug and start to treat him with clozapine, taking the chance that he had been receiving a different drug during the study. Doses were continuously increased and his mental status began to improve dramatically as the dose reached 300 mg per day. Clozapine was ultimately increased to 375 mg per day with good results. Mr. Manson tolerated the new medication very well and was discharged after three weeks.

Mr. Manson looks back on his stay in the hospital very critically.

"I felt well cared-for," he states, "but it was a mistake to go there — a very strange experience. I am glad to get out of there. If you're not crazy when you go in, you are crazy when you get out."

Follow-up after Hospitalization

Following hospitalization, it was clear that Mr. Manson's care needed to be changed. Concerning his psychiatric treatment, Dr. Miller decided that the medication with clozapine should be continued. Clozapine belongs to the group of so-called atypical antipsychotics, which work well for a broad range of patients. They are at least as effective as typical antipsychotics like haloperidol, but not as likely to cause the symptoms of rigidity and tremor that result from interference in the regulation of the dopamine balance in the brain or to worsen tardive dyskenesia. Clozapine is probably the most effective drug for many severely ill patients but its use is complicated by the risk of a severe reduction in white blood cell count and dangerous neuromuscular effects. Nevertheless, for Mr. Manson, clozapine remained the only therapeutic option because of its ability to reduce the symptoms of patients with tardive dyskinesia without worsening that condition. After his hospitalization, Mr. Manson steadily improved as his doses of clozapine were increased and finally stabilized at 500 mg a day. He is followed carefully with blood tests every week for adverse effects of the drug.

Mr. Manson decides to join a therapy group, which meets every two weeks at the Freedom Trail Clinic. In these therapeutic meetings, patients discuss their experiences with schizophrenia and the treatment of their mental illness. Other changes are necessary in Mr. Manson's medical follow-up by his primary care physician. During his stay in Arbour Hospital doctors discovered that he has diabetes. His blood glucose values were not alarming, but high enough for them to prescribe the oral medications metformin, a blood glucose reducer, and rosiglitazone, an insulin sensitizer. His high blood pressure was treated with lisinopril, an ACE-inhibitor, and his reflux esophagitis was treated with omeprazole, a drug that inhibits gastric acid secretion.

Since his discharge from the hospital it is obvious that Mr. Manson needs help to function in everyday life. His social worker requested a visiting nurse who now comes to Mr. Manson's home once a day to give him his medication, check his blood sugar level, and make a short psychiatric assessment of his current condition. MassHealth, the same Massachusetts Medicaid insurance that pays for his inpatient and outpatient psychiatric care, pays for this service.

Financial Problems

While his psychiatric and medical condition improved, a new financial problem confronted Mr. Manson. After he left his job in 2001 he received a civil service retirement from the army, but he also applied for Supplemental Security Income (SSI). SSI is a federal income supplement program funded by general tax revenues. It is designed to help aged, blind and disabled people who have little or no income and provides cash to meet basic needs for food, clothing and shelter. The current benefit rate for an individual at the time was $579 per month. Nobody could recall how it happened, but Mr. Manson was erroneously determined to be eligible for SSI. The mistake was discovered after he had received several payments from SSI and he was told to pay back $9000. The social worker at the Freedom Trail Clinic helped to make an arrangement that he has to pay back $100 a month for a period of 90 months. Considering his monthly retirement income of $1000 and his expenses for rent ($475), payment for Medicaid ($66.60), co-payments for medication, the costs for the diabetes care unit ($97) and the back payment of $100, it is not surprising that Mr. Manson is in tight financial circumstances.

Improvement

Mr. Manson continually improves under the treatment with clozapine. He does not have any psychotic episodes and becomes less disorganized. Seroquel, an atypical antipsychotic, is added to his medication to treat his insomnia. After he had panic attacks, especially in small rooms and in the morning between 3 and 5 o'clock, Dr. Miller prescribes clonazepam, an anti-anxiety drug, and diazepam, commonly known as Valium. With this medication, the symptoms of Mr. Manson's mental illness are controlled sufficiently and he is able to live his life as independently as possible. The residual symptoms of his schizophrenia, in particular mild thought disorder and mild disorganization, seem to affect him only a little. Asked about the greatest wish he has for his future, Mr. Manson answers, "I wish that my back pain would go away."

Part III

Sweden:
Liberal Political Climate
and Comprehensive Health Care

Part III

Sweden:
Liberal Political Climate
and Comprehensive Health Care

7

Swedish and US Health Care Systems Compared

Miriam S. Wetzel, PhD

"All public power in Sweden proceeds from the people."

First sentence in the Swedish Constitution [1]

The Country

Sweden has a lot going for it.

It is by any measure a first-world country with bustling cities, rich natural resources, and a highly literate population.[2] The products of its manufacturing and service industries are valued around the world. Having overcome a slowdown in the 1990s, the economy has stabilized and unemployment has settled down to an estimated 5.6 to 6.6%.[3,4] As a consequence of the ongoing global economic crisis, which is having its effect even on Sweden, economists predict that it may increase to as much as 10% in 2010. With an average per capita income of $34,780 in Purchasing Power Parity, Sweden is among the top nine percent of the world's countries.[5]

Sweden's geographic area of approximately 450,000 square kilometers (173,700 square miles) is slightly larger than the state of California. In spite of its northerly location, the climate is surprisingly moderate, especially in the southern part, because of the influence of the Gulf

Stream. The northern 15% of Sweden is above the Arctic Circle where the sun never sets for part of each summer and the winter nights are 24 hours long and extremely cold.[6] Eighty-three percent of the 9.1 million people in Sweden live in urban areas.[7] By comparison, in California there are 9.9 million people in Los Angeles County alone and more than 35 million in the entire state.[8]

Culture and Politics

Sweden has a long and proud history dating back to the seventh and eighth centuries when Swedish merchant ships plied the seas of the known world. Its history is not without conflict with its Scandinavian neighbors and other European countries, but in modern times Sweden maintained neutrality during both World Wars and has not been involved in armed conflict since 1814. Its government is a parliamentary democracy with a constitutional monarchy. King Carl XVI Gustaf is the formal head of state but the country is ruled by the Government, headed by the Prime Minister and accountable to the 349-member Riksdag. Members of the Riksdag are chosen by popular election every four years.[9] In 1995 Sweden joined the European Union[10] after much debate and some controversy but ultimately rejected the Euro as their form of currency in favor of retaining the Swedish krona (SEK).[11]

Life in modern Sweden is much like that in other developed countries. Swedish culture is deeply rooted in family, religion, and national holiday celebrations. Swedes enjoy sports of all kinds, especially outdoor sports and activities that bring them in close proximity to nature. Swedish citizens also enjoy a full range of music, film, art, and literature.[12] In Sweden schooling is compulsory from age 7 to 16. The government pays for appropriate education at all levels including vocational and academic programs after upper-secondary school for students who qualify for it.[13] Sweden boasts 39 institutions of higher education, including the famous Karolinska Institute.[14]

The political climate in Sweden is decidedly liberal, with the Social Democratic Party predominating for most of the years since 1932.[15] Since the election in 2006 however, Prime Minister Fredrik Reinfeldt has led a coalition of four center-right parties. Reinfeldt received the Bachelor of

Science in Business Administration and economics from Stockholm University in 1990. He came up through the ranks of the Moderate Party since his student days when he was a member of the Executive Committee of the Young Moderates. He held minor positions in Stockholm governance and became a member of the Riksdag in 1991 and chair of the Moderate Party in 2003.

Postwar prosperity fueled Sweden's welfare policies, which continue to provide a wide range of social benefits for Swedish citizens. These include government-provided daycare for children from 2–6 years of age, generous sick leave and disability benefits, long-term care, old age pension, and health care.[16]

Health Care in Sweden

With its long-standing social welfare policies, health care in Sweden is considered a responsibility of the government and is paid for almost entirely out of tax money. Principles of solidarity mandate that medical care be provided equally for every citizen according to need. From the patient's perspective, this means there are physicians, nurses, clinics, and hospitals to turn to in case of illness or medical concerns and the government will heavily subsidize the cost. The health care provider of first choice is a family physician or General Practitioner (GP) located in the geographic area where the citizen resides, but since January 2003, Swedish people are free to seek health care anywhere in the country.[17] Furthermore, they can choose to go directly to a specialist without a referral from a GP.

Along with General Practitioners, the **primary level** of health care in Sweden includes local health clinics staffed by physicians, physiotherapists, midwives, and district nurses. General Practitioners are mostly salaried employees of the county councils. To become a GP, Swedish physicians have to pass five years of training in family medicine or "*allmän medicin*." The district nurses are authorized to evaluate, treat, and prescribe medications for children or adult patients. As part of this system, free clinics are provided for prenatal care and health care for children. Vaccinations, health check-ups and consultations are free of charge for all children up to 18 years of age. There are social and health services to enable elderly and disabled persons to continue to live in their own homes as long as possible. Those who cannot stay at home may live in nursing homes or subsidized apartments with access to nursing services 24 hours a day.[18]

The hospital system provides the **secondary level** of health care in Sweden. An entirely different group of physicians staffs the hospitals. The patient's own GP has no responsibility for treatment and care in the hospital. As we see in the case of Professor Bruun (An Up and Down Course)[19] choosing your own physician is not the norm in the hospital. However, when the patient, Professor Bruun, was dissatisfied with one of his physicians, he turned to "personal connections" to have him replaced with a physician he trusted.

Many hospital clinics offer both outpatient and inpatient care in specialty areas such as surgery, medicine, and radiology. Eight regional hospitals provide a wider range of specialists and treat the more rare and complicated diseases and injuries.[20] Sweden has seen an upward trend in the number of specialists compared to GPs[21] even as the number of outpatient visits greatly increased. Day surgery and many other tests and treatments are now available outside the hospital but still require the services of specialist physicians. Specialists are usually salaried employees as well.

The concept of Integrated Care has been growing in Sweden. This involves cooperation between county councils and municipalities to provide for the needs of the elderly. Local hospitals, health centers, and social services work together to coordinate this care.[22] This is especially advantageous to patients with chronic conditions that require regular monitoring and occasional inpatient treatment.

Comparisons with US Health Care

In both the United States and Sweden, health care is provided by a wide array of physicians, nurses, and adjunct medical professionals. The GP is the mainstay of medical care for many citizens in both countries but reliance on the GP is not as great in Sweden as in some European counties since citizens can go directly to a specialist. A referral to see a specialist may be required in the US under certain insurance plans, or in a

Health Maintenance Organization (HMO) but other plans allow the patient to see a specialist without a referral. In the United States a GP may follow the patient and provide care in the hospital, however the "hospitalist," or hospital-based physician is an idea that has been borrowed from European countries and is gaining favor in the US. In the US one of the hospitalist's primary duties is to keep the patient's GP informed about the patient's treatment and progress.

Health care in the US is paid for by a combination of public (government) and private resources, but private insurance predominates. Sweden's population is covered by tax paid health care provided by the government, however required patient fees typically pay for approximately three percent of the cost so it is not entirely free to the individual.[23] It is common for the county councils to contract and pay for as much as 10% of services from private health care providers and this arrangement is steadily growing.[24] The Swedish government health care system is comprehensive and compulsory, so there has been little need for private insurance. In 2003 only about 2.3% of the population had supplementary insurance.[25] However, in Sweden as in Denmark and Germany, the role of private or supplementary insurance is increasing.

Sweden's spending for health care as percent of GDP has held steady around nine percent for several years (9.1% in 2007). The per capita expenditure in 2007 was $3,323 (US$ Purchasing Power Parity), less than half that of the United States at $7,290.[26] Many Americans envy Sweden's universal health care but are not enthusiastic about the huge tax increases it would require, especially in the face of an economic downturn. The public health insurance programs of Medicare for the elderly, Medicaid for low income and disabled people and CHIPRA health coverage for

Table 7.1. OECD Health Data 2009. June 2009[27]

Sweden Public Expenditure	81.7
Sweden Private Expenditure	18.3
United States Public Expenditure	45.4
United States Private Expenditure	54.6

Public/Private Expenditures for Health Care as Percent of Total Health Care 2007.

children have steadily grown in scope, but still largely leave out middle class working Americans.[28]

Organization of Swedish Health Care

How is Sweden's comprehensive system of health care organized to provide for every citizen? The Swedes have developed a fairly straightforward organization for delivery of health care by establishing clear lines of responsibility that follow the three major organizational levels of the government: state, county councils, and municipalities. Swedes also pay taxes at these three levels from which health care is paid. The national social welfare and solidarity philosophy is expressed in the mandate for the health care system as stated in the Swedish Health and Medical Services Act of 1982.

> "Health and medical services are aimed at assuring the entire population of good health and of care on equal terms. Care shall be provided with due respect for the equal worth of all people and the dignity of the individual. Priority shall be given to those who are in the greatest need of health and medical care. (Section 2, "Goals").[29]

At the **State** level, the Ministry of Health and Social Affairs has the responsibility to carry out this mandate. This agency analyzes the state of health and medical care in the country, develops new legislative proposals for health care and social welfare, negotiates with the county councils and municipalities who must carry out the health care plans, and works to meet the objectives set by the Riksdag (Swedish Parliament). Several agencies assist this ministry.[30]

National Board of Health and Welfare (SoS) — Oversees implementation of government policies related to health and social services. Evaluates health services to see if they fulfill the intentions of the central government.
The Medical Responsibility Board (HSAN) — Investigates complaints about care or treatment of patients.
Swedish Council on Technology Assessment in Health Care (SBU) — Reviews scientific data and provides information to guide decision-making.
Medical Products Agency (LMV) — Approves medical products. Ensures access to safe and effective products of high quality. Unlike

other governmental agencies, this agency is funded by charges to manufacturers.

Pharmaceutical Benefits Board (LFN) — Decides which pharmaceuticals are to be included in health benefits and determines price of these products. It recommends generics whenever possible.

Agencies under the Ministry of Health and Social Affairs have a great deal of autonomy. The government sets the general role and responsibilities and provides resources. The agency is free to decide how to use these resources to implement its mission.

The 21 **County Councils** comprise the next level of organization of Swedish health care. They are responsible for primary care and hospital care including public health and prevention measures. They are grouped into six geographical regions and are responsible for health care, education, transportation, culture, and regional development in areas with populations as large as 1.9 million.[31] The eight regional university hospitals where a high level of specialized care is offered and most teaching and research takes place are located in Gothenburg, Uppsala, Lund, Malmö, Linköping, Umeå, Örebro (no university but a high-level hospital), and the Karolinska Hospital in Stockholm.[32]

In addition there are 66 county hospitals and over 1000 health centers.[33] The County Councils can also purchase or contract for services from private companies, voluntary organizations and foundations. These purchases vary widely among the counties but have increased from a total of slightly less than SEK 12 billion in 2001 to SEK 14.7 billion in 2005.[34] These expenditures are mainly for the purchase of outpatient services and represent just under 10% of the county councils' net costs for health and medical care, excluding dental care.

Sweden's 290 **municipalities** are responsible for care beyond the hospital and primary care setting.[35] Half of the municipalities have agreed with the county councils to be responsible for the care of elderly and disabled people living at home, including the mentally disabled.[36] Many services are provided to enable people to remain in their own homes, which is considered to be the most desirable setting for their care. When the local community is unable to assume the care of a patient who has been approved for discharge from the hospital, it is still the community's responsibility to pay for the care of that patient while he or

she remains hospitalized.[37] This sometimes causes conflict over financial resources between the county councils and the local authorities. One
of the tasks of the Swedish Association of Local Authorities and
Regions is to mediate such conflicts and to clarify the rules that apply to
both the patient and the care provider.[38] Health care workers are union-
ized, which provides them with an organization to bargain collectively
with the government.[39]

A Day at Vardcentral

This first-hand account of a day in the Swedish health care system, written by one of the medical students participating in the US-EU-MEE
student exchange program in 2001, illuminates details of the system from
the perspective of health care personnel. Names have been changed.[40]

A typical day for a GP is to arrive at the office around 8 am and for
half an hour take phone calls that have been previously screened by one
of the nurses on phone duty. According to Dr. Erik Nilsson, a GP at the
vardcentral in Sodra Sandby, a few patients may also confer with him by
email. After receiving calls, Dr. Nilsson attends to patients until approximately 5 pm. In some areas of the country, the GP has an additional role
of traveling within the district to attend to acute problems, which have
been triaged to him by the central emergency service.

The district nurse has a similar work schedule, and depending on the
place of employment, she or he may also travel within the district to
respond to health care needs in patients' homes or travel to other health
care centers to confer with other district nurses or physicians. After 5 pm,
the vardcentral is closed and patients' records are not accessible until the
following day. Patients have no access to the GPs and district nurses after
normal working hours.

The numerous responsibilities of the GPs and district nurses often put
a strain on those practicing in the vardcentral. According to Nurse Alice
Olsson, when she worked as a district nurse, she had so many responsibilities that she was not able to perform her duties effectively. When her
complaints were not satisfactorily addressed by the politicians, she quit
her position as district nurse. She added that sometimes "the people
who are working with the [health care] administration are not listening.

The politicians think [health care] is like a machine, but ill people, they are not machines."

Nurse Olsson suggested that the GPs sometimes feel the same stress. Since the government officials don't increase the funding for centers based on patient load, she says, "there is a problem for the good doctors because all the patients want to go to them and if you're a good doctor, you just get more tired, you don't get more money."

The result of the increasing workload and inadequate compensation has led many nurses and physicians to leave their practices and find employment in other areas such as the pharmaceutical industry. Moreover, because there are fewer health caretakers, there is less of a focus on preventive medicine because there are not enough resources and professionals to support widespread screening programs."

For some people many things have already moved too quickly in Sweden's health care system while for others change moves too slowly through the political process. Some significant changes have taken place since this US-EU-MEE student's experience in the vardcentral. By 2003 Sweden had adopted a system of electronic health records that made information available to health care providers if a patient enters a hospital after clinic hours.[41]

OECD data shows Sweden ranking fairly evenly with Norway and Denmark, and ahead of the US in the number of physicians per 1000 population from 1996 to 2004. There were more nurses per 1000 population in Denmark than in Sweden or the US in the late 1990s but Norway consistently ranked ahead of the other three. By 2004, Sweden's numbers began to catch up but they still had slightly fewer physicians per 1000 population than Norway and Denmark (3.4 versus 3.5 and 3.6) but more than the US, which had 2.4. By 2004, Sweden had considerably fewer nurses than Norway (10.6 versus 14.9; see Tables 7.2 and 7.3).[42] Comparisons with Germany are also interesting. OECD data for the number of nurses in the US from 2003–2005 are not available.

Paying for Health Care in Sweden

In 2005 Sweden spent SEK 175 billion (approximately USD $27 billion) on health care and services, including a subsidy on pharmaceuticals.

Table 7.2.   Practicing physicians per 1000 population — Density/1000 pop.

	1996	1998	2000	2002	2003	2004	2005
Denmark	3.2	3.2	3.3	3.4	3.4	3.6	
Norway	2.8	2.7	2.9	3.4	3.4	3.5	3.7
Sweden	2.9	3.0	3.1	3.3	3.3	3.4	
Germany	3.1	3.2	3.3	3.3	3.4	3.4	3.4
United States	2.2	2.3	2.3	2.3	2.4	2.4	2.4

Source: OECD Health Data 2007, July 2007.

Table 7.3.   Practicing nurses per 1000 population — Density /1000 pop.

	1996	1998	2000	2002	2003	2004	2005
Denmark	7.0	7.2	7.5	7.6	7.5	7.7	
Norway		9.8	10.3	14.2	14.4	14.9	15.4
Sweden	9.6	9.7	9.9	10.2	10.4	10.6	
Germany		9.2	9.4	9.6	9.7	9.7	9.7
United States	7.9	7.9	8.0	7.9			

Source: OECD Health Data 2007, July 2007.

This represented 9.1% of GDP — a spending level that has remained fairly constant since the early 1980s. This expenditure is financed from the following sources:[43]

Local taxation by county councils	71%
State contribution	16%
Patient fees	3%
Sales, contributions and other sources	10%

Patient fees and co-pays represent a small but important part of the revenue stream. They lessen the tax burden and act as a mild deterrent to overusing services. In January 2007 exchange rates, hospitalization costs the individual patient SEK 80 ($12) per day. Consultation with a primary care physician is SEK 100–150, ($15–22) with higher co-pays for consultation with a specialist. The county councils set the fees for this outpatient care hence they may vary slightly from county to county. There is a cap of SEK 900 ($132) per year for medical consultations. When this amount has been paid, all further consultations for the rest of the year are free of charge, counting from the date of the first consultation. Likewise, no one has to pay more than SEK 900 per year for prescribed medications, making the total cost for consultations and prescriptions SEK 1800 ($264) per year.[44]

Taxes

Clearly, providing a wide range of social services, including health care for all citizens requires a strong financial commitment. The people and government of Sweden make this commitment in the form of some of the highest taxes in the world.[45] Taxation in general is not easy to understand, and Sweden's tax system is no exception. In addition to tax on ordinary income, there are corporate taxes, capital gains taxes and the Value Added Tax (VAT) on goods and services. There are complicated restrictions and exemptions. Individual earned income tax is set by the "municipality of residence" at rates ranging from 29 to 35%. There is no uniform tax rate across the country but the National Board of Health and Welfare and the Swedish Association of Local Authorities and Regions are working to establish a system for comparing and evaluating goals and results. This should help county councils and municipalities to manage and streamline health care and provide the public with more easily accessible information.[46]

An additional tax of 20–25% is levied on income over SEK 327,600 per year (in 2007), the US equivalent of about $51,000. Add to this, taxes of around 30% on interest, dividends, and capital gains and the Value Added Tax (VAT) of 25% on purchases (lower rates on food and certain other essentials) and it is easy to see that the Swedish people bear a heavy tax burden. The government has discontinued the tax that was imposed on personal wealth above SEK 1.5 million for single people and SEK 3.0 million for couples and replaced the present real estate tax with a low property-related charge in 2008.[47]

The people of Sweden have been accustomed to high taxes for a long time and expect that they will receive many services from the government in return for the investment of a large part of their income. As one US-EU-MEE exchange student put it, "...most still believe in the system and would advocate raising taxes or shifting more government money to health care rather than cutting any support or services." He also mentions that the younger population is not quite so confident and realizes that with the increasing costs of health care, the system is not sustainable without raising taxes.[48]

Even government policymakers acknowledge that taxes are at the maximum and cannot go higher without repercussions. Sweden has already experienced some unintended consequences from the heavy tax burden. High taxes are thought to cause wealthy citizens to shelter money outside the country to avoid the wealth tax and the previous additional marginal tax on income over SEK 327,600. By some estimates, as much as SEK 974 billion (about $151 billion) is sheltered abroad.[49] During the 1990s when the Swedish economy was struggling, public revenue (taxes) represented more than 60% of the Gross Domestic Product. Since 2000, this percentage has gradually decreased but is still high at 56.3% in 2007. By comparison, in the US in 2000, public revenue as percent of GDP was 35.9%, and in 2007, 34.6%.[50]

When taxes are at a high level, as in Sweden, there is the danger that young college graduates and other workers will lose the motivation to work or will seek careers outside the country. Working across countries is seen as a trend that has increased since Sweden joined the European Union. Some people were concerned about a "brain drain" throughout the early 1990s when the number of physicians and nurses per 1000 population in Sweden declined as these professionals sought better working conditions and situations where they could keep more of their earnings. A number of qualified physicians left the country for better salaries in Norway, the UK or other European Union countries; however migration has decreased during the past few years.

High taxes on businesses have also curtailed entrepreneurship in Sweden.[51] Thirty-four of the one hundred companies that hire the most workers are run by entrepreneurs, but none of these companies was founded after 1970.[52] Although the present government has made some constructive reforms designed to increase incentives to work rather than live on government allowances, more could be done to create a better business climate. For example, mandatory overtime pay rates increase by about 70% on weekday evenings and 100% on weekends. This makes it difficult for restaurants and retail stores to afford to be open at those times but they still keep very generous daytime and evening hours.[53]

Other Tax-Supported Social Programs

Parental benefits

It is not only health care that has kept Sweden's taxes high, but its other generous social programs as well. Parents are eligible for an extensive list of benefits that include a child allowance of SEK 1,050 per month for all children up to the age of 16. A supplementary amount is paid to families with two or more children. Maintenance support may be extended up to age 20 if the child is studying in compulsory school or upper secondary school.

A total of 480 days of paid parental leave is available and may be taken by either parent any time until the child's eighth birthday. This leave is available to the mother 60 days before her expected due date.[54] During the first 390 days, the paid benefit is equal to 80% of salary up to a designated ceiling. Parents with low income or no income at all are paid at the basic level of SEK 180 per day for 390 days. Other parental benefits include care allowance for a sick or disabled child, a government grant of SEK 40,000 to assist with inter-county adoption and a housing allowance for households with children living at home, depending on the number of children and the household income.[55]

Pensions

Taxes also help to support a generous pension plan. Sweden was the first country in the world to establish a government-run pension system. By 1998, the tax-based entitlement program was running into financial difficulty because of economic and demographic changes. As a solution, the Swedish government offered partial privatization to the workers.[56] The first contributions to this Premier Pension Fund were made in 2000.[57] In this two-tiered system, the total contribution is 18.5% of gross earnings, shared by the individual and his or her employer. Sixteen percent finances the first tier, or income pension (known as the PAYG system), which pays a benefit based on a worker's earnings. Years spent in military service, child rearing, and higher education also count toward pension and years of residence in Sweden is factored into the payout formula. The other 2.5% is put into an individual, self-directed retirement account. The government guarantees a basic minimum pension for individuals with low or no earnings.[58]

Swedish officials realized that the former tax-funded pension system was not sustainable for the same reasons that threaten the US Social Security system. With people living longer after retirement and a shrinking workforce, payout would soon surpass incoming funds. They also noted that the system was inherently unfair. Workers contributed over their entire working lifetimes but their pensions were calculated only on their 15 years of highest earnings. This tended to redistribute income from mostly low-income workers to those with shorter work histories and higher earnings.[59]

In the new system, instead of being calculated on years in the workforce, the pension is based on the amount of taxes a worker has paid into the system. In addition, investments from the privatization contribution will have the opportunity to gain value over time. A separate account is set up for each worker where he or she can see the account grow. Women are expected to qualify for their own pensions without a spousal benefit.[60] With more women in the workforce the government needs to supply a reliable source of day care. Most Swedish women put their children in government-run day care at age one or one-and-a half and go back to work.[61] One critic estimates that a typical child in Sweden will have 275 adult caretakers by the time he or she is six years old.[62] The lack of women at home means they are also not available for the care of sick or elderly family members.

When partial privatization of pensions was first proposed, some lawmakers were opposed but ultimately legislators from the right and the left united in support of the new system. Sweden's experience has proven that it is possible to change a huge government entitlement. According to Göran Normann, Ph.D, president of Normann Economics International and an associate professor of economics at the University of Lund, among the many benefits Sweden has experienced from these changes are increased incentive to work, increased national savings, a flexible retirement age, lower taxes and less government spending. He says, "The reforms in Sweden could be a model for US lawmakers as they grapple with the problems of Social Security."[63]

Sick leave

One of Sweden's greatest problems during the 1990s and into the beginning of the twenty-first century was the growing disinclination of its citizens to work. In October 2003, Kristina Persson, the deputy governor of Sweden, emphasized this point, saying:

> "Finally, the decisive factor for the labour supply is how many hours we work. The number of hours worked has fallen recently for several reasons: overtime has declined, part-time work has increased and absence to care for [one's] own children has also risen. But the single biggest reason and consequently the most serious problem in Sweden is sick leave. Both the number and length of absences due to sickness have risen sharply in recent years, thus entailing a reduction in working hours per employee. ...our demographic situation will require measures that result in a higher average number of hours worked, a larger number of workers ... and an increase in immigration. This assumes that we want to keep or enhance our welfare system."[64]

In a survey of 20 countries, the OECD reported that Sweden had the highest number of working days lost because of sickness.[65] The report stated that on a normal day, nearly a fifth of the potential workforce in Sweden is on sick leave or receiving a disability benefit. The 2007 edition of the Statistical Yearbook of Sweden noted that the number of sick days doubled in the five years between 1997 and 2002, from 47,573,000 to 110,805,000 annually before showing a decrease in 2003,[66] which has continued thereafter.

The government set a target of halving the number of sick days by the year 2008. Other western European countries also have generous sick leave, but by all measures, Sweden tops the charts (see Figure 7.1). It is

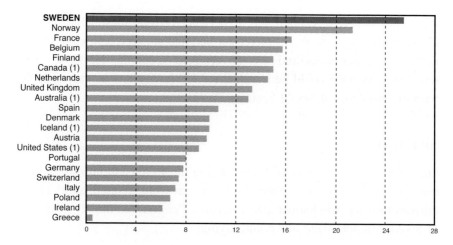

Figure 7.1.   OECD Economic Review of Sweden 2005.[67]

Working days lost per full-time equivalent employee per year, 2004.

not uncommon for workers in Sweden to be on sick leave for a number of years at 80% of salary. Bertil Thorslund, a caseworker at Sweden's Social Insurance Agency is quoted as saying, "If the sick leave levels in Sweden really were an indicator of how sick we are, we would be facing a plague here."[68]

Stress, anxiety, depression and a condition called "dejection" accounted for 33 to 40% of time taken off from work in 2006. When Prime Minister Fredrik Reinfeldt proposed to institute a law that would limit paid sick leave to three weeks for people suffering from "mental burnout" he was met with widespread criticism, causing the plan to be shelved.[69]

Typically many workers use long-term sick leave as a route to early retirement. By taking this path they receive a higher pension when they turn 65. In June 2005, the Swedish daily paper *Aftonbladet* quoted official numbers stating that 500,000 people in Sweden were on early retirement with 68,000 of them between the ages of 20 and 40. According to *Aftonbladet* computations, by the time all 500,000 reach age 65, Sweden will have paid out 700 billion kronor in compensation.[70]

The government is taking action to make it worthwhile for people to work. In 2002 the disability pension system was reformed and renamed "sickness compensation," for persons aged 30–64 and "activity compensation" for those aged 19–29. Activity pension is granted for a limited period of time, at most three years.[71] The OECD published specific recommendations that would help the Swedish government to curb the use of sick leave and early retirement. They recommended a "mutual obligations" approach, putting greater responsibility on the sick person, the employer, and the social insurance office.[72] Requests for sick leave would be more carefully scrutinized and not so readily granted, recipients would be required to participate in vocational rehabilitation, and the continuing need for sick leave would be periodically reassessed.

Efforts to Control Health Care Costs

Rising health care costs are a global problem affecting the US, Sweden and almost all other industrialized countries. While some of the major problems of an aging population, a decreasing workforce and the escalating cost of medical technology will only be addressed over time, in the past decade both Sweden and the US have looked for immediate ways to cut costs. For example, outpatient care and day surgery have greatly increased, thus allowing a reduction in the average length of inpatient stays and the number of acute care hospital beds (See Tables 7.4 and 7.5).[73] While these changes seem small, when applied across the population they have an important impact.

Both countries have increased the use of non-MD health care providers. Sweden's district nurses are a good example. The US is seeing more use of nurse practitioners and physicians' assistants in the rapid care

Table 7.4. Average length of in-patient stay — days.

	1996	1998	2000	2002	2003	2004	2005
Germany	12.9	11.7	11.4	10.9	10.6	10.4	10.2
Denmark	6.7	6.7	6.2	6.0	5.8	5.6	5.4
Sweden	7.5	6.6	6.4	6.2	6.1	6.0	6.1
United States	7.5	7.1	6.8	6.6	6.5	6.5	6.5

Table 7.5.   Acute care beds per 1000 population.

	1996	1998	2000	2002	2003	2004	2005
Denmark	3.8	3.6	3.5	3.4	3.3	3.1	
Germany	7.3	7.0	6.8	6.6	6.6	6.4	6.4
Sweden	2.8	2.6	2.4	2.3	2.2	2.2	2.2
United States	3.3	3.1	2.9	2.9	2.8	2.8	2.7

Source: OECD Health Data 2007, July 07.

clinics that are becoming increasingly available.[74] Pharmaceutical expenses are lower in Sweden than in most OECD countries. Low prices for the public are thought to be the reason rather than a low level of use. In 2002, Sweden instituted a pricing and reimbursement policy that features a cost-effectiveness analysis of drugs and requires the use of the lowest priced generic alternative.[75]

In 1990 a new approach to health care in Stockholm — the Stockholm Model — drew international attention. It featured public-private cooperation, consumer choice, and performance-based financial incentives for providers. The adoption of Diagnosis Related Groups (DRGs) had a dramatic effect on lowering costs and increasing efficiency in Sweden's hospitals. Prior to that time, hospitals were costing the County Councils more and more and delivering less and less as waiting lists grew longer. With the adoption of DRGs, hospitals were paid according to what they really delivered, not what the budget dictated.[76] This gave hospital managers an incentive to improve performance and productivity. In 1990 the Stockholm plan lowered costs, improved efficiency and reduced wait times in the Stockholm area.

Economic Turnaround

To keep and enhance their welfare system and control a growing deficit, since the late 1990s Sweden has adopted bold market-economy type reforms. Widespread deregulation and regulatory reform helped to encourage competition and boost productivity. Prime Minister Frederik Reinfeldt ran for election in 2006 on a platform called Alliance for

Sweden, which emphasized reducing unemployment. In a speech at the London School of Economics he said,

> "No employment–no opportunity for people to obtain a livelihood for themselves and their families. No employment–no progress. No employment–no welfare services, no schools, no childcare and no elderly care."[77]

From the experience of Sweden it is clear that no government, even in a wealthy country, can meet unlimited demands for health care and other social services with inevitably limited resources. Providing those resources rests squarely on the shoulders of working men and women. As Sweden adopts market-based solutions and the US moves in the direction of more government provided care, the two countries can learn a lot from each other.

Acknowledgments

We gratefully acknowledge the contribution of US-EU-MEE students Ylva Andersson Carlsson, Rotonya McCants Carr, Kim Gosai, Malin Inghammar, Aliyah Sohani, Peter Tang and Kavid Udompanyanan in the preparation of this chapter. Special thanks to Rotonya McCants Carr for the account of a day at Vardcentral. We also thank Stefan Lindgren, M.D. for mentoring the US students in Sweden, for his careful reading of the Swedish chapter and his helpful suggestions.

8

Cases Written by US Students in Sweden

Case 24: It's Lucky We Found It*

Rotonya McCants Carr

Lying on the examining table, Niklas Nilsson is quite unfazed by the unusual request to be interviewed by a stranger trying to learn about the Swedish health care system. He is a 41-year-old businessman who was diagnosed with colon cancer in the fall of 2000. "It was a lucky thing we found it," he said. Reacting to the confused look on my face, he added that the discovery of the cancer was almost by chance.

"My system wasn't going well," he said in an embarrassed way. "My only symptoms were gas and some stomach problems. Occasionally I had 'fresh blood,' but I thought this was caused by the hemorrhoids with which I was diagnosed some years ago. The blood did not alarm me because I'd seen it before," he explained.

In answer to my questions he said he didn't have any weakness or weight loss; nor did he notice a change in the shape of his stool. He only said that sometimes he had loose stool, and sometimes he had hard stool. Otherwise he felt fine. Even the left groin pain he had been having for about a year did not disturb him. He attributed all of his symptoms to "too

---

*This case was written by Rotonya McCants Carr when she was a medical student at Cornell University and participated in the US-EU-MEE program at Lund University, Sweden in 2001.

much milk or coffee," but when he traveled to places like South America on business where he noted the coffee was actually much stronger, he tended to feel better.

"I thought it might be stress, since I felt better when I was away from home," he continued. "After all, I had the responsibility of my company and my employees, and at the same time I was diagnosed with cancer, I found out my fiancée, Inga, and I were expecting a baby. Imagine that, a first baby at my age!"

Mr. Nilsson admitted that had it not been for his having a fiancée who is a physician in training, he might not have gone to see the doctor about his symptoms.

"For years I rarely saw a doctor. I led a relatively healthy lifestyle, exercising two or three times a week, but I saw no reason to visit the doctor regularly. As a child, everyone is 'in the program' and you are taken care of. As an adult, there is no program and you have to look out for yourself. Some larger companies require their employees to get yearly check-ups, but smaller companies like mine usually do not."

I asked when he had last seen a doctor before his diagnosis of colon cancer.

"It was five years ago, when I was diagnosed with hemorrhoids, but my last complete physical exam was two years before that when I had the required medical exam for flight certification, and before that it was at the age of 17 when I last saw a doctor for an examination for military service."

So, it was on advice from his fiancée, Inga, that he decided to see his local general practitioner (GP). His examination was positive only for hemorrhoids and the GP ordered routine laboratory studies at that time, which came back normal. He also had a negative endoscopy and rectoscopy.

"My GP would have stopped there but Inga insisted I have a further work-up because she was afraid I might have polyps like my father did. My GP was persuaded, reluctantly, to send me for a barium enema study, which I got approximately two weeks later."

It was this test that showed the cause of Mr. Nilsson's vague symptoms: a 5 cm left flexure stricture consistent with a left upper quadrant tumor. Getting this test was the "lucky thing" about which he spoke at the start of the interview.

Two weeks after the results of the barium enema, Mr. Nilsson saw surgeons at Helsingborg Hospital. His operation date was set for September 28, 2000, another two weeks later. Pre-operatively, Mr. Nilsson had a colonoscopy, which showed two 1 cm polyps in the descending colon, which were excised and shown to be adenomas with moderate dysplasia. He also got a pre-operative ultrasound of the abdomen, which showed a normal liver.

"By that time I had plenty to be stressed about," Mr. Nilsson continued, "but I wanted to know all I could about my disease. Inga graduated from medical school and will continue her training after a few months of maternity leave. She brought home medical books and together we read everything we could find about colon cancer."

"When I had my surgery and was told I had a 'left hemicolectomy,' I understood that this meant that a part of my left colon was removed. The specimen was sent to pathology and was also sent to Lund for a genetics study since I am younger than the normal age for colon cancer and I have a known family history of colon polyps."

"During the operation, a 1 cm nodule was also excised from my liver. When Inga asked my surgeon at Helsingborg, Dr. Svensson, what his initial gut feeling was about the nodule, he replied, 'I don't think it's anything significant.'"

One week later, however, the pathology report not only read that Mr. Nilsson had adenocarcinoma of the colon, but also that the nodule excised from the liver was in fact consistent with a metastasis from the colon.

"This finding was really bad for my frame of mind," Mr. Nilsson stated, "as I had been encouraged by Dr. Svensson's opinion before the final pathology results returned that the nodule appeared benign."

Because no one at Helsingborg performed liver resections, Mr. Nilsson had to go somewhere else for a partial liver resection. He decided on the Lund University Hospital for this procedure. One week after he received news of his metastasis, Mr. Nilsson met with a liver surgeon at the Lund University Hospital. At this time Mr. Nilsson, having read a great deal about his illness, requested a PET scan pre-operatively to look for other metastases.

"There was much resistance to this idea," Mr. Nilsson recalls, "but because I had the financial means to pay for the procedure and a fiancée with connections in the medical field, I was able to get the PET scan in Copenhagen, Denmark just one week later. This test was, of course, extremely important for my peace of mind."

The PET scan showed that there was increased uptake between the right and left lobes, consistent with the surgical findings, and that there was no increased uptake elsewhere in the body. Dr. Hans Jansson, a general surgeon at the Lund University Hospital, said that Mr. Nilsson was the first patient at his hospital to get a PET scan for this indication; but now more colon cancer patients have been referred to Copenhagen for pre-operative PET scans. Mr. Nilsson also got both CT and MRI before having his liver resection, exactly one month after his first surgery. Results of both studies were consistent with the PET scan findings.

On November 8, 2000, Mr. Nilsson underwent a wedge resection of the liver with 1.5 cm margins. He received peri-operative and intra-operative ultrasounds. Intraoperatively, small granules were found on his colon, but they were negative for malignancy. There was also some inflammation seen below his spleen, but pathology showed only fat necrosis. Both of Mr. Nilsson's surgeries were without complication and required average hospital stays of 5 days each.

On November 22, Mr. Nilsson was started on neoadjuvant chemotherapy with 5-flurauracil (5-FU) for 12 cycles and was receiving his 10th cycle during our initial interview. In Sweden, the Duke's classi-fication system is used. A "Duke's A tumor" is limited to the mucosa, a "Duke's B1" extends into the muscularis propria but not the serosa, a "Duke's B2" penetrates the bowel wall but does not extend to the lymphatics or distantly; a "Duke's C" involves regional lymph nodes; and a "Duke's D" represents distant metastatic disease.

The decision for chemotherapy was made because although locally, his cancer was a Duke's stage B, he had a solitary metastasis with nega-tive lymph nodes making his clinical scenario more like a Duke's stage C. Both the surgeons at Helsingborg and Lund agreed that Mr. Nilsson's presentation was not consistent with a true metastatic process. According to Dr. Jansson, he felt that the solitary nodule in the liver was more likely to have been caused by the escape of one cancer cell than the progressive spread of disease. Therefore, he felt comfortable treating Mr. Nilsson as a Duke's C patient. As a Duke's C patient, adjuvant chemotherapy with

5-FU, leucovorin, and oxiplatin had been established to increase survival by as much as 50% in a published study by Giachetti, *et al.* (*Annals of Oncology* 10; 1999: 663–669).

The method of delivery of the chemotherapy was also discussed. Mr. Nilsson had the option to either receive his chemotherapy as an inpatient or to receive infusion therapy as an outpatient. For Mr. Nilsson, there was no debate. It made the most sense for him to receive the infusion therapy so he could spend more time at home with his fiancée and newborn son. The regimen consisted of 12 cycles of two-day therapy every two weeks. On each of the two days, he received a bolus injection at the clinic in the morning. The rest of his chemotherapy was delivered over 22 hours as an outpatient via an implantable portacath. After the completion of his 12 cycles, Mr. Nilsson will have a follow-up PET scan to assess the effectiveness of his chemotherapy. Other surveillance measures have yet to be determined, as he does not represent the typical patient with colon cancer.

Speaking to Mr. Nilsson about his illness gave me some insight into his character. He seemed careful to convey that he did not have much difficulty with his diagnosis and disease course. Perhaps most interesting was how he described this process as a "change" in his life.

"All my life, life has been changing," he said. "I like change. The only time I really worried was in the beginning when I didn't have any information. Once Inga helped me to find information and become actively involved in my care, I worried very little — literally only moments of each day. Suddenly it drops into your consciousness and you deal with it and then you're normal again."

This way of dealing with his illness in some ways mirrors Mr. Nilsson's life course. Born in a town in Skåne just north of Lund, he is the only male of four children and describes his childhood as "protected." He went to school in his hometown and in Gothenburg when he was young and later continued his formal education in Lund at the University of Lund and the Lund Institute of Technology. He studied physics and was about to defend his dissertation when he had an idea to start his own company. He didn't enjoy the topic of his thesis very much and saw his company as the root of his true career happiness.

So, for 12 years, he has sustained a successful company that employs a few other people and whose purpose is to "develop optical spectroscopies for control of metallurgic processes" — quite a mouthful. In layman's terms he explains that it means using light emissions to gain information about different types of metals including steel and copper. His company is active in various parts of the world. He does not consider himself a workaholic, but says that he is "focused and intense when working." He seems to have always had challenges; but more significantly, has been able to surmount them. Even his hobbies can be described as somewhat intense: skiing and sailing and flying, for which he had that flight medical certification years ago, but has never been able to pursue as a private pilot because of the high cost in Sweden.

Besides all the difficulty he faces with his illness and his work, Mr. Nilsson is quite involved with the care of his son who was born just eight weeks prior to our first interview. This new priority in his life has partially influenced the decision by his surgical team in Lund to treat him aggressively, according to Dr. Jansson, offering him therapies that have only been shown to be efficacious in colon cancer patients whose disease is not exactly representative of Mr. Nilsson's.

I was invited to visit Mr. Nilsson at his home. Watching him with Inga and their newborn son, I understood the decision to treat him with all that was available. He seemed rejuvenated when spending time with his family despite his feeling somewhat weary and unclear of thought after receiving the first part of his 11th chemotherapy cycle earlier that day. Suddenly, the small reminder of his illness (which was the pouch he wore around his waist to hold the chemotherapy drug) faded in importance as I watched him and his fiancée care for their son. I wished the best for him, with a complete recovery and many happy years ahead.

Sweden and US Contrasts

Colon cancer is a disease that interests me and also was a good example in which to observe the differences in health care in Sweden and the US. There are several steps in the development of colon cancer including genetic mutations and chromosomal deletions, disturbances of epithelial proliferation, microadenoma development, polyp development and finally cancer development. Both the activation of oncogenes and the inactivation of tumor-suppressor genes have been implicated in colorectal cancer.

Additionally, in the familial type, such as Mr. Nilsson's, inherited germline mutations have been identified. This is why it was important for his excised polyps to undergo genetic analysis.

Early discovery of these polyps is very important. Although countries differ on screening policies, the diagnosis is done universally by endoscopy or barium radiography. In Sweden, there is limited availabilty of colonoscopy, so barium radiography is more commonly used, although Dr. Jansson told me that he expects a shift to colonoscopy in the next five years or sooner.

Another difference between Sweden and the United States is that in Sweden people are not urged to get screened for colorectal cancer. This policy, however, may change soon as physicians are meeting in Stockholm this year (2001) to discuss the results of screening studies completed in Denmark. Some physicians in Sweden are not in favor of widespread screening because of the additional strain it would impose on the already long waiting lists. One of the doctors said, "...because we already have 1000 people on the waiting list, and to this we would add many more with screening...education of patients and doctors is the key...or if you can find risk groups, that is much better." For now, most patients with colorectal cancer are diagnosed just as Mr. Nilsson was, that is after being seen for specific complaints including rectal bleeding, weakness, abdominal discomfort, and change in bowel pattern.

In Sweden, although the process of diagnosis may move slowly, once a presumptive diagnosis is made, referral to a colorectal surgeon and subsequent surgery happen relatively quickly, as they did with Mr. Nilsson. Exploration of the rest of the bowel and inspection and palpation of the liver are also part of the surgery. In Sweden, intra-operative ultrasound is also used for examination of the liver, as was seen in Mr. Nilsson's case.

In Sweden, patients who have had surgery for colorectal cancer are followed with a post-op check one month after surgery. This meeting offers a chance for the patient to ask questions as well as have an examination for operative complications. Approximately 3–6 months after surgery, a colonoscopy is performed to check for missed tumors. For Dukes C patients who have received chemotherapy, the colonoscopic surveillance is performed after completion of the chemotherapy cycles.

In general, surveillance after curative resection is a much-debated issue. Even among institutions in Sweden where so much seems to be regulated by the government, there are disparities. For example, at the University of Lund, patients with "clean colons" after surgery are sent back to their general practitioners for continuous follow-up with yearly or every six-month liver function tests and carcinoembryonic antigen (CEA) tests, depending on the severity of the stage. Abnormalities require a referral back to the surgeon. At Helsingborg Hospital, surgeons do not use serial tests for follow-up. Neither center uses serial CTs because of studies in Sweden that have shown no benefit of CTs as a follow-up tool, according to Dr. Svensson.

The lack of a consensus for follow-up of colon cancer patients can prove quite confusing to patients. In Mr. Nilsson's case, his follow-up regimen is largely dependent on the center where he receives his care. Currently, the plan for him is still being discussed but will include following him with another PET scan after completion of his chemotherapy.

Case 25: Taking it Easy in Landskrona*

Aliyah Sohani

It was in mid-December, about four months before I met him, that Mr. Ericsson began to notice a difference in his health. At first he didn't think that anything was wrong because his symptoms were so minor, and he didn't feel he needed to visit a doctor.

Mr. Ericsson had reached the age of 63 in tremendously good health. Besides an injury to his knee in a motorcycle accident during his late teenage years and an appendectomy in his twenties, he was never ill. He had one chronic condition; lower-back pain had been bothering him for several years now, and more so in the last several months. He took a daily dose of naprosyn, an anti-inflammatory and analgesic medication, but it wasn't helping the pain as much as it used to. For this reason, he had taken early retirement in June from his job as a technical manager at a construction machinery manufacturing company.

Retirement

Mr. Ericsson was with the same company for 14 years and felt sad to leave his colleagues, many of whom had become friends. He worked very hard

---

*This case was written by Aliyah Sohani when she was a student at Harvard Medical School and participated in the US-EU-MEE project at Lund University, Sweden, in the spring of 2001.

all his life, in various construction and repair jobs since the age of 19. He felt that in light of his worsening back pain, it made sense to retire early and "take it easy." Besides, he and his wife had taken out private pension insurance for just such an occurrence and were now looking forward to enjoying a life of hobbies and traveling without any financial worries. When they reach the official retirement age of 65, they will also receive their pensioner's income from the Swedish government, as mandated by its comprehensive social welfare legislation.

At age 63, a few months into early retirement, Mr. Ericsson was enjoying a more relaxing life and looking forward to spending Christmas with his wife, mother, daughter and two young grandsons. This was when he first noticed the cough. It was a dry cough that irritated the back of his throat. Although it was accompanied by occasional chills, he didn't think much of it. He had visited his former company's doctor just the previous month, in November, and had a complete physical exam and blood tests. He was told that he was in the best of health and had nothing to worry about. Not being one to complain about little things, Mr. Ericsson decided not to go to see a general practitioner at his local health center about his cough. He just wanted to enjoy a nice holiday with his family.

Trouble Ahead

The cough persisted through the holiday period into the New Year and became more bothersome. One morning in mid-January when Mr. Ericsson began coughing up blood he knew something was definitely wrong. He and his wife both began to worry and he decided that he must see the doctor. He chose to go to a general practitioner (GP) at his local health center in Landskrona, a town in the southern region of Sweden known as Skåne.

At the clinic in Landskrona that same day, the general practitioner, whom Mr. Ericsson was meeting for the first time, performed a physical exam, and ordered blood tests and a chest x-ray. He heard some distant lung sounds on the right but the blood tests revealed normal values. The chest x-ray, performed three days later, was normal. He told Mr. Ericsson that the abnormal lung sounds could be caused by his 50-year smoking history. Since the chest x-ray was normal, he felt that Mr. Ericsson was healthy and could go home. Mr. Ericsson was relieved by this news.

Mr. Ericsson's symptoms did not get better over the next few days — in fact, they got worse. He continued to cough up blood more frequently and in larger amounts, sometimes up to two or three times a day. It was worse when he was lying down — he would cough and have difficulty breathing. He began sleeping on two, then three, then four pillows, until eventually he could only sleep sitting up.

It was during this time that he began to suspect that something was quite wrong with him. A few of his friends in his social circle and at work had received a diagnosis of lung cancer. Many were current or former smokers. Mr. Ericsson himself felt that he had quite a mild smoking habit compared to some of his friends. He had begun smoking at the age of 12, and had smoked one to two packs a day until the age of 28. He did not quit entirely then, but limited his habit to social events where he would smoke a few cigarettes while having drinks. In the recent past, he only smoked two to three cigarettes, five or six times a year.

Mr. Ericsson returned to the same GP at the local clinic two weeks after his first visit in greater physical and emotional distress. The doctor, upon hearing Mr. Ericsson's further history, ordered another chest x-ray, including an additional oblique view where Mr. Ericsson turned fifteen degrees to one side. On this view, a small round 1.5 cm infiltrate in Mr. Ericsson's right lung could be seen, raising suspicion for cancer.

Is it Cancer?

Mr. Ericsson was told of the chest x-ray results by the general practitioner in his office. The doctor began approaching the possibilities in a round-about way, not mentioning the word "cancer" at first. Mr. Ericsson's greatest fear wasn't the diagnosis itself. From seeing the same symptoms in his friends and colleagues, he strongly suspected what it would be. He asked the doctor, "Do I have cancer?"

"That is a possibility," the doctor replied.

Thinking immediately of his two young grandsons, Mr. Ericsson asked the next logical question, "How long do I have to live?"

"That question can be better answered after a few more tests and a consultation with a lung specialist. I want you to see one as soon as possible."

He returned home to his wife to tell her the news.

Mr. Ericsson was put on a waiting list for computed tomography (CT) of his chest, which was to be performed locally in Landskrona. While he was awaiting this test, his GP made a referral for him to see a lung specialist and gave him a choice of whom to see. In theory, he could choose any specialist he wished in any region of Sweden, even without a referral. The general practitioner recommended two larger, regional hospitals, both some distance away, but still in Skåne. One was at the Lund University Hospital, about 35 kilometers away and the other was a hospital in Helsingborg, closer to Landskrona. Despite the proximity of the hospital in Helsingborg, Mr. Ericsson chose to see a lung specialist in Lund. He chose Lund University Hospital because it was an academic center affiliated with a university medical school, and Mr. Ericsson felt that this would offer him better quality care.

While Mr. Ericsson was waiting to see the specialist, the chest CT was performed. He had to wait nine days after the second chest x-ray because of the queue for CT and the limited number of local scanners. The chest CT was more revealing than either of his previous chest x-rays. It showed a centrally located tumor on the right between the trachea and the spinal column. The tumor was large, compromising the right main bronchus and pushing the esophagus to the left. There was complete atelectasis of the right lung, meaning that the alveoli, or tiny air sacs in his lung had collapsed. There was also a separate 2.5 cm nodule located toward the back, close to a vertebra in his spine, likely a local metastasis. The chest CT showed that the lymph nodes running along the esophagus and the trachea were involved. The CT included views of the liver, which did not show any distant metastases. Because of the very central location of the tumor, it was understandable why it had not been seen on the initial chest x-ray. The round infiltrate seen on the oblique view of the second chest x-ray likely was a local metastatic nodule.

Referral to a Specialist

The Department of Lung Medicine at Lund University Hospital received the referral letter two weeks after the second chest x-ray and four days after the CT was performed. His case was given an appropriate level of priority and Mr. Ericsson was put on a waiting list to see a specialist.

Fifteen days later, he met with a specialist at Lund. He was quite surprised at this short waiting period, as so many reports on the television spoke of the notoriously long waiting periods to see specialists in Sweden. Mr. Ericsson met with Dr. Alexandra Karlsson at Lund University Hospital, who reviewed his history, x-ray and CT results, and performed a physical exam. Since his first appointment with the GP, his symptoms had worsened markedly. She found that he was short of breath and had very low exercise tolerance. The physical exam detected no lung sounds on the right side. He was scheduled for a bronchoscopy, which would provide a visual image of the interior of his major airways. Dr. Karlsson also gave him instructions to discontinue the naprosyn for his low back pain, as its other effect as an anti-clotting agent might exacerbate his hemoptysis.

Mr. Ericsson returned to Lund the next day for the bronchoscopy, which showed total obstruction of the right main bronchus with tumor containing coagulated blood, an appearance confirming the diagnosis of cancer. The mass was fragile and bled easily. For this reason, no sample was taken for pathology. Because of his advanced stage and the very central location of the tumor, Mr. Ericsson was told that he was not a candidate for surgery, which would involve elaborate tracheal reconstruction. However, another option was available. Lund University Hospital had one of the few lung medicine specialists skilled at performing interventional laser bronchoscopy. A laser beam would be targeted towards the tumor, burning it off, allowing at least the majority of it to be removed from the lung. It would not be a cure, but a palliative treatment designed to extend life and help with his symptoms. It would also remove the majority of the tumor, though many cancer cells would still remain.

Because of the specialized nature of laser bronchoscopy, it was performed only one day a week at the outpatient clinic. Mr. Ericsson therefore had to wait nine more days for the laser bronchoscopy to be performed. He was glad, in retrospect that he had chosen Lund University Hospital for his specialized care, because the hospital in Helsingborg did not have a laser bronchoscopist and he would have had to wait even longer to have the treatment if he were not already a patient at the hospital. By the time laser bronchoscopy was performed nearly eight weeks had elapsed since his first visit to the general practitioner in Landskrona. Mr. Ericsson's symptoms were quite severe because of the growing tumor obstructing his right main bronchus. He was very short of breath and he was not able to walk very far without severe difficulty breathing. He continued to cough up blood and continued to be able to sleep only sitting up. He had also lost seven kilograms in the intervening weeks.

During the laser bronchoscopy, the bronchoscopist removed as much of the tumor as possible, burning it off in fragments. Once this was done, it was clear why Mr. Ericsson had experienced symptoms of shortness of breath and low exercise tolerance. His entire right lung was filled with blood that had come from the tumor. This blood was emptied from his lung at the completion of the procedure.

Diagnosis and Laser Treatment

Tumor fragments were sent to pathology, where they were fixed and stained for a microscopic tissue diagnosis. The pathologist, Dr. Jan Larsson, looked at Mr. Ericsson's tumor under the microscope and found that it contained cyst-like artifacts or fragments of tissue. Many of the fragments contained tumor cells, which had large, irregularly shaped nuclei of different sizes. The cells themselves did not appear to be forming glandular elements, and there was evidence of intercellular bridges between the cells. This appearance was typical of a poorly differentiated squamous cell carcinoma of the lung, a type of non-small cell carcinoma. The combined results of the chest CT, bronchoscopy and pathology revealed the size of the tumor, the type of lung cancer, and evidence of separate tumor nodules within the same lung. The mediastinal lymph nodes on the same side were also involved. All of this evidence showed Mr. Ericsson's cancer to be at a fairly advanced stage.

After the laser resection of the tumor, Mr. Ericsson felt considerably better. He was no longer short of breath, and he could once again walk at a normal speed and distance. The next steps in Mr. Ericsson's care involved chemotherapy and radiation therapy. Dr. Karlsson would remain primarily involved in his care, though Mr. Ericsson would meet with a radiation oncologist to plan for the radiation therapy. He would also have a follow-up bronchoscopy, because the tumor could begin to grow again in the same location, causing renewed symptoms of lung obstruction.

The multiple appointments created a dramatically different life from the one Mr. Ericsson had previously enjoyed. He actually felt quite well compared to how he had been feeling before the bronchoscopy, so the idea that there was cancer growing in his lung seemed odd to him. He felt fortunate to have his wife and his daughter close by for support. He was fearful for his future, knowing that his time with his grandchildren was limited. However, he had great trust in Dr. Karlsson and the other specialist doctors, and believed that their expert advice was really the best. He felt hopeful, as he believed that treating the cancer with combined laser resection, chemotherapy and radiation therapy would provide him with an extension of his life.

His treatment with chemotherapy began three days after his laser bronchoscopy. He was given the drugs gemcitabine, vinorelbin, and carboplatin. His wife accompanied him to the appointment. He received his chemotherapy in a special infusion unit known at Lund University Hospital as "Ward 6." Patients arrived at the hospital in the morning, received their chemotherapy intravenously, and departed in the afternoon the same day. This allowed them to continue to be treated as outpatients and have their blood drawn at their local health centers in the community. After his first chemotherapy treatment, Mr. Ericsson continued to feel better and began to gain back some of the weight he had lost. Though he had been warned of symptoms of nausea after the treatment, he actually felt well except for a period of low appetite immediately afterward.

Currently, Mr. Ericsson is receiving chemotherapy every week. He will have a total of four treatments and then be re-evaluated for the possibility of further treatments. He is also on a waiting list for radiation therapy. His initial meeting with the radiation oncologist is scheduled for five weeks after he first met with Dr. Karlsson. If all goes according to plan he will receive his first dose of radiation ten days after this appointment. The wait time for radiation therapy has been a source of frustration to Mr. Ericsson. Though the radiation treatment facility in Lund is the largest one in the southern part of Sweden, it has such a high demand that there is a waiting list for up to one month or even longer for patients to get treatment.

Wait Times But Exemplary Care

Despite the wait time to receive radiation, Mr. Ericsson finds the care he is receiving at Lund University Hospital to be exemplary. The physicians and nurses there are very involved and very caring. He feels that they have answered his questions forthrightly and planned his treatment carefully. He has essentially obtained all the information about his illness from them, not feeling the need or the desire to consult other sources such as books, media or the Internet. The hardest part of all, he believes, is the lack of control he feels as a patient. All his life, he has been in control of his career and family decisions and has been able to make these decisions on his own. It is certainly an odd sensation to have decisions now made by other individuals.

From Mr. Ericsson's point of view, the doctors know best and he trusts them and their expertise. Additionally, he finds great irony in the fact that he has worked hard all his life to provide for his family and his future retirement, and now that he has reached the age when he can finally take it easy, he is hit with a diagnosis involving such life-altering circumstances. He is positive about his future, hoping that after chemotherapy and the eventual start of his radiation treatments, he will gain back enough strength to be able to travel with his wife to Hungary in the next two months.

Case 26: An Up and Down Course*

Peter Tang

It was 4:30 in the morning and nature was calling again — the third time tonight. "These trips to the bathroom are becoming bothersome," Professor Bruun thought sleepily as he left his warm bed, "I'd better make an appointment with Dr. Bergman."

At age 67 the Professor had recently retired as a Professor of Nordic Languages at Lund University. These days he was spending more time on the golf course, working on his book, and visiting his grandchildren. He lives with his wife, Marianne, who works at a book publishing company. They have been married 40 years.

During this whole year of 1996, Professor Bruun noticed his voiding problems becoming more severe. The flow was not as strong and he would have to go to the bathroom many times during the day and several times at night. Marianne noticed, too, when her sleep was interrupted by his nocturnal trips and urged him to see his doctor. Dr. Bergman, his internal medicine doctor, knew of Prof. Bruun's problems and had already arrived at a working diagnosis of benign prostatic hypertrophy (BPH).

---

*This case was written by Peter Tang when he was a student at Weill Medical College of Cornell University and took part in the US-EU-MEE medical student exchange at the Lund University Hospital, Lund, Sweden in 2000.

A digital rectal exam earlier this year revealed a mildly enlarged prostate. A Prostate Specific Antigen (PSA) test was not often done in 1996, so none was ordered at that time.

The next morning, instead of heading for the golf course, the Professor called his local health center and received an appointment with Dr. Bergman for two weeks hence. Under Sweden's universal health care system, he knew he could choose to make an appointment with a urologist without a referral, but he preferred to first see Dr. Bergman. He had been seeing him for the past few years after his previous doctor retired. For doctor's visits the Professor pays 80 Swedish kronos ($9 US dollars in 1996) but there is an annual deductible of 800 SEK ($87 US dollars) after which primary care visits are at no charge for the rest of the 12-month period.

Dr. Bergman knew the Professor well. He had diagnosed him with Type 2 diabetes mellitus seven years ago and is pleased that he can control it by diet. Five years ago Professor Bruun had a mild stroke which led to the discovery that his blood was "hypercoagulable" or prone to clot. He has been on 75 mg of aspirin every day since that discovery. Professor Bruun is active and in good health except for slightly high cholesterol, psoriasis, and hypertension for which he takes a beta-blocker.

After hearing how the voiding problems were getting worse, Dr. Bergman examined the Professor only to discover the same physical finding as at his last visit. Dr. Bergman recommended a consultation with the urology clinic at the University Hospital of Lund, which is one of the nine regional hospitals where specialized care such as neurology, urology, pediatrics and plastic surgery is offered. Since Dr. Bergman is one of the many salaried doctors in Sweden employed by the county councils, he has no financial incentive to delay referring Prof. Bruun to a specialist.

All employees at the hospital are salaried and there are government-set global budgets so there is no financial incentive on the part of the employees or the hospital to treat patients at a rate higher than they already do; thus the queues for medical care can become quite long. Patients referred to the urology clinic are assigned a priority — high, moderate, or low. A patient suspected of BPH is considered low priority and may have to wait half a year to be seen at the urology clinic. Those with suspected prostate cancer will usually be seen within one to two weeks. At this time Professor Bruun is referred for urinary problems and not necessarily prostate cancer so he is given an appointment at the clinic in six weeks, in November 1996. His care will now be in the hands of the hospital doctors — "hospitalists" — and Dr. Bergman will have no further role. He will eventually receive a report from the hospital.

The Regional Hospital — Initial Visit

The first urologist Prof. Bruun meets in the clinic at the University Hospital of Lund, on rectal exam finds a slightly enlarged prostate that feels homogeneous, or the same throughout. However, a PSA test is done and four days later the results show that his PSA level is abnormally high at 24 ng/ml (normal: <4 ng/ml). The urologist calls Professor Bruun and explains the possibility of cancer and that the next step should be a transrectal ultrasound (TRUS) to detect masses and perform biopsies.

Prof. Bruun knows that he may see different doctors at the urology clinic, or even be operated on by a different doctor, although they try to maintain continuity of care. Patients are reassured that all the doctors are of equal competence and surgical skill and have the same philosophy in management, though in reality there may be slight variations from one doctor to the next. He is therefore not surprised to find that he is scheduled to see a different doctor, Dr. Per Hegstrom, at his next appointment.

On examination Dr. Hegstrom finds a hard prostate especially around the apical or top area on both sides but more on the right. Clinically, he makes the diagnosis of a T3 tumor, one that has grown outside of the prostate capsule. The Transrectal Ultrasound (TRUS), which is done in the clinic, shows suspicious changes in the outer zone of the capsule. Biopsies are done and Professor Bruun comes back with his wife, Marianne, a week later for the results. They are told that he has prostate cancer and the pathology reveals a grade two to three, moderately to poorly differentiated lesion. This finding, along with his elevated PSA test, prompts a bone scan to detect any spread to the skeletal system.

After a week of anxious waiting, Professor Bruun and Marianne find that fortunately there is no spread. When he gets the bone scan results, Dr. Olson, another urologist, explains the different options available to the professor. If his cancer was contained within the prostate, being T1 or T2, radical prostatectomy or external beam radiation could be offered as definitive treatments but the only options now were: (1) Observation or watchful waiting, (2) Gonadotropic releasing hormone (GNRH) analogue, (3) Antiandrogen therapy, (4) Total androgen blockage (choice 2 and 3 together), or (5) External beam radiation as part of a research study. The last option is an experimental procedure where T3 tumors without lymph nodal spread are given external beam radiation. However, no lymph node spread must be proven by pelvic lymphadenectomy in which the pelvic lymph nodes are removed and tested for cancer spread.

Professor Bruun opts for inclusion in the study and is scheduled for lymphadenectomy on January 14, 1997. He is admitted to the hospital the night before and Dr. Linhart comes to introduce himself as he and another doctor will be doing the surgery. The operation goes well but the results are disappointing. There is metastatic spread of the tumor to the lymph nodes on both sides. Dr. Olson is the next to see Prof. Bruun in clinic and tells him the disappointing news. The only medical option is now hormone therapy, which is palliative — total androgen blockage with GNRH (gonadotropin releasing hormone) analog. Casadex, an antiandrogen is started on January 30, 1997.

Initial Response

Professor Bruun's initial response is encouraging, but soon he embarks on a roller coaster ride. His PSA in April is 1.6, down from 24. In November it is 2.1. However by September of 1998 his PSA has jumped to 21. It is decided to remove the antiandrogen with the hope of a hormone withdrawal effect, which occurs in 10% of patients. In these patients antiandrogen removal induces a paradoxical drop in PSA and by implication, shrinkage of the tumor. This maneuver fails in Professor Bruun and his PSA is up to 42 in January 1999.

At this visit Professor Bruun is scheduled to see one of the residents who admits to the Professor that he does not know much about prostate cancer. Professor Bruun is quite upset with this and demands to be seen by only one physician, Dr. Eliasson, the head of the Urology Departments at the University Hospitals of Lund and Malmo, and one of the national experts on prostate cancer. With some personal connections, Professor Bruun secures Dr. Eliasson as his physician.

On February 2, 1999, Professor Bruun has his first meeting with Dr. Eliasson. This time the Professor has come prepared with multiple Internet articles. Fortunately, Dr. Eliasson is familiar with all this work and more. The Professor is much relieved and is confident he is in good hands. His PSA is now 44 and Dr. Eliasson decides to continue the GNRH analog and start Estrocyt, which is estradiol and mustard gas. This chemo-hormonal drug has been reported to have a response rate of 35% in patients.

Seven weeks later, Professor Bruun is admitted to the emergency room for diarrhea, weight loss, fatigue and fever. Estrocyt is suspected to have caused these symptoms and it is discontinued. In April of 1999 his PSA has reached 50. A discussion with the oncologists offers no additional therapies.

Back Pain

In June, Professor Bruun calls Dr. Eliasson and tells him he has started to have lower back pain. "Do you think it's the cancer?" asks the Professor.

"I'm not sure," Dr. Eliasson replies. "You should see your general practitioner to start the evaluation."

Instead, Professor Bruun decides to see a private orthopaedist who orders an x-ray of the lower back and finds only degenerative changes. The private orthopaedist prescribes some anti-inflammatory medications.

By August, 1999 Professor Bruun's pain is worse and his PSA level is 81. Up until this point in his illness Professor Bruun has been fully active and not debilitated by his disease. He has been able to continue to play an occasional round of golf and to enjoy his grandchildren's visits. Now he can barely get out of bed because of his back pain. Marianne is a great source of physical and emotional support, but she is very worried.

Dr. Eliasson is suspicious of bone metastases and decides to order a bone scan and MRI with contrast agent. The bone scan reveals uptake in T7 to T10, T12, all of the lumbar spine, and the left sacroiliac joint. Radiation treatment is started and Prof. Bruun is prescribed Tylenol and dextroproxyphene (a centrally acting opioid).

A New Treatment

By October 1999 Professor Bruun's PSA is 159. The MRI shows tumor impinging on the L1 to L2 nerve roots and tumor growth outside the dura, the outermost membrane covering the spinal cord, at the levels of L1-L2-L3, L5-S1. With the rising PSA and the lack of alternative therapies Dr. Eliasson has few options available. He has heard that some hormone treatment-resistant prostate tumors may respond to yet another more experimental treatment. He recommends an octreotide scan to detect octreotide receptors. This could help to determine if Professor Bruun might respond to treatment with octreotide, a synthetic drug similar to the natural hormone, somatostatin.

Professor Bruun and Marianne trust Dr. Eliasson and agree with his recommendation. They anxiously await the appointment for the scan. In the meantime they have some serious discussions about the amount of time Professor Bruun may have left. They determine to fill it with the things that bring them the most pleasure — time with the grandchildren and some limited travel as the Professor's medical condition permits. The results of the scan come in November and show receptors centrally in the abdomen, distal thoracic spine, and proximal lumbar spine.

Octreotide analogue is started. In late November Professor Bruun's PSA has dropped to 45 and he is in no pain. By March of 2000 his PSA is 10. A new octreotide scan shows regression of earlier changes in the abdomen. Professor Bruun is continued on the octreotide analogue injections and GNRH analogue. He is back to full activity, but no one is sure how long this treatment may last. He and Marianne are taking life one day at a time and trying not to worry too much about the future.

Case 27: The Kidney is King*

Kavid Udompanyanan

Something is Not Quite Right

Thomas's story began when he was only eight months old. He was brought to the hospital by his parents because he refused to eat. While this was a common enough complaint, the pediatrician who saw him felt that something wasn't quite right with Thomas and sent for some routine lab tests, though she really wasn't expecting anything abnormal. Unfortunately, the lab results came back showing that Thomas's kidneys were in acute failure and he was placed on dialysis and given antibiotics immediately. He recovered from this bout in a few days and was sent home apparently healthy.

Over the next three and one-half years, Thomas grew as any normal child. He learned to walk and talk and play with his older brother without any sign of health or developmental problems. The doctors who had seen him finally concluded that he had had a case of hemolytic-uremic syndrome (HUS). But slowly, Thomas's health began to decline at a steady and insidious rate. His feeling of being not quite well never really went away, even after a full night's sleep. He tired faster than the other kids in school and frequently got sick.

---

*This case was written by Kavid Udompanyanan when he was a student at Harvard Medical School and took part in the US-EU-MEE program at Lund University, Sweden in May, 2002.

Finally, his family took him to get a complete physical and the doctor discovered something very strange. Despite the progress of the rest of his body, Thomas's kidneys were not growing–they were still the same size as they were when he was a baby. Scarring, which started when he had HUS, had continued slowly all the while. His kidneys were still functioning and had managed to sustain him until then, but as his body grew larger, demands on the renal filtration system increased to the point where he could no longer effectively cleanse his own blood. The demands on his kidneys needed to be reduced and the doctor suggested a low protein diet. Thomas loved milk and eggs, but they had to be dramatically decreased in his diet along with meats. He did manage, however, to live a relatively normal childhood for four more years.

A Downhill Course

When Thomas was eight years old, the doctors that he had been seeing for regular check-ups saw that his condition was again worsening. Toxins and waste products were building up in his blood and they had to consider peritoneal dialysis. Thomas reluctantly agreed and was scheduled for minor surgery to place a catheter through his abdominal wall, allowing access to his abdominal cavity. This allowed him to drip a two-liter bag of dialysis solution into his abdomen, keep it there for a few hours while waste products filtered out from the blood, then drain it out again. This cycle was repeated several times a day and sometimes even at night, but it gave him freedom from being hooked up to a dialysis machine.

Peritoneal dialysis is a relatively new concept that first entered common use for End Stage Renal Disease (ESRD) patients in the 1970s. Home dialysis has been shown to cost much less than institutional dialysis in Sweden, which saves the entire health care system money. It also frees up doctors, nurses and other resources for other needs. However, it is not quite as effective as hemodialysis and requires some remaining kidney function. At least, with Sweden's single payer health care system, Thomas does not need to worry about the cost. Swedish residents feel that health care is a right. All their lives they have paid high taxes, ranging from 30–50% income tax, varying by county, plus a 25% value added tax (VAT) on goods and products, so they feel they are entitled to a return of that investment through services from the government. In the United States as well, patients with end stage renal disease or needing dialysis are eligible for financial aid under Medicare.

Even with peritoneal dialysis, Thomas was not totally well. Where he used to be a relatively active child, he now became sullen, quiet and a homebody. At an age when kids are beginning to learn to play sports and making new friends with their teammates, Thomas focused on video games or watching TV because he tired easily with any physical exertion. What he really needed was a kidney transplant, but the waiting list for a non-critical patient was at least two to three years and neither Thomas nor his family felt they could wait that long. Of course, there is one way to get around the list: get a donated kidney from a living donor.

Finding a Donor

With high hopes, his family was crossed matched — father, mother, brother, sister — to see if they would be able to donate a kidney but his dad was the only one who did not have a positive rejection reaction. So, when Thomas was nine years old, he received a new kidney. The operation seemed to be successful. After waking up, both Thomas and his father felt well and they were optimistic. But two days later, Thomas again felt weak and after checking his blood, the doctors realized that the kidney was not functioning despite the cross matching beforehand and all the care they had taken during the operation. They had no choice but to remove the kidney. Thomas considers this the first of the 'mistakes' the doctors made, which have built his anger towards medicine.

Thomas then continued peritoneal dialysis and went on the transplant list, resigning himself to a long wait. In Sweden, as in the United States, everybody is given the opportunity to sign up for organ donation when they receive a driver's license. While many Swedes accept, there is a strong cultural belief about being buried as a "whole person" with all organs intact. Even Thomas's family members who have seen what he has gone through refuse to donate their organs after death.

During this time, Thomas followed a relatively normal routine, going to school when he could, but staying home quite often. Amazingly, after only three months, his family received a call telling them a kidney was available. They quickly rushed to the hospital for preparations and within a few days, Thomas had a new kidney. Again, the family was optimistic and went home speaking of plans to return the equipment for the peritoneal dialysis.

But the same immune system that kept the rest of his family healthy once again turned on Thomas and in the space of a month, his doctors could see that he was rejecting this new kidney as well. Slowly, but surely, the organ was being sealed off from the rest of his body. This is where Thomas says the second mistake happened. Thomas said of the doctor who was taking care of him, "He did not care about me, only about keeping the kidney going." Whether this was true or not or what the reasons were behind the doctors' actions, this is how Thomas viewed the situation.

A Regimen of Drugs and Steroids

Thomas began an intense regimen of massive immunosuppressive drugs and steroids. These drugs undermine the immune system and are used to stop, or slow, rejection of transplanted organs. By taking them Thomas stopped his body's assault on his kidney and stayed off dialysis. But this did not come without cost. Steroids are powerful drugs working at the foundations of the endocrine and immune system that regulates the entire body. They are life saving in many circumstances but also have many unwanted side effects including the increase and redistribution of body fat, increased susceptibility to infections, thinning of bones, water retention and some psychological effects.

At the same time, doctors gave Thomas growth hormone in an attempt to stimulate his development. Shortly after receiving the medication, Thomas came to the hospital with nausea, vomiting and headache — classic signs of increased intracranial pressure. The combination of growth hormone with his immunosuppressive drugs seemed to set off a reaction that caused a buildup of pressure in his brain. Thomas began to have problems with his vision. Everything blurred or sometimes shifted out of focus when he turned his head. As the day passed the symptoms worsened and at times his vision would fade so that he was unable to see anything but a bright or dark blur. The pressure that was building up in his skull was compressing his optic nerve and causing these problems with his vision.

Thomas never knew what really caused the cerebral edema but he blames it on his medications, and consequently on his doctor for not watching the drug interactions carefully. The growth hormone was stopped immediately and high doses of cortisone were given to halt the cerebral edema. While this worked to reverse his vision loss and other symptoms, the side effects of the steroids were building up. The combination of all of his medications made Thomas physically fat and ungainly and emotionally unstable. When doctors tried to reduce his cortisone dose, he suffered blindness and headaches — they were stuck in a catch-22. At his worst, Thomas was unable to walk and had to be pushed around in a wheelchair.

At the age of 13, Thomas began to have thoughts of suicide. He felt he had a horrible existence and often was tempted to take many of his pills and just fall asleep. He had few friends and while his family was supportive, they had their own lives to lead and often he was left at home alone for long periods of time. Eventually his doctors realized that Thomas's quality of life was so poor that he was thinking of hurting himself and knew they had to change his treatment plan. A neurosurgeon placed a shunt in Thomas's brain–a diverting tube that would allow excess fluid to drain to a different location in his body. Without the threat of fluid buildup and blindness, Thomas's steroid medications could be decreased. Nephrologists also concluded that his transplanted kidney was not serving its purpose and removed his second graft. Thomas was able to stop many of his medications and begin hemodialysis.

Hitting Bottom

The period of time after Thomas began hemodialysis was the worst for him and he was the most depressed he had ever been. Despite being off steroids and immunosuppressive drugs, the side effects of the medications were still affecting him. He now also lost three days a week to the dialysis machine watching his blood being pumped in and out through clear plastic tubing. He was unable to attend school regularly and eventually stopped going entirely. He lost the few friends he had, who moved on to other things and places.

It was an improvement in his life when the doctors switched him to overnight dialysis at home. Much of the cost of in-hospital dialysis goes to overhead and salaries for health care workers. This puts added strain on the finances of the hospital but luckily for Thomas and other dialysis patients, except for the copayment and the per diem fee at the hospital, the rest of the bill was covered by the public health care system.

Thomas described the routine of his life on dialysis like a roller coaster ride. "At the end of one dialysis treatment in the morning I feel drained in spite of having slept all night hooked up to the dialysis machine. I go through the morning, eating and taking it easy. By afternoon I feel better and stronger. From then until evening I am feeling pretty good. I can go out with friends, walk without becoming exhausted and have dinner at a restaurant, although I have to watch what I eat and drink. That night I am tired and sleep comes quickly."

"The next morning is still good but already I am starting to feel a bit off. A bloated feeling follows me around and I have a slight ache in the back of my skull. I notice that I can't do as much before I tire. By lunch I no longer want to leave the house and I begin to feel a bit toxic and nauseated as the metabolites build up in my system. The day ends with resting in bed and pulling the hemodialysis machine out of the closet to begin another session at night."

Thomas once said, "I am a perfectly ordinary 14-year-old trapped in the ugly twisted body of an eight year old." One of the side effects of renal disease is slowed growth and Thomas was barely 4.5 feet tall. He spent most of his days watching movies and playing video games. Lord of the Rings and Star Wars were among his favorite movies along with his Playstation II console. "Movies and games," he said, "help me to forget where I am and let me escape to another place." Although he was not of legal age, someone he knew bought him alcohol and he began drinking when he had nothing else to do. If he had continued like this, there surely would have been a point where he would have ended his own life.

A Little Progress at Last

Luckily, Thomas's doctors began to work with changes in his dialysis, in the hopes that they could somehow stimulate his growth. After many regimens, they switched him to daily night dialysis and reduced some of his other medications. Miraculously, it worked. He began to grow and eventually went through puberty. He grew taller and his voice became deeper. He lost weight and was able to walk more on his own. His mood picked up and he became more optimistic.

One of his happiest days was when he grew taller than Sara Pedersen, the head nurse of the home dialysis unit at Lund University. She says that he had "a grin from ear to ear" for that entire day. Over the years, Thomas had developed a friendship with Sara and they would sit during his dialysis sessions and talk about anything and everything. He also began going to school again, though to a different campus for students who weren't able to learn as fast as others. There he also did part time work as a locksmith in the school workshop — a job that gave him a sense of accomplishment and pride.

Two years ago when he turned 18, Thomas decided that he wanted more independence and moved out of his mother's house. He got himself an apartment although he continues to go to his mother's every other night because he cannot do hemodialysis alone. It seemed like the worst was over.

One More Twist of Fate

At first he didn't realize what was happening. It's quite possible that his seizures started earlier and they were unnoticed, but his first observed seizure was when he was in the hospital at age 18. During these periods, he would blank out, just for a few seconds and lose touch with everything. When his consciousness returned, his body would be shaking just slightly and it would take him a few minutes to recover. He thought it would improve over time; after all, someone did open up his skull to operate on his brain and he was on many medications. But the seizures did not stop and Thomas was diagnosed with absence epilepsy. This type of epilepsy is characterized by a type of seizure where one 'spaces out' for a short time and often recovers after only a few minutes of disorientation.

Thomas thought that as long as he took his medications, the epilepsy would be under control, until he had a seizure and drove his family's car off the road. He was not injured but since that day he has not gotten behind the wheel. He also must have someone watch him while doing his dialysis routine at home. One time he had a seizure after pulling out his dialysis needle and he lost quite a lot of blood. For now it seems his epilepsy is under control but he is careful not to place himself in any situation that could be dangerous if he blanks out. The doctors have found an "epileptic focus" in the left temporal lobe of his brain. They are now working on seizure control with medications but have not decided whether more aggressive measures, i.e. surgery, may be needed.

Thomas has settled into a simple routine. Two years ago he finished with school and now he spends most of his days at home with his movies and games. He has made a few new friends and when they are around, they hang out and go out to eat. On weekends, they try to take day trips to the lake or sea and just enjoy themselves. But Thomas has never been farther from his home than Stockholm because he must be back to his hemodialysis machine every forty-eight hours. In the summer he is looking forward to going to his father's farm to work with the animals alongside his grandfather. His family continues to be very supportive and are always there for him if he ever needs help. His sister often brings her two kids over to his apartment because they love to hear Thomas tell them stories. He no longers considers hurting himself. He says, "I love my family too much for that."

Thomas is also looking for a job. While he receives a disability check from the government every month, it does not cover more than his rent and food. Luckily, his medical expenses are low because of the Swedish social insurance but he wants to work because he wants to be productive and is frustrated with sitting at home all day. He isn't sure what he is qualified for but will try anything. He has also considered going back to school so he can add to his resumé. He continues to come to the hospital about once a month either for some extra dialysis or for infections. He has overcome his fear from his previous transplants and is now on the kidney transplant list once more. He yearns to be free of the yoke of dialysis and is willing to risk another chance at having a functional kidney. He has also begun creative writing at home, mostly fantasy and fiction, however, his latest writing project is a story of his own experiences as a patient.

9

Cases Written by Swedish Students in the US

Case 28: Learning the Hard Way*

Kim Gosai

Mrs. Kline

When I met Helen Kline in September 2003, she was in New York City for an appointment with Dr. Goldman, a physician in the Cornell Gastroenterology and Hepatology Group practice at New York Presbyterian Hospital (NYPH). Waiting for Dr. Goldman, we chatted for a few minutes. Mrs. Kline told me that she lives in Connecticut outside New York City, but with city traffic being what it is, an hour and a half's journey from NYPH. Still, she is willing to make the trip because of her faith in Dr. Goldman.

She is a 67-year-old woman who owns a real estate business and has been widowed for 20 years. She has three grown children, two daughters who are married and live in New Jersey and a son who is a physician. Today her son has business at the hospital and drove her to her appointment.

When Dr. Goldman arrived he invited me, with Mrs. Kline's permission, to sit in on the interview. I was a little puzzled that the purpose of the visit seemed to be to discuss further treatment of her hepatitis. Dr. Goldman seemed doubtful about resuming treatment because apparently Mrs. Kline had suffered a great deal from the side effects of the medications the last time.

---

*This case report of two patients was written by Kim Gosai when she was a student at Lund University and took part in the US-EU-MEE project at Weill Medical College of Cornell University in 2003.

"This time will be different," Mrs. Kline assures Dr. Goldman. "I will stay on the Calexa and fight the side effects."

The matter is not entirely settled and they agree to meet again soon to make a final decision. In the meantime, Dr. Goldman wants up-to-date lab results on Mrs. Kline's liver function tests and hepatitis C viral count.

Mrs. Klines' son, Dr. Sherwin Kline, arrives and she introduces us saying, "Ms. Gosai is here to study US health care. You can start by filling her in on the details of my illness while I go to the lab."

"Five years ago I became very worried about my mother," Dr. Kline began. "She is usually full of energy, running her real estate business and keeping up with her civic interests — she's on the local chamber of commerce board of directors and the town planning committee — but at that time she started to complain of feeling continuously tired. Two years previously, in 1996, she was diagnosed with osteoporosis and started taking Evista, a selective estrogen receptor, as you probably know. The osteoporosis didn't seem to slow her down and didn't really account for her constant fatigue."

"Finally, my mother decided to tell me the whole story," he continued. "In 1990 she went to the Red Cross to donate blood and the blood tests that are done routinely showed that she had hepatitis C. She was referred to a local medical center near our home in Connecticut where she still receives her primary care. At the time she was diagnosed she did not show any symptoms of hepatitis, but by 1998 her liver enzymes had started to rise and she was experiencing extreme tiredness."

Dr. Kline read the question that was on my mind and continued.

"The source of infection was thought to be my father. He travelled to India and Southeast Asia on business and was never immunized against hepatitis. He was diagnosed with hepatitis C before he died, but my mother never spoke of it."

"I'm a cardiologist," he continued, "but after I knew about my mother's diagnosis of course I began to follow her case closely. As a medical student, you may be interested in some of the details. In 2000, she had a liver biopsy, which showed mildly active inflammation and septal fibrosis (grade II, stage 2). By now, her transaminases were increased (AST 78, ALT 90, ref. 10–45 IU/L), and the hepatitis C viral count was above one million copies/ml (ref. <1,620 copies/ml). It was time to start treatment. I did some research to find the best hepatitis C specialist and found Dr. Goldman here at NYPH."

At this point, Mrs. Kline returned from the lab and said, "Enough information for now. I'll explain American health insurance to Ms. Gosai when we meet next week."

True to her word, when we met again she told me that her business as a private realtor went well so she was able to afford private health insurance. Unfortunately, the insurance did not cover any pharmaceutical costs. A one-year anti-viral treatment with pegylated interferon and ribavirin costs $25,000. Luckily, Dr. Goldman has been involved in a research project focusing on this treatment for several years so Mrs. Kline was offered the opportunity to participate in the study, and thus got the medicines free of charge.

She started on a one-year treatment in March 2001. At first everything seemed to go well; her viral count was negative after three months of treatment, and at the six-month check-up no viral RNA was found. However, after half a year she started to feel severe side effects such as general malaise, headaches and depression, and could hardly find the energy to get out of bed in the morning. Dr. Goldman prescribed the SSRI anti-depressant Celexa, but Ms. Kline felt this only made things worse and did not continue the medication. Since the side effects seemed to be caused mainly by the interferon, the interferon dose was lowered. Mrs. Kline noticed no effects from this, and chose to end the treatment seven months after she had started. Soon thereafter she felt her energy increasing to the same level as before the treatment.

The side effects had made it difficult for Mrs. Kline to work, and she thought it was a good time to retire since by then she had reached the age of 65 and became eligible for Medicare, a federal health care program, which replaced her private insurance. Since Medicare covers less than the private insurance she had while working, she subscribed to a secondary "Medigap" insurance policy as a supplement to cover certain expenses.

After discontinuing her treatment, Mrs. Kline's transaminases were normal, as was her viral count. Unfortunately she relapsed towards the end of 2001 and her liver and viral values increased again. Still, she felt no symptoms besides fatigue. A second liver biopsy was done in April 2003, which showed some progression compared to the first biopsy (grade II, stage 2–3). Her viral count and transaminsases were still elevated. At this time Dr. Goldman told her that his opinion was 60% pro-treatment and 40% against. In any case, Mrs. Kline wanted to wait until after the summer for treatment, so it was that I first met her at Dr. Goldman's office in September 2003.

I asked Mrs. Kline how the disease has affected her life.

"Since I have been off treatment, the only way it has affected my life is that I am often tired and need to take a nap in the afternoon. I am happy that my insurance lets me see any doctor I choose, and I am grateful that my son is a doctor and has helped me to find a good specialist. I feel safe with Dr. Goldman, and even though there are doctors closer to my home, I will continue to travel the one-and-a-half hours to New York City to see him."

I asked if her illness had caused her any financial difficulty.

"My illness has not had any effects on me financially so far, thanks to the free medication I received in the study I took part in, and my private insurance, which covers co-pays and deductibles. However, one future problem could be that the ribavirin and interferon would not be paid for by the study if I take the treatment again. I hope that Medicare will pay for the medications, but I am not sure this will be the case."

I asked if she would like to see more of her health care costs covered by Medicare.

"Yes, of course, but not at the price of paying higher taxes."

Mr. Montero

The two patients I met in New York were a good study in contrasts and a good introduction to the US health care system. Actually, to someone accustomed to the single payer system in most European countries, it hardly seemed to me like a system, but rather a widely diversified array of types of health insurance.

I met Ricardo Montero the week after I met Mrs. Kline. He is a patient of Dr. Isaacs, a gastroenterology fellow at NYPH. Before I met Mr. Montero I only knew that he was a 54-year-old man of Mexican descent who lives alone in a small apartment on Staten Island.

Mr. Montero greeted me warmly and immediately noticed that I was surprised that he was in a wheelchair.

"Don't be surprised. You haven't made a mistake and ended up in the Orthopedic Department," he laughed. "I'll tell you the story from the beginning."

"I was born in the United States to migrant worker parents in 1949. We went back to Mexico and I lived there until I was 20 years old. Then I came back to the US as an adventuresome young guy and worked in the restaurant business, in landscaping — anything I could find. I worked 'off the books' because I did not believe in paying taxes. I was married briefly but that ended in divorce. Fortunately, we did not have any children."

"I finally ended up working in construction for small companies outside of Manhattan," he continued. "After a few years I began to have serious lower back pain. Up until this time I really had no need for medical care, so it didn't seem to matter that I didn't have an "official" job and was not covered by workers comp or any other insurance. Gradually I was unable to work and it was clear that I needed to see a doctor. The construction companies I worked for were not willing to help for fear of getting in trouble themselves, but I was able to prove my US citizenship, since I was born here. In due time, I was covered by Medicaid and was seen by orthopedic surgeons at another hospital in New York that will remain nameless."

"The doctors told me that I had a herniated disc and needed lower back surgery. They told me there was a chance that I would be a paraplegic afterwards, but I could not live with the pain, so in 1985 I went ahead with the surgery. As predicted, the lower half of my body became paralyzed and I will be in a wheelchair the rest of my life. Actually, I have had a lot of help from social services and rehabilitation through Medicaid, so I can manage to live by myself and get around on public transportation."

I thought that was quite remarkable and admired Mr. Montero's cheerful outlook, but he could see that I was still puzzled about his present illness.

"So you are still wondering why I am here seeing a gastroenterologist. In June 1999 I started to feel tired all the time. I went several times to the hospital where I had my back surgery but they didn't do a very thorough examination and sent me home. A friend of mine had been hospitalized at

New York Presbyterian Hospital (NYPH) and received good care. He recommended that I come here instead."

"I followed my friend's advice and went to the emergency unit at the NYPH. There they found that my potassium levels were high and my sodium levels were low. I was admitted to the hospital. I stayed here for seven days, and they finally diagnosed me with adrenoleukodystrophy."

Remembering my classes in genetics and endocrinology, I realized that this was a hereditary disease marked by adrenal atrophy and abnormality of the cerebral white matter.

"While I was there," Mr. Montero continued, "they also found that I had hepatitis C."

Later, when I had a chance to look at his medical records I noted that he had a viral load of 900,000 (ref. <1,620 copies/ml) at that time. All liver related laboratory values were normal, and he showed no symptoms beside fatigue. He was started on cortisone and has not reported tiredness since then, which may indicate that the fatigue was mostly related to the adrenal problems. The source of his hepatitis infection was possibly a blood transfusion during his back surgery in 1985 before stricter screening measures were put into effect for blood donors.

There was still more to Mr. Montero's story.

"After I was discharged," Mr. Montero continued, "I went for follow-ups to an endocrinologist and a gastroenterologist at NYPH. However, after the tragedy in New York on September 11, 2001, I stopped coming to these appointments. I lost friends that day and I did not want to come to Manhattan. Instead I went back to the other hospital, where this year I had a liver sonogram, which showed normal results. At my last visit, my doctor told me that the hospital had no specialist trained to deal with my adrenal dystrophy. He suggested that for further treatment I should go back to NYPH, where I had been diagnosed. I contacted NYPH, and got appointments within a month with both an endocrinologist and a gastroenterologist."

So it happens that this current visit to a gastroenterologist at NYPH is the first time Mr. Montero has visited Manhattan since September 11, 2001. Dr. Isaacs, a fellow in gastroenterology is seeing Mr. Montero today. He concludes that Mr. Montero still shows no symptoms of liver involvement, and that there is no reason to suspect that cirrhosis has begun. Recent tests show a viral load of 800,000 and a slightly elevated ALT, but otherwise normal laboratory results. Dr. Isaacs considers it likely that Mr. Montero will be a good candidate for treatment. He orders viral genotyping and a new ultrasound of the liver. If the hepatitis tests show genotype 2, Dr. Isaacs plans to start treatment without a prior liver biopsy, since the success rate is 80% with this genotype. If it is genotype 1, for which the treatment is less likely to succeed, a liver biopsy will be done first.

I ask Mr. Montero to tell me more about how he manages his daily life.

"Since I have been unable to work, I receive Social Security income," he replies. "This amounts to $535 a month; just enough to survive on. Thanks to Medicaid, I don't pay anything for my doctor visits or for any tests. I take several medicines; Florinef (cortisone) for my adrenal disease, and Fosamax (biphosphonate) and calcium to prevent osteoporosis. For my back pain I use Vicuprofen (opioid analgesic and NSAID combined) and Oxycontin (opioid analgesic). For these prescriptions I pay only a small co-pay."

Mr. Montero feels that he receives very good care at the NYPH. He trusts the doctors and believes they are among the best in the country. He says that now he wouldn't go to any other hospital, even though it takes him one-and-a-half hours to get to NYPH. He is thankful that Medicaid pays his health care bills, and does not know how he would have obtained medical care otherwise. The only negative aspect he can think of is that he cannot see any doctor he chooses as a Medicaid patient. Mr. Montero believes in paying taxes now.

"I learned the hard way," he concludes.

Contrasts

I realized that I had gotten a glimpse of two widely contrasting aspects of health care in the United States. When Mrs. Kline was working, and before she turned 65, she had private indemnity insurance. She chose that type of plan because she was free to choose the doctors she wished to visit. She was able to afford the monthly premiums, which were higher than in an HMO (Health Maintenance Organization) where she would have been limited in her choice of doctors. Her insurance also permitted her to visit any specialist without having to be referred by a primary care physician, and therefore she had no insurance problems when she started seeing

Dr. Goldman. No drug costs were covered at that time, but with the addition of the Medicare Prescription Drug Plan in 2006, most prescription drugs would now be covered. She would need to check to see if very expensive or experimental drugs such as interferon and ribavirin would be included.

Because Mr. Montero is unable to work and lives on Social Security he is eligible for Medicaid, which takes care of almost all his health care costs. Each state can influence the design of its own Medicaid program, resulting in differences from state to state. According to federal law, Medicaid is required to cover hospital care, nursing home care and physician services, among other things. Mr. Montero's prescription drugs cost him only a nominal fee.

Both Mrs. Kline and Mr. Montero are pleased with the level of care at NYPH, which is considered to be one of the best hospitals in the US. Mr. Montero is convinced that he could not receive better care, and is pleased that he gets appointments quickly and gets all the care he needs. Still, one disadvantage he experiences is that not all physicians accept Medicaid patients. He has to travel a long distance to reach a teaching hospital where he can be sure of getting good care with doctors he trusts.

One segment of the American population that was not represented by either Mrs. Kline or Mr. Montero is the large number of uninsured and underinsured people in the United States. The reasons for this situation are varied and complex. This group is made up of workers whose employers do not offer health insurance, low-paid workers who cannot find affordable insurance, and citizens who, for whatever reason, do not choose to spend money on insurance.

The American population values personal freedom highly, and their attitude towards government and taxes is more suspicious than in most other countries. This has characterized Americans since the establishment of the first colonies and is also reflected in the views of Mrs. Kline and Mr. Montero. Mrs. Kline is unsure that she would like to pay higher taxes even if this meant increased Medicare coverage. Mr. Montero was initially unwilling to pay taxes at all, but changed his attitude now that he has benefited from public health insurance. Both emphasized the importance of being able to choose their health care providers. This emphasis on freedom of choice in American culture may help to explain why the American health care system differs from that of many European countries.

Case 29: Living with HIV*

Malin Inghammar

Facing the News

Somehow Helen Wright had known for a long time that she was HIV-positive. The possibility first dawned on her that horrible night in September 1991 when she had to take her boyfriend to the hospital after they had been smoking crack together. She remembered the cold feeling inside when she realized the reason the nurses could not find any veins from which to draw blood was that he was an intravenous drug user. She was frightened and angry that he had not told her. They had actually had unprotected sex together once a couple of weeks before. That was the same night she got pregnant with her daughter, she later found out. She remembered having had a terrible flu some weeks after that.

But still, it was a real shock, sitting in front of the doctor that day in April 1994 in the pediatric department at Dartmouth Hitchcock Medical Center to hear that her 22-month-old daughter's severe nosebleeds and failure to thrive were caused by HIV-infection. It was even more devastating to hear that Helen herself had probably been the "source of transmission." She felt like there was ice-cold water running down her back.

---

*Malin Inghammer wrote the story of this patient when she was a student at Lund University, Sweden, and participated in the US-EU-MEE program at Harvard Medical School in 1999.

Helen was beside herself with grief and apprehension. She answered the doctor's questions as accurately and completely as she could: that she was 29 years old, that she had been using drugs since she was in high-school, mostly cocaine and crack the past few years, occasionally cannabis and alcohol but never any IV drugs. She had also sold sex for drugs. She told him that there was nothing additional in her medical history except for seasonal rhinitis, genital herpes and genital condyloma a couple of years earlier. She had never had TB or syphilis.

Helen had been tested for HIV twice: once in 1991, which was negative and the second time just after the delivery of her daughter. That test was as part of a study of the native incidence of HIV. To exclude biased selection everyone was tested anonymously. No one was given the results even if they turned out to be positive.

As a basic work-up at this appointment in 1994 the doctor ordered a pulmonary x-ray and a PPD (tuberculosis test), which turned out negative. She tested negative for CMV-antibody and toxoplasma serology but she was IgG positive for toxoplasma, indicating that she had been exposed at some time. She was offered pneumoccoccal immunization and a flu shot. To assess her HIV infection the doctor ordered a CD4 count. At that time it measured $580/\mu l$.

Hopeless and Hitting Bottom

The doctor went on and on talking about prognosis, possible means of treatment, immunizations, how she had to protect other people from infection, that she had to stop using drugs and so on but Helen heard little of it. Both her daughter and her six-week-old son were in foster care, she was out of work, she had no place to stay, and she believed she was going to die anyway, so why should she care. She had all the perfect reasons not to change her way of living.

The following six months she used drugs more and more but getting high was somehow not the same. She tried to compensate for the lack of euphoria by using even more. Out of work and shelter she sold sex walking the streets of the town where she lived and slept with her dealers. She slowly sank lower and lower into the mire of guilt, low self-esteem and fear of death. Somewhere in the back of her head she heard her doctor telling her that above all she had to stop using drugs.

When Helen was arrested for prostitution in February 1995 what was left of this once beautiful, happy, strong young girl was a 31-year-old homeless wreck with no self-esteem at all. Both of her two children were in foster care; her daughter was HIV-positive while her son was luckily negative. Her CD4 count had dropped from 580/μl to 242/μl in seven months and now Helen faced the charges for prostitution.

Turning Around

After a short trial Helen spent two months in a state prison for women, waiting to be transferred to another institution for an eleven-month drug rehabilitation program. Once there she began the difficult process of dealing with guilt, acknowledging she was an addict but also trying to accept herself as she was, understanding that she was still worth something and starting to look forward to the future. She learned how to deal with problems instead of running away from them and how to set goals that she could accomplish. She finally realized that her health was seriously threatened and given the one positive fact that her son was uninfected she decided to absolutely quit using drugs.

Although still incarcerated, in the rehabilitation facility she could wear her own clothes and use make-up and her daughter came to visit her once a week. During this time she joined the NA (Narcotics Anonymous) and a Bible circle to help to deal with her darkest times. Her doctor referred her to an infectious disease specialist to get a specialist's opinion on treatment. As early as July 1994, after her first visit, she was put on the antiretroviral drug AZT (zidovudine) but she didn't comply until being imprisoned. She became severely anemic after some months on AZT, with a red blood count of 6.7, shortness of breath and continuous burning pain in her hip, probably from problems with her bone marrow production. She eventually needed a four-unit blood transfusion.

The AZT was switched to ddC, another nucleosideanalogue. Two PAP smears showed abnormal cervical cells and a cone biopsy performed shortly afterward confirmed the diagnosis of cervical carcinoma *in situ*, a fairly common complication of HIV in women. She was to be followed up by PAP smears every three months with this care administered by a gynecologist outside prison.

During this period she began dealing with the fact that she had to take control of her situation and of her disease. To educate herself she researched and wrote a paper on HIV. She joined the ABC quilts movement and together with women all over America she made quilts for the benefit of children with HIV. While being an addict her primary interest had always been herself but by making these quilts she got a sense of community and togetherness that she had been lacking for a long time.

In prison she became close friends with several of the other women. On her last night in prison she disclosed her HIV status, hoping they would see that she too had her cross to bear. She was relieved although some of the inmates were upset and didn't want to see her again. They thought she was going to die and not seeing each other again would save them all the pain of missing a friend.

The real struggle began once she was out of prison. She found a part time job and a fairly cheap apartment. With many years of living on the edge, getting used to an ordinary life with a regular job, an apartment and paying bills was really hard. She was learning not only to be a mother but the HIV-positive mother of an HIV-positive child as well as staying absolutely clean from drugs. Because her income was so low she qualified for Medicaid.

Covering Health Expenses

This federal and state public insurance program covered all medical expenses for her and her daughter. The upper limit of income to qualify for Medicaid in New Hampshire at that time was $1190. She could have had her drug costs covered by the state drug reimbursement program for people with HIV but that would not have included any doctors' visits or additional medication such as antibiotics and medications for her sinus and nasal conditions.

Helen had to carefully monitor the number of hours she worked each month and any extra income she got from peer counseling so she would not exceed the $1190 limit. She could not save money in a bank account and some months she had to spend all her extra money so she would not lose Medicaid. Her mother officially owned the car she used to get around when she did peer counseling. Every doctor's visit cost $100 and a regular CD4 count cost $60. Medications ran around $3000 monthly. In total the yearly medical expenses for Helen and her daughter were around $40,000. She also got food stamps every week and some subsidized childcare.

Reaching Out

Helen chose to disclose her HIV status only to some of her closest friends but did not tell any one at work or any of her neighbors. When her daughter started school she told the school nurse and they had a meeting with some of the teachers involved to avoid future conflicts with students or their parents. Helen got involved with the local Narcotics Anonymous and Alcoholics Anonymous organizations and did peer counseling in a family support group. It was her way of dealing with all her feelings of hopelessness and desperation and by doing this she felt she got the support she needed to continue.

In November 1996 her CD4 count had dropped to $280/\mu l$ and her viral-load, now possible to measure, was 99,700 copies/ml. Her doctor found it necessary to change her drug regimen to Zerit (d4T), along with 3TC (Epivir) both nucleosideanalogue-reverse transcriptase inhibitors. These drugs are generally well tolerated except in some people who may develop peripheral neuropathy on d4T. Helen tolerated it well, however she developed increasing nasal problems with constant nasal congestion and recurrent episodes of sinusitis. She thought it might be a consequence of having snorted all that cocaine. She tried several antibiotic treatments for sinusitis and upper respiratory tract infections. The symptoms were difficult to control even with a corticoid nasal spray and an albuterol bronchodilator.

The Battle for her Son

Helen felt she had sorted her life out fairly well, and now wanted her son back home. She was allowed visiting time one hour every month and her first step was to get those hours increased to five hours every weekend.

This turned out to be very hard to implement because the foster mother always found excuses not to bring him, such as his having a cold and being dangerous to Helen and her daughter. There was always an excuse and at one point she hadn't seen her son in almost three months. She decided to try for custody of her son.

Helen could show the court that she was able to stay clean and that she took the best possible care of her daughter but still the case was dismissed in August 1996 for reasons she could not understand. She had the strong feeling that the real reason was that she was HIV-positive and her son was not. Discrimination of HIV positive people is against the law and so Helen decided to appeal. With the help of the local AIDS service organization she found a lawyer who was willing to take her case *pro bono*.

The case was dismissed once again in June 1997 for very vague reasons. Helen became more than ever convinced that the combination of a judge with prejudices against HIV-positive mothers and a foster mother who had bonded with Helen's son made her lose the case. This was an extremely difficult period for her. She lost several pounds of weight and had daily tension headaches. She had to tell herself over and over, "You are not going to make me use." Settling down again after all this hassle she could at least be very proud of having stayed away from drugs.

Keeping HIV in Check

Helen's CD4 count was steady during this period but the viral load began rising slowly and in April 1997 it measured 2196 copies/ml. Protease inhibitors had just become available at that time and she was put on nelfinavir (Viracept) 1000 mg by mouth, twice a day, in combination with the nucleosideanalogues she had had before.

Helen tolerated the medications fairly well and generally took them very faithfully. She administered her daughter's drugs religiously and that helped her to remember her own. When measured in June 1997 her CD4 count was 484 and her viral load was undetectable at less than 500 copies/ml. She saw her infectious disease doctor fairly often because of all the complicated HIV-related issues and she considered her to be her main doctor even though she had a primary care physician, whom she seldom saw. Her nasal problems, for example, were more or less the concern of her infectious disease doctor and all of her cervical cancer follow-up was taken care of by a gynecologist. Helen's daughter saw a doctor on the pediatric HIV team at Dartmouth Hitchcock Medical Center. Their two infectious disease doctors worked together to get a family perspective on their care.

Before she started taking the protease inhibitor Helen had slightly elevated plasma cholesterol and LDL counts but on nelfinavir therapy these counts increased even more. After a year she had developed an obvious peripheral lipodystrophic syndrome, losing muscle and subcutaneous fat on her limbs and face and adding more on her hips and belly. This worried her doctor, especially since Helen had a strong family history of high cholesterol and heart disease. The natural history of the disease with people on protease inhibitors was not known so in December 1998 when her fasting cholesterol measured 350 and LDL count 252 Helen's doctor decided to prescribe the cholesterol lowering drug, Lipitor 10 mg a day.

Since she was doing so well on antiretroviral therapy her doctor also began worrying about her hepatitis C infection. That hadn't been a big problem before but now when the prognosis of the HIV infection had radically changed it was time to consider what to do about the hepatitis C. Her liver function tests had been waxing and waning over the last months but she had no clinical evidence of advanced liver disease. Quantitative hepatitis C viral load was measured and a liver biopsy was planned for the near future to decide whether to treat Helen with Interferon and Ribavirin. There were no guidelines available at this time but all data suggested that it would be worth trying to eradicate Hepatitis C even for people with HIV.

In December 1998 Helen's CD4 count measured 531/µl and her viral load was 1030. She discussed the advantages and disadvantages of changing therapy with her doctor since with a detectable viral load a development of resistant strains could be expected in the long run. Helen's viral load was still rather low though, and she tolerated the current regimen well. As a change would not necessarily lead to better effects, they decided together that she was to stay on the drugs she had and that they would do a more frequent viral load check-up than the usual three month interval.

Living in the Real World

Helen had chosen to tell her daughter about their HIV disease a year earlier when her daughter had started to ask questions about why she had to go to the doctor so often and why she had to take so much medicine. Helen argued that if one is old enough to ask one is old enough to know. She felt much relief afterwards but still worried about her daughter telling other people who might not be the people Helen would have chosen to tell. Just recently her daughter told some friends at school, which made Helen agitated when she found out. Helen was still afraid of being stigmatized and that her daughter would encounter problems at school. Helen then decided to see someone for counseling and support.

Helen now lives as normal a life as is possible with HIV. She tries to take one day at a time even though she has her "HIV days" when life isn't too happy. She works part time but she hardly ever relaxes in her spare time. Just managing her own and her daughter's disease with all the medication and different doctor's visits takes a huge effort. If mistakes are made by the agencies that administer Medicaid, Helen has to go through a lot of red tape to justify everything retrospectively. She spends a lot of time peer counseling for other HIV positive people and she even runs a family support group and is active in the local Narcotics Anonymous. She got her four-year medallion for being clean last year. More than anything she would like to have her son back, especially since her life is stable. The unfair trial still feels like a deep scar inside her, but she hasn't given up yet.

Helen says with a smile, "God did not choose the easiest path in life for me, but at least he made me strong enough to walk it."

Case 30: For a Better Life*

Ylva Andersson Carlsson

Flavia Nazzaro

Seated in front of me is a small, thin 47-year-old woman. You could describe her as petite. She speaks softly in heavily accented English although she has been in the United States for nearly 35 years. She has tears in her eyes as she tells me, "I do not want another operation. I have had enough!"

Flavia Nazzaro was born in the Dominican Republic. When she was 12 years old her parents and the entire family of six children came to the United States "to get a better life," she whispers. Flavia was the eldest child.

"Are you afraid of having more chemotherapy?" I ask.

"No, the chemo has never been a problem," she replies. "I lost all my hair but that was really nothing. I never felt sick or anything. I am scared of the surgery itself — the anesthesia. At least now I have good life insurance for my daughter. I have signed up for a small insurance policy so she will have some money when I am not here anymore. It costs $45.00 a month. I cannot afford anything more expensive, but it is good insurance."

*Ylva Andersson Carlsson wrote the story of this patient in 2001 when she was a student at Lund University, Sweden, and participated in the US-EU-MEE exchange at the Weill Medical College of Cornell University, New York City.

As for me, I am a medical exchange student from Sweden and Mrs. Nazarro is my assigned patient. Little by little she tells me her story. Throughout childhood, both in the Dominican Republic and after she moved to the United States, she had recurrent episodes of high fever and stomach pain.

"I never went to a doctor for this," she explained. "My family could not afford it. After a few days the fever would fade and the pain would go away. One of my father's brothers, my uncle, also had some kind of stomach problem but it was never discussed in my family."

Emergency Operation

"One day when I was sixteen and still in high school," she continues, "I felt a terrible pain in my stomach and started to vomit blood. Someone at school drove me to the Emergency Room of the nearest hospital. By the time I got to the hospital I was bleeding from the rectum also. They immediately took me to the operating room."

"That was your first operation?" I asked.

"Yes. They took out a large polyp that was causing the bleeding, as well as part of my colon. I needed a lot of blood during the operation and afterwards I was severely anemic. I only weighed 75 pounds at the time."

"That must have been a difficult experience for a sixteen-year-old," I commented.

"It was difficult in so many ways. I had dreams and plans for the future. I wanted to go to the local community college and become a licensed practical nurse — maybe eventually become an RN (Registered Nurse). Those plans all vanished into thin air after that first operation."

"Were you able to go back to high school after the surgery?"

"Yes. For awhile I got very depressed and my recovery was slow but the school gave me some help at home and I was able to rejoin my class and graduate two years later."

"What sort of medical care did you have after this first surgery?" I asked.

"I really had no follow-up care. No one in my family could speak English very well and no one at the hospital spoke Spanish in 1970. We were not given any information about what was wrong and why this had happened to me. My father only had a part-time job and the family did not have any health insurance."

"Was your health better after your operation?"

"Not really. I had a lot of problems with diarrhea during this time and had to take painkillers because of frequent stomach pain. I now know that those medicines were also bad for my stomach. Anyway, I did manage to get a job as a salesgirl in a store when I was 19. Then disaster struck again."

"What happened?"

"I had a new episode of terrible, persistent stomach pain and a lot of rectal bleeding. This time they took me to the Emergency Department at Elmhurst Hospital, one of New York City's public hospitals. There I had a second operation. They removed three large polyps."

Diagnosis

"This time I had a very nice doctor from India. He took time to explain what was happening. He pointed out the dark spots on my lips and inside my mouth that I had had since I was a little girl. He explained that these spots, along with my other symptoms, could be a sign of a disease called Peutz-Jeghers Syndrome."

"It must have been a relief to at last have some explanation of your illness."

"It was. After that I read all I could find about Peutz-Jeghers Syndrome and understood what was happening to me much better. I understood that it is a hereditary disease that causes the polyps and other gastrointestinal problems. It can cause lung and gallbladder problems, too, but luckily I have escaped these. I was also told that I am at much greater risk for colon cancer because of the Peutz-Jeghers Syndrome."

"Do your sisters or brother have any of the Peutz-Jeghers symptoms?"

"My sisters are all healthy but my brother has the black-pigmented spots on his lips and inside his mouth and I am sure my uncle has had intestinal problems similar to mine."

"How was your health after your second surgery?"

"I was weak and anemic after my operation but the nice doctor from India followed me closely in spite of the fact that I had no insurance and could not pay. I went to see him every two weeks until I moved to

Queens. I actually did pretty well for the next several years and I only had one episode at age 24 when I had another bleeding polyp removed at Bellevue Hospital. My parents and all except my sister two years younger than me eventually went back to the Dominican Republic but I decided to stay and make a life for myself. I met and married a man who was also from my home country and in 1987 I found out I was pregnant."

A Happy Event and More Troubles

"My daughter is my whole life. I am very fortunate to have her. When I was eight months pregnant, during an ultrasound check-up at Bellevue, a huge polyp was visible on the screen. A C-section was performed and at the same time as my daughter, Olivia, was born they also took away the polyp. Although she was born one month early she did fine. That was my fourth operation."

"I can understand why you are reluctant to have more surgery."

"My health was not my only problem. Unfortunately, my husband was killed in a traffic accident when Olivia was three years old and we were left by ourselves. She is 14 now."

Medicaid

"After my husband died we moved into a one-bedroom apartment in Queens where we have lived ever since. A friend told me about the out-patient clinic in Queens where they accept uninsured people and help you apply for Medicaid. It usually takes about two months for a Medicaid application to go through but there are ways to get it quicker. I enrolled in a Medicaid managed care program, which does restrict me from seeing any doctor I choose but it pays for my prescriptions. I have to pay a co-payment, which can be hard."

"Have you ever found it impossible to pay the co-pay?" I asked.

"Yes, more than once I have not gotten the prescription filled because I did not have the $30–$40 for the co-payment but after we qualified for Medicaid I was at least able to have regular check-ups with a Primary Care Physician at the outpatient clinic at New York Presbyterian Hospital."

Primary Care Physician

"Do you see the same physician for your regular check-ups?" I asked.

"Yes. Dr. Romero is my Primary Care Physician. He is the person I turn to first if anything goes wrong. If I need to see a specialist he will arrange it."

I was glad that Mrs. Nazzaro had access to this basic care. If she has an emergency, such as she had in high school, I knew that all hospitals in the US with an Emergency Department are obliged to take care of anybody, with or without insurance."

"Finding Dr. Romero is a big help," Mrs. Nazzaro continued, "but it was not the end of my medical problems."

"What happened?" I asked.

Another Devastating Diagnosis

"By the beginning of 1998 I was slowly losing weight. I was getting more and more tired and had rectal bleeding from time to time. In December 1998 Dr. Romero discovered I was severely anemic. I had a positive Fecal Occult Blood Test and he sent me straight to the Emergency Department at New York Presbyterian Hospital. A colonoscopy and a CT scan were done that same day. Because of Medicaid, my expenses were all paid. The diagnosis was recto-sigmoid cancer."

"That must have been a shock."

"The worst part was that I would have to face surgery once again. I had horrible memories of waking up from anesthesia after my previous operations and I dreaded going through that another time."

More Surgery and Chemo

From Mrs. Nazzaro's medical records I learned that she received preoperative radiation and after one month she agreed to surgery and went through a hemicolectomy to remove the entire left side of her colon. The tumor was a Stage II, Dukes' B, two centimeters in size, moderately differentiated. Her lymph nodes were negative for cancer, but diffuse, benign adenomatous polyps were seen throughout her colon. Afterwards she received five cycles of chemotherapy with 5-FU and high dose Leucovorin, the treatment of choice at that time.

"How did you manage with the chemo?" I asked.

"The chemo was not a problem, even through I lost my hair and had constant diarrhea. The operation was the worst part. Again I went through the horrors of coming out of anesthesia. I did not feel sick from the chemo afterwards and that was the most important thing for me because I needed to continue to be a mother to my young daughter. We live in a rough neighborhood and I am constantly fearful for her. She has had some difficulties in school, but she has decided she wants to go to college after high school," Mrs. Nazzaro says with pride in her voice. "I am looking into possible schools now while I still have the energy."

Life's Everyday Difficulties

"Our daily life is difficult just now," Mrs. Nazzaro continues, "because my sister's daughter, my niece, and her baby have moved into our tiny apartment. The four of us in a small one-bedroom apartment make things very crowded and brings about many tensions and conflicts."

"How long will she stay?" I ask.

"Every month she says she needs just one more month to find an apartment of her own, but she has already been with us almost four months. It's hard to turn down a relative who needs help," she sighed, "but I think it is making my health problems worse."

"How is that?" I ask.

"In the last two weeks I have started to have heart palpitations as well as anxiety attacks. Dr. Romero says it is probably caused by the stress in my life. Because of my frequent diarrhea it is hard for me to keep a job. I work in the mailroom in my apartment building a few hours a week but I don't earn much. Fortunately, my government-subsidized rent is only $25 a month (this is 2001) and I receive a government support check of $500 a month but it is still very hard for two people to get by on this in New York City."

Living with Peutz-Jeghers

I knew that living with Peutz-Jeghers Syndrome could be difficult under any circumstances. This disease can cause polyps throughout the intestines. If they do not bleed they may cause no problems but this is usually not the case. Mrs. Nazzaro has had a lot of problems with anemia so it is likely that she has had bleeding polyps. Her diet is severely restricted. She cannot eat fruit with peelings, such as apples, and she cannot drink orange juice. She can only tolerate low-lactose milk and has to make sure all her food is cooked properly. It is hard to get enough fiber on this diet. At the moment her hemoglobin is good and her cholesterol is also in a good range.

"My anemia and cholesterol are probably under control because of my strict diet," she says. "I have been on a constant diet since I was diagnosed with Peutz-Jeghers Syndrome. It's hard to stay on it, though. Sometimes I cannot resist eating something I shouldn't have and I usually pay dearly for it."

"What happens?" I ask.

"I get very bad diarrhea and I am forced to stay home, close to the bathroom, for a day or so."

I note in Mrs. Nazzaro's medical records that she is now in menopause and having problems with severe hot flashes. The chemotherapy and radiation she received may have brought on this slightly early menopause. She also takes the antacid Zantac for occasional dyspepsia and her left kidney is atrophic because of obstruction from renal stones. Her only symptoms from this condition are frequent urinary tract infections. All of her difficult health experiences have made Mrs. Nazzaro sometimes want to avoid doctors. Her PCP keeps a close watch on her to make sure she keeps appointments for her follow-ups and necessary biopsies.

"I am extremely happy with the care I get in the outpatient clinic of New York Presbyterian Hospital," she tells me. "Everybody treats me nice there, not as if I am nobody as staff in other places have in the past. My doctor really listens to what I have to say."

Looking to the Future

Mrs. Nazzaro's daughter Olivia has not yet had any gastrointestinal problems but she has the black-pigmented spots around and inside her mouth that can indicate that she, too, has inherited Peutz-Jeghers Syndrome. She will be checked with a colonoscopy at age 18 or earlier if she shows any symptoms.

"I want to make sure she has these exams," Mrs. Nazzaro says firmly. "I don't want her to have to go through what I have had to. Now that we are on Medicaid, the cost will be covered. That is a great relief, and now that I have arranged for life insurance, I feel that I have done all I can for her future."

Mrs. Nazzaro goes for regular check-ups by her PCP every two or three months. She has a colonoscopy every year, which usually reveals polyps that are removed. At her latest colonoscopy in November 2000, a large, flat, tubulovillous adenoma was discovered. Because of its shape and size it could not be safely removed through the colonoscope. Dr. Romero, as well as the colonoscopist and the surgeon, were concerned that it could become cancerous in the near future. They all advised surgery to have it removed, along with margins of normal tissue. This is the recommended surgery that is the subject at the beginning of our conversation.

Mrs. Nazzaro is adamantly against another operation. She has recently gained a little weight and is in no pain.

"I have gone through enough," she says. "Now I want to wait and see how it goes."

Part IV

The United States Health Care System

10

The US Health Care System

Miriam S. Wetzel, PhD

> *"Every system is perfectly designed to achieve the results it gets"*
>
> *Paul Batalden, MD*[1]

In comparison to Denmark, Germany and Sweden, the US health care system may seem like no system at all. Instead it is a conglomeration of private, public, and charitable organizations and institutions, which provide health care through what has been called "a confusing maze" of hospitals, clinics and individual physicians. This is further complicated by the fact that the 50 states administer important elements of health care, such as Medicaid, and SCHIP (State Children's Health Insurance Program), resulting in a certain amount of variation from state to state. The fundamental difference is the lack of universal health insurance managed by the government. The free-wheeling American system has grown up over the years alongside a democratic government that leans strongly toward individual freedom and choice.

The American system has roots in the earliest settlements in the New World. Many historians credit William Bradford with saving the Plymouth Colony by giving each family its own plot of land and thus introducing the free enterprise system to North America. When the colonists abandoned their original plan of communal agriculture,

Bradford reported that, "The women now went willingly into the field, and took their little ones with them to set corn, which before [they] would allege weakness and inability..."[2] A strong free market economy eventually grew from this reliance on the initiative of the individual and the American entrepreneurial spirit.

US Health Insurance Basics

Although a few health insurance plans were offered in the US during the Civil War, the idea of group health plans originated in 1932 with Blue Cross and Blue Shield.[3] Until that time most medical expenses were paid for by what is now called "fee for service." When someone got sick and called the doctor or needed to go to the doctor's office or hospital, they paid the bill. In rural areas many country doctors were paid with chickens, garden produce, firewood and venison. Mothers of large and small families learned to treat common illnesses with home remedies and avoid an expensive trip to the doctor.

During World War II wages were frozen by the United States government. Unable to pay employees higher salaries, employers began to offer health insurance as a bargaining chip to attract needed workers. By the time the war was over, much of the workforce had come to expect this benefit.[4]

Unlike Germany, Denmark, and Sweden we think of the private rather than the public sector as playing a much larger role in paying for health expenses in the United States. Actually, according to data from the Organisation for Economic Co-operation and Development (OECD), expenditures in the US are more nearly equally divided between private (55.3%) and public (44.7%).[5] The OECD notes, "despite a dominant private sector, US public spending per capita on health remains higher than in most other OECD countries."[6] These countries include Switzerland, Canada, France, Germany, Denmark, Sweden and the United Kingdom — all countries with universal health care.

US Safety-net Insurance

Medicare and Medicaid are the two primary social insurance programs in the United States. Medicare provides health insurance for citizens over 65 and

Medicaid is the medical insurance program for low income and needy people. These programs originated in 1965 as Title XVIII (Medicare) and Title XIX (Medicaid) of the Social Security Act Amendment.[7] Originally Medicare included insurance for people with end-stage renal disease. In 1972, it was expanded to include people younger than 65 with permanent disabilities who meet certain qualifications.[8] Coverage was added later for several other diseases as well. If an individual qualifies for Medicare and full Medicaid coverage, most health expenses are paid.[9] These programs are financed by mandatory contributions from employers and employees, tax revenues, premiums paid by beneficiaries, deductibles and co-payments.

Medicare and Medicaid account for the largest government outlay for health care. In 2007 Medicare cost $431.2 billion, representing a growth rate of 7.2% and the cost for Medicaid was $329.4 billion, at the "relatively normal" growth rate of 6.4%.[10] By 2008 total Medicare spending was $468.1 billion and total expenditure for the Medicaid program was $356.3 billion.[11] In addition to Medicare and Medicaid, the Department of Veterans Affairs and the Railroad Retirement Board provide insurance for certain segments of the population. Other government health care programs include the Federal Employee Health Benefits Program (FEHBP) for members of Congress and other retired federal employees and their families[12] and TRICARE for active-duty service members, retirees, and dependents. There are also Tribal Health Programs and Urban Indian health Programs run by the government Indian Health Service.[13]

Almost all US workers, including federal employees and members of Congress, pay a percentage of their salary to the Social Security fund for old age, survivor, and disability benefits known as the Federal Insurance Contribution Act (FICA). Exceptions are employees of the Railroad Retirement Board and state employees such as teachers with other benefit plans. The amount of FICA tax is determined every year based on the rise in the yearly average wage of American workers. For 2009 the percentage was 6.2% and the taxable wage base was $106,800, up from $102,000 in 2008. Employers also contribute 6.2% and the government contributes the same amount for persons receiving social security. Employers and employees each pay a Medicare tax of 1.45% (total 2.90%) on total earnings.[14]

Medicare

Medicare is a federal health insurance program, consisting of Parts A, B, and since 2006, Part D (prescription drug coverage). It is basically the same anywhere in the US. Medicare covers almost every American above 65 years of age, persons below the age of 65 who are on kidney dialysis or have had a kidney transplant, and people with disabilities who are receiving Supplemental Social Security Insurance (SSI), after a two-year waiting period.

Medicare Part A is hospitalization insurance and covers most inpatient care, critical access care, hospice care, some home health care and a certain number of days in a skilled nursing facility after a three-day stay in a hospital. Part A is free for Americans above age 65 if the recipient or his or her spouse had Social Security-covered employment and paid Medicare taxes for a sufficient length of time to be eligible for Social Security benefits. If they did not pay these taxes, they may still be able to buy into Part A.[15]

Medicare Part B is medical insurance. It covers physicians' services and outpatient hospital care. It also covers certain other medical services that Part A does not cover, for example some of the services of physical and occupational therapists, and certain home health care. Part B also helps to pay for covered services and supplies when they are *medically necessary* — that is when they are recommended by a doctor and they:

- Are needed for the diagnosis or treatment of the medical condition
- Are provided for the diagnosis, direct care and treatment of a medical condition
- Meet the standards of good medical practice in the local area
- Are not mainly for the convenience of the patient or the physician.[16]

Recipients of Medicare Part B each pay a monthly premium of $96.40 per month (2008 to 2010), which is deducted from their Social Security checks. The amount may be higher for people who did not sign up for Part B when they first became eligible. It is increased up to 10% for each 12-month period they could have had Part B but did not sign up for it. These people will have to pay this extra amount as long as they have Part B.[17]

In his paper on the US-EU-MEE project, Danish student Jacob Thyssen suggested that an income-based scale of payment could go a long way toward equalizing coverage for all US citizens.[18] US lawmakers devised such a plan and put it into effect on January 1, 2007. For the first time, monthly premiums for Part B were based on a sliding scale according to annual income. In 2009 the highest monthly premium was $308.30 for a single individual with annual income above $213,000 or couples with a combined income above $426,000.[19]

Part C Medicare Advantage plans[20] are options approved by Medicare and offered by private insurance companies. These plans operate more like HMOs (Health Maintenance Organizations) or PPOs (Preferred Provider Organizations). Usually the patient will have to agree to receive medical care from an approved network of providers. Often the monthly premiums are less than for the Original Medicare Plan, and there are some that have no premium beyond the normal Medicare Part B premium. There are many different plans and the details can be found in the Department of Health and Human Services booklet, *Medicare & You*, which is sent each year to every Medicare recipient.

Medicare Part D. In January 2006, Part D, prescription drug coverage was added to Medicare benefits.[21] This was the first major change in Medicare since its beginning in 1965. Private insurance companies provide the coverage and patients pay a monthly premium, which varies according to the plan chosen. In the first year of Part D coverage, so many variations of costs and benefits were offered that many people found it difficult to understand the whole scheme or to find the right one to meet their needs. Some people were dismayed to discover a gap in coverage, dubbed the "donut hole."[22] When expenditures for prescription drugs reach a certain amount, the patient pays the entire cost until the amount reaches a higher limit. At that point the individual is eligible for "catastrophic coverage." Extra financial help is available under certain circumstances if a person is eligible for both Medicare and Medicaid.

Medicaid[23] is a joint federal and state program that helps with medical costs for people in the US with low incomes and limited resources. Although it is a national program, each state controls its own Medicaid policies. Congress and Centers for Medicare and Medicaid Services (CMS) set the main rules for the program but the individual states tailor them to the specific needs of their citizens. Policies for eligibility, payments, and services covered can vary from state to state. Each state has its own name for its Medicaid program, for example MassHealth in Massachusetts and MaineCare in Maine. Participation by the states in the Medicaid program is not mandatory, but since the early 1980s, every state has had a Medicaid program. Funding is by block grants from the Federal government, which are then administered by the states.

Eligibility for Medicaid is based on income and personal financial resources. In some states, Medicaid may provide coverage for nursing home care, home care, and outpatient prescription drugs not covered by Medicare. Sometimes the individual must spend down personal assets to qualify for Medicaid.

Medicare and Medicaid go a long way toward providing health care for more than 50 million Americans, but like the Social Security system it is not designed to provide for every health care need. For Medicare recipients there are co-pays, deductibles and exclusions. To cover these expenses many Americans buy private supplementary "medigap" insurance or pay out-of-pocket.

Medicare is not strong in preventive measures such as physical exams, and hearing and vision tests. It covers only one screening examination, including EKG, within the first twelve months of receiving Medicare coverage[24] and pays for only a limited amount of laboratory blood tests for cholesterol or other blood abnormalities unless disease is suspected. It does, however, pay for and encourage certain screening examinations such as a yearly mammogram, PSA test for prostate cancer, and colon cancer screening.

Children's Health Insurance Program

In addition to Medicare and Medicaid, the State Children's Health Insurance Program (SCHIP) was launched in 1997 to provide funds to help states expand health care coverage for more than five million of the nation's uninsured children.[25] It was designed to provide health insurance for children in families who earn too much to qualify for Medicaid, but not enough to afford private insurance.

SCHIP was renewed in 2007 at its original funding level after a bitter fight between congress and President Bush who objected to policies of states that have greatly expanded the program to include adult parents and to insure children in families earning more than $82,000 a year. On February 4, 2009, President Obama signed into law an expanded program for children's insurance, now called CHIPRA (Children's Health Insurance Program Reauthorization Act of 2009). It establishes funding from FY 2009 to FY 2013[26] at a higher rate.

US Health Care Changes

Public debate in the US about health care seems to be rising to a fever pitch but actually it has been accelerating for several decades. Costs have been increasing steadily since World War II, fueled by funding from the National Institutes of Health for research and the establishment of Medicare and Medicaid for consumers. In the1980s costs rose precipitously as a percentage of GDP (Gross Domestic Product). For example, in 1980 health care costs represented 8.8% of GDP and by 1988 they had risen to 10.8%. The profitability of companies and their ability to compete in international markets was adversely affected by these high costs and it was clear that this rate of growth was not sustainable.[27]

The public became alarmed at this situation. Workers were afraid to change jobs for fear of losing health insurance, which was not a portable benefit. Hospitals and medical schools that had expanded during the time of plentiful postwar resources from the 1960s to 1980s were now having trouble meeting expenses. By the 1990s there was an oversupply of hospital beds and there was talk of an oversupply of doctors as well, especially foreign medical graduates.[28] The era of seemingly unlimited resources for health care was at an end. As the influence of the medical establishment weakened, third party payers in the form of insurance companies and large for-profit health care corporations emerged and gained power. They demanded, and got lower prices. Competition for patients became fierce.[29]

DRGs

In 1983, when the government established "prospective payment" for Medicare patients, a whole new era of cost containment began. Hospitals were paid for patient care on the basis of a list of 467 Diagnosis-Related Groups (DRGs). Private insurance payers soon adopted a similar system. If a patient's care cost less than allowed by the DRG, the hospital made money; if it cost more, the hospital lost money.[30] There had never been a payment system with incentives like this to move patients in and out of the hospital as quickly as possible. Suddenly, speed and efficiency became important, leading to derogatory terms such as "drive-by mastectomy" and procedures that were so devoid of human interaction as to be almost humorous. In one university-affiliated teaching hospital, pre-operative instructions directed the patient on the day of surgery to proceed to a designated empty room, go to the phone on the desk and dial a certain number and a voice on the telephone would give instructions as to undressing, leaving belongings, and proceeding to the operating room area.[31]

Competition for patients needing tertiary care was especially strong. Medicare and third party payers paid a premium for the care of these costlier patients. Academic medical centers formed networks with smaller hospitals, sometimes a considerable distance away, with the promise that tertiary care patients would be sent to them. Hospitals gradually adapted to the demands of the DRG system but it was a difficult time for clinical medical education. Now there were only two types of patients in the hospital: those who were very ill and those who were in and out in a very short time, or had day surgery and never were admitted to the hospital. Medical schools turned to teaching in clinics and physician's offices to make up for the hospitalized patients who were no longer so readily available.[32]

HMOs

There were other challenges on the horizon, especially for academic medical centers. In response to escalating prices, health maintenance organizations (HMOs) gradually gained ground. Health care at a defined level was provided for people who joined an HMO and paid a monthly fee. As prices continued to climb, it was reassuring to HMO members to know what their basic health care would cost. There were various types of HMOs, each with fees set according to different levels of service and choice of providers.

HMOs had the benefit of hiring from a supply of well-trained primary care doctors and specialists and sending patients to well-established hospital systems, but at first did not contribute to the costs of medical education, research, or caring for indigent people. As employees of HMOs, physicians who had enjoyed teaching as a part of their professional lives now found there was no time to teach. Eventually alliances were formed by some HMOs with nearby medical centers and more equitable arrangements developed. With an incentive for keeping people well and out of the hospital, HMOs were theoretically better at providing routine maintenance and preventive health care than fee-for-service plans.[33]

After the announcement of President Clinton's proposed health care plan in 1993, membership in HMOs exploded, going from 9 million in 1980 to 50 million by 1995. Primary care physicians acted as gatekeepers and recommended specialists only when necessary. Accordingly, the demand for primary care physicians rose as did medical student choice, with 14.4% of medical students seeking primary care residencies in 1992 and 27.7% in 1995.[34] HMOs kept their medical staffs as lean as possible and demanded a high level of productivity. With increased hiring of physician's assistants and nurse practitioners, for the first time some doctors found themselves facing unemployment and some specialists worked as primary care physicians. Prior to this time there were approximately 240 doctors per 100,000 people in the US but HMOs managed with 100 to 140 doctors per 100,000 members.[35]

During the 1990s, there were complaints about HMOs denying care and putting profits before patients. Case managers were hired and had a lot of power over medical decisions but they were not always medically trained. Patient-doctor relationships suffered under the time constraints and accelerated pace of medical care.[36] With more government oversight, and criticism from the public, eventually a sort of equilibrium was reached. HMO managers realized that it was good business to become more "user friendly;" point-of-service and out-of-network treatment options allowed for more choice and market forces gradually brought the number of hospital beds and physicians in line with need.

The Clinton Health Plan

The Clinton health plan, presented to Congress by President William Clinton on September 22, 1993, was the first major attempt to reform the US health care system since Medicare and Medicaid. It promised health care for everybody provided mainly by employers and the government through private health maintenance organizations closely regulated by a network of public organizations called health care alliances.[37] At first it seemed to meet with approval, but after a year of debate in Congress and by the public, Senator George Mitchell announced on September 26, 1994 that health care legislation was dead.[38]

No doubt there were many factors that led to the demise of the Clinton plan. During the year of debate, polls showed that it lost the support of the middle class. Middle class people didn't think they would gain anything from it and thought they would lose some benefits they already had.[39] Other concerns reflected the basic mistrust of Americans in government and the fear that this plan would create a huge bureaucracy and squander large sums of money through the health care alliances. Underlying the objections was a sense of dissatisfaction in the way the plan was crafted by a task force of 500 led by First Lady Hilary Rodham Clinton.[40] There was little input from the medical profession on the task force, reinforcing mistrust and opposition by physicians and the American Medical Association. The plan ran to more than 1000 pages and was probably never adequately understood by either Congress or the public. A final death knell was sounded by the fact that legislators who favored health care reform did not wholeheartedly support the Clinton plan and came up with a total of 27 alternate plans.[41] In polls the public expressed the sentiment that the government should work to make the health care system better but should not destroy the parts that were working well. One real or perceived threat was the fear that everybody would be forced into a government-run plan, even if they were perfectly satisfied with their health care.[42]

US Health Care Costs

With a rate of increase of 44.7% in per capita spending since 1995, the escalating cost of medical care is a serious concern in the United States.

Some predict that US health care spending will double over the next decade to $4.1 trillion a year with the government share of the cost reaching 50%.[43] Social Security, Medicare and Medicaid make up about 40% of annual US government expenditures. These are mandatory programs; required by law. They are also known as entitlements because the American people have become increasingly dependent on them and feel entitled to them. These expenditures could escalate rapidly in the next decade as 78 million "baby boomers" (born between the years of 1946 and 1964) are expected to retire.[44]

Health care costs have risen faster than GDP (Gross Domestic Product) in the United States since the 1960s.[45] This rise is reflected in the increased cost of health care insurance purchased by both employers and individuals. In 2006 the cost began to moderate slightly from its highest annual increase of over 14% in 2003 but still outpaced inflation and other consumer prices by a wide margin.[46] The percentage of GDP spent on health care in the US has been consistently higher than in Germany, Denmark, Sweden and other European countries (See Table 10.1).[47]

The US has also had the highest expenditure per capita for health care among OECD countries (See Table 10.2).[48] This figure has risen steadily and in 2006 was more than twice the amount spent per capita by Denmark, Germany and Sweden.

The usual explanations fail to completely explain why the cost of health care goods and services and the salaries of some specialists and administrators have increased so much more rapidly than the cost of living in the US. Donald Berwick of the Institute for Healthcare Improvement and others continue to work to develop better systems in hospitals and medical practices and to stem the tide of paperwork, much of it imposed by the government.[49]

Table 10.1. Total Health Expenditure as % of GDP.

	1999	2000	2001	2002	2003	2004	2005	2006	2007
Germany	10.3	10.3	10.4	10.6	10.8	10.6	10.7	10.5	10.4
Denmark	8.5	8.3	8.6	8.8	9.3	9.5	9.5	9.6	9.8
Sweden	8.3	8.2	9.0	9.3	9.4	9.2	9.2	9.1	9.1
United States	13.5	13.6	14.3	15.1	15.6	15.6	15.7	15.8	16.0

OECD Health Data 2009, November 2009.

Table 10.2.   Total Expenditure on Health per capita, US$ PPP.

	1999	2000	2001	2002	2003	2004	2005	2006	2007
Germany	2592	2671	2808	2937	3088	3162	3348	3464	3588
Denmark	2281	2378	2521	2696	2832	3055	3352	3357	3512
Sweden	2129	2283	2508	2697	2829	2950	2958	3124	3323
United States	4450	4704	5053	5453	5851	6194	6558	6933	7290

OECD Health Data 2009, November 2009.

Michael O. Leavitt, the US Secretary of Health and Human Services from 2005 to 2009 has said that the increasing burden of health spending on the US economy is unsustainable.[50] Better ways must be found to provide an adequate level of insurance for the elderly and the most needy Americans. President Obama announced that $635 billion would be set aside in the 2010 federal budget to help finance health reform. During the spring of 2009 he frequently stated that, "The Recovery Act puts us on a path to modernize the health care system and deliver better care while reducing unnecessary costs." He specifically mentioned three paths to this goal:

- Computerizing American health records in 5 years
- Developing and disseminating information on effective medical interventions through comparative effectiveness research
- Investing in prevention and wellness

He says this program of health care reform will be financed by rebalancing the tax code, aligning incentives toward quality, promoting efficiency and accountability, and encouraging shared responsibility.[51] After a major political debate, Congress passed the Patient Protection and Affordable Care Act (PPAC) in March 2010, calling for reforms in insurance coverage and health care policy to be implemented over four years.[52] The act was passed by congress despite polls indicating that a substantial majority of the American public did not agree with this reform. The estimated public and personal cost impact of PPAC remains the subject of vigorous debate. Projections range from a modest cost saving to a major cost increase approaching a trillion dollars.

What Are We Getting for Our Money?

In the US, as in other countries, the increase in health care costs is fueled by the aging population, increased demand for health services and increased cost of new health care technology. David Cutler, Ph.D., of Harvard University says the real question is whether we are getting our money's worth from medical technology. He says "current health technologies on average return $4 in approximate life value for every medical dollar spent."[53]

A Kaiser Family Foundation report details the technological advances in the treatment of heart disease from 1980 to 2000 and the resulting decrease in mortality from 345.2 to 186.0 per 100,000 persons. They cite other examples of remarkable advances in the treatment of pre-term infants and formerly fatal diseases such as diabetes, AIDS, and end-stage renal disease.[54] These advances come at a price. No matter whether US health care is paid for by a universal health care plan administered by the government or by a combination of public and private plans, working men and women will bear the burden. Already US taxes weigh heavily on the country's middle class.

Still Looking for Solutions: The Uninsured and Underinsured

The United States receives bad press for its well-publicized 45.7 million uninsured (15.3% of the total population in 2007, according to official numbers available from the US Census Bureau).[55] This number crept up by 1% a year from 2000 to 2004 as a slight economic downturn forced more people out of work and into lower paying jobs and fewer employers offered insurance. The number of uninsured actually decreased slightly from 2006 to 2007. The full effects of the serious economic downturn of 2008 are yet to be seen. In 2007 the US Census Bureau reported that the number of uninsured had been overstated by nearly two million since 1995 because of a computer programming error.[56] The uninsured, give or take a few million, is still too high and is the subject of much debate and concern.

Who are the uninsured and why are they uninsured?

According to the Kaiser Foundation, more than 70% of the uninsured are in households that have at least one adult who is employed full-time. An additional 12% are in households with a part-time worker.[57] Some workers may be employed by companies that do not offer insurance, or if they do, the employees cannot afford their share of the insurance premium. Small companies in particular may not be able to afford to offer insurance. Self-employed workers or those in part time occupations and entry-level jobs are more likely to lack insurance. Other individuals may be between jobs and lack insurance for only a few months; when a tally is taken they are counted among the uninsured. Others have different priorities for their money and choose not to buy insurance. The largest group of uninsured adults is in the 19–29 year age range.[57] Many of these largely healthy young adults do not see the point in paying for a product they do not feel they need. Foolhardy as this may be, in a free society, individuals are free to make foolish choices. In addition, an estimated 1.8 million disabled workers aged 50 to 64 who qualify for Social Security Disability Income but must wait 24 months to qualify for Medicare are counted among the uninsured.[58]

It may be surprising that according to US Census figures, in 2007 more than one third of the uninsured in the US lived in households with annual income of $50,000 or more and almost 20% were from households with income of $75,000 or more. The percentages in Table 10.3 are based on 45.7 million total uninsured. According to census figure estimates, approximately ten million are not US citizens.[59]

The high cost of health insurance in the US provides a partial but not wholly satisfactory explanation for people with moderate income lacking health insurance. There is no doubt that there is a need for more affordable health insurance for working middle class families. According to the Kaiser Foundation, since 2001 premiums for family coverage have

Table 10.3.   Household Income of Uninsured in the US, 2007.

Household Income	Uninsured (in Millions)	Percent of Uninsured
Less than $25,000	13.5	29.5
$25,000 to $49,999	14.5	31.7
$50,000 to $74,999	8.5	18.6
$75,000 or more	9.1	19.9

US Census Bureau Current Population Report issued Aug. 2008.

increased 78% while wages have gone up only 19%. In 2008, Kaiser lists the typical annual health insurance premium for a family of four as $12,680.[60] An annual income of $50,000 to $75,000 is not considered unusually high in many parts of the country and would require careful budgeting to afford coverage at this rate. There is often a huge jump in price between insurance for an individual and for a family, with no in-between price for couples without children. This may influence young married couples to pass up insurance in favor of other purchases.

The Commonwealth Fund reports that 6 million uninsured children and two-thirds of uninsured poor parents already qualify for Medicare, Medicaid, or SCHIP but are not enrolled.[61] Why are they not enrolled? The government has stepped up educational outreach and enrollment efforts to help reduce this number. This problem is greater in the southern and western part of the US. Forty percent of those who are eligible and are not enrolled are Hispanic, 37% are white, and 18% are black.[62] While the children who were born here are US citizens and are eligible for public health insurance, many live with adults or parents who are not legal US citizens. Most new immigrants are not eligible for Medicaid during the first five years in the US and undocumented persons are eligible only for emergency services. Parents who are in the US illegally may not want to draw the attention of the authorities by registering their children.

In every society there is a small number of individuals who do not access the services available to them, whether because of apathy or lack of ability to navigate the bureaucracy or for other reasons. Ulrika Nordin writes in *The Magazine of the International Red Cross and Red Crescent* Program.[63]

> "Even in Sweden's super-regulated society, there are thousands (nobody knows how many) undocumented persons who do not qualify for health care from the government. These are people who have not registered with the government for a variety of reasons, so have no state identity number. As in the US, they are entitled to emergency care but nothing more."

In the US there are an estimated 10 to 12 million undocumented workers, many of whom may be in a similar situation. The Rand Corporation found that 68% of undocumented immigrant adults they studied in 2005 had no health insurance.[64] They calculated that this could account for about one-third of the increase in uninsured adults from 1980 to 2000. While accurate figures are difficult to verify, there is no doubt that this group has an impact on the number of uninsured, especially in the border states of California, Texas, Arizona and New Mexico.

In a report for an organization called *Insure the Uninsured Project*, Lucien Wulsin called covering 800,000 undocumented workers "the most politically difficult decision facing the Governor and state legislature" [of California].[65] Health care for illegal immigrants is reportedly costing Los Angeles County $30,000,000 per month.[66] In Arizona, Mexican nationals can call for a US ambulance and be admitted to the US under the "compassionate entry" policy. This costs hospitals such as the Copper Queen Community Hospital in Bisbee, Arizona hundreds of thousands of dollars in uncompensated care, although since 2005 the US government has reimbursed part of the cost.[67]

Too often US citizens and non-citizens alike rely on hospital Emergency Departments for primary care. The Emergency Medical Treatment and Active Labor Act (EMTALA), a Federal law passed in 1986, gives any US citizen, and those who live in the US but are not US citizens, the right to receive emergency care regardless of ability to pay.[68] This is sometimes cited as proof that there is health care on demand in the United States. The problem is that this is not optimal care, nor perhaps even good care for several reasons.

First and foremost, according to EMTALA, doctors in Emergency Departments are only required to examine, screen and stabilize the patient, and transfer him or her to another facility if necessary and appropriate. Second, this is expensive primary care because it is provided in an inappropriate setting, with high tech equipment and highly trained personnel, when treatment for an earache or sore throat could be more effectively and efficiently provided in a General Practitioner's office or in one of the new "Minute Clinics" increasingly available in the US.[69] The third major reason that Emergency Department care is inferior for this purpose is that there is no mechanism for follow-up and there is no time for education to promote healthy behaviors. The mission of the emergency room is to provide necessary acute care and the person who comes for routine care interferes with that mission.

The Underinsured

And finally, there are the underinsured in the US. They are defined as "people who have insurance but whose medical expenses (excluding insurance premiums) total 10% or more of their post-tax income or 5% or more of their income if it is below 200% of the federal poverty level." According to this definition, a 2003 study by the Agency for Healthcare Research and Quality found that 17.1 million Americans under age 65 were underinsured, including 9.3 million with employer-based insurance.[70]

The primary causes of underinsurance include:

- Loss of workplace insurance
- High cost of insurance premiums
- Plans that have high deductibles and reduced benefits.

Some programs meant to reduce the number of under- or uninsured have had unexpected consequences. For example in Maine, the state government-subsidized insurance plan, DirigoChoice, is financed partly by an assessment on private insurance companies, which in 2007 amounted to $34 million.[71,72] Disagreement about this "offset" has caused many insurance companies to leave Maine and has resulted in some of the highest insurance premiums in the United States, making it harder for many people to afford coverage.

Insurance Linked to Employment — Good or Bad?

The majority of people in the US who have health insurance get it through their jobs. The number of employers offering insurance to full-time workers was on a downward trend from 2004 to 2006 but remained steady at around 60% from 2007 to 2008.[73] The connection between health insurance and employment has both positive and negative aspects.

Offering a good health insurance plan helps companies attract and maintain a stable workforce, which benefits the company, workers, customers and the economy as a whole, but not every worker qualifies for employer-provided insurance. In some companies there is a waiting period or a requirement for a minimum number of hours worked to qualify for health insurance. Some employees cannot afford their share of the insurance premium depending on how much it is subsidized by the employer. The employee's share of the premium doubled since 2000.[74] There is criticism of a tax advantage for employer-provided health insurance compared to insurance purchased by individuals because the amount the employer pays is not taxed while in some instances the individual must purchase insurance with after-tax money.

Making Insurance More Affordable

The Medicare bill of 2003 paved the way for Health Savings Accounts, designed to make health insurance more affordable for working families. These plans combine low cost, high-deductible insurance for catastrophic coverage with a health savings account in which pre-tax dollars up to an annual limit may be deposited to pay for health care expenses. This money earns interest and grows tax free. Some plans also cover preventive services. The deductible amounts seem quite high but subscribers are protected from catastrophic health care costs and can benefit from staying healthy. Participation in these plans has been growing slowly but steadily, from about 4% of covered workers, or 2.7 million people in 2006 to about 5% or 3.8 million people in 2007.[75]

In addition to helping solve the problem of affordable insurance, Health Savings Accounts hold the possibility of changing the way Americans think about paying for their health needs. Instead of being insulated from the cost of health care by a third-party payer, the cost is apparent to the consumer who will benefit directly by finding the best value for the money. As Americans become accustomed to exercising more control over health care decisions and taking more individual responsibility for paying for health care, the hope is that choice and competition will help to curb medical inflation.

A 2006 report, "Making Consumerism Work: A Practical Guide for Transforming Healthcare" by SHPS, Inc., found that "people covered by consumer-driven health plans are 50% more likely to ask about the costs of treatments when making choices, and more likely to choose lower-cost options. They are more likely to seek care at lower-cost urgent/convenience care clinics than in hospital Emergency Departments, 30% more likely to get annual physicals and 20% more compliant with disease management regimens."[76] Transparency in pricing in the medical market-place is essential to making these plans work. Hospital Corporation of America, the nation's largest hospital chain, has begun to post prices for procedures in some of its 165 US hospitals.[77] Other hospitals and medical practices are expected to follow suit.

The federal government has provided some money to the states to develop their own innovative insurance plans. All residents 18 and older in the state of Massachusetts have been required to purchase insurance that meets certain basic requirements since July 1, 2007 or face a penalty. The penalty is based on age, income and family size and can be as much as $1068 per year.[78] The number of uninsured in Massachusetts has declined but the program has been more expensive than anticipated although the federal government reimburses 50% of the cost.

Tennessee Governor Phil Bredesen's CoverTN plan started April 1, 2007 and was designed to provide basic low-cost health insurance for small business and uninsured working people. It costs employees around $60 a month, with the employer and the government paying a similar amount. Tennessee also offers insurance programs for people with serious pre-existing medical conditions and pregnant women and children as well as prescription drug coverage for people who do not have it. Enrollment is suspended when the program reaches its budget limit[79] and some criticize the program for putting people at risk because of inadequate coverage.[80] The Dirigo program in Maine that was hailed as an example of effective state-run programs has enrolled only about ten percent of intended beneficiaries and is considered by many to have fallen far short of expectations.[81]

Ingenuity

Innovative ideas for making US health care more available and affordable are springing up in the form of quick care clinics. MinuteClinic pioneered by Rick Krieger in the Minneapolis-St. Paul area in 2000 quickly grew to 87 walk-in clinics that are being widely imitated.[82] By 2010 the number expanded to 560 clinics in 25 states located in CVS drugstores. Baylor Health Care System teamed with MedBasics to launch a series of clinics located in Metroplex Food Stores. TakeCare and RediClinic are other chains that have opened in the Chicago area, the southwest and other locations. Wal-Mart, Walgreen's, Kerr Drug and other stores announced plans to offer low-cost prescriptions and establish thousands of low-cost, walk-in clinics in shopping malls and retail stores. These clinics are staffed by nurse practitioners who can competently diagnose and treat 25 to 40 common medical conditions and write prescriptions. Fees range between $39 and $75. They are open weekends and evenings and do not require appointments.[83]

Besides offering convenience and affordability, these clinics are helping to bring about changes in the health care system. The American Academy of Family Physicians urged its 94,000 physician members to expand office hours and same-day appointments. Larry Fields, the physician head of AAFP said, "Hopefully, we'll be able to compete."[84] Grace-Marie Turner writing in the *Wall Street Journal* says, "Take note, Congress. The market is providing cheaper medicine."[85]

Time will tell if the quick care clinics will thrive. Clayton Christensen, a professor at the Harvard Business School and author of *The Innovator's Dilemma* (1997), *The Innovator's Solution* (2003), and *The Innovator's Prescription* (2009), thinks they are exactly the kind of innovation that will be the impetus for change. They are similar to other "disruptive technologies" that have gone in a new direction and made peoples lives better by "commoditizing" a service or product and making it more affordable and accessible.[86] Christensen states that "Hoping our hospitals and doctors become cheap won't make health care more affordable and accessible but a move toward lower cost venues and lower cost caregivers will.[87]

Outcome Measures

Outcome measures such as life expectancy and infant mortality are often used as indicators of the quality of a country's health care system. On these indicators, the United States is frequently pointed out as ranking lower than other OECD countries (see Tables 10.4 and 10.5).[88] These are rankings we are not proud of, but not everyone agrees that longevity is a particularly valid indicator of a country's quality of health care. Many factors such as diet, lifestyle, substance abuse and cultural customs, have a profound influence on health and longevity.

Table 10.4. Life expectancy; Total population at birth — Years.

	1996	1998	2000	2002	2003	2004	2005	2006
Germany	76.9	77.6	78.2	78.5	78.6	79.2	79.4	79.8
Denmark	75.7	76.5	76.9	77.1	77.4	77.8	78.3	78.4
Sweden	79.0	79.4	79.7	79.9	80.2	80.6	80.8	80.8
United States	76.1	76.7	76.8	77.2	77.5	77.8	77.8	77.7*

OECD Health Data 2009, July 2009.

*US value for 2006 not available from OECD. Data from CDC, National Vital Statistics Reports, Vol. 57, No 14.

Table 10.5. Infant Mortality — Deaths/1000 Live Births.

	1996	1998	2000	2002	2003	2004	2005	2006
Germany	5.0	4.7	4.4	4.2	4.2	4.1	3.9	3.8
Denmark	5.6	4.7	5.3	4.4	4.4	4.4	4.4	3.8
Sweden	4.0	3.6	3.4	3.3	3.1	3.1	2.4	2.8
United States*	7.3	7.2	6.9	7.0	6.8	6.8	6.9	6.7

OECD Health Data 2009, July 2009.

*US data based on birth weight greater than 500 gms. Other countries use higher birth weight.

Dr. David Asch, executive director of the Leonard Davis Institute of Health Economics and the Eller Professor of Health Care Management and Economics at the University of Pennsylvania notes that in the US we are frequently reminded that we spend more on health care than any other country and achieve population health outcomes lower than other industrialized nations. "The much more complicated reality," he says, "is that what we really have is an extremely broad distribution of health care costs and spending across segments of the population and an extremely broad distribution of health care outcomes across the population. ... The averages tell you nothing in a country like ours."[89] Others have pointed to the higher rate of homicides and accidents in the United States — not an admirable statistic, but one that tends to cut young lives short and skews the longevity curve. Some researchers have shown that when these causes of death are removed, the US rises to the top of the list for life expectancy.[90]

There are also problems with using infant mortality as a marker of the quality of health care compared to other countries. In the US, all infants weighing over 500 grams are included in the calculations. Other countries use a higher minimum birth weight, which raises the chances of viability and makes US data less comparable. Advances in obstetrical care have made it possible for infants in the US to be born alive at lower and lower birth weight and gestational age. These infants, along with children born to teenaged mothers, to mothers addicted to cocaine, and to illegal immigrant mothers who may not have had adequate prenatal care all contribute to the US infant mortality rate but do not necessarily indicate a poorer quality of health care[91]; see Table 10.5.[92]

Culture, Politics, and Health

The whole issue of health care has become a major political area of contention in the US. On one hand, some think that free market forces can bring about needed improvement.[93] With less rather than more government intervention, they contend that competition will reduce costs and improve the quality and availability of care. They point out that health care and economics are very closely related and the US system has produced a vibrant economy and major medical advances that are sought after by patients from all over the world. Critics point to the need to improve accessibility and patient satisfaction and decrease medical errors, costs, and waste.[94] Some people believe that governmental regulation is necessary to achieve these goals.

In the summer of 2009, President Barack Obama and the Congress have focused intense energy on a viable health plan for the United States. The topic dominated TV and radio and even the *New England Journal of Medicine* weighed in weekly online and in print with opinions.[95,96] The question sometimes seemed not to be what was best for the American people, but who could win the struggle. One *NEJM writer* questioned whether it was important to consider "American Values" in redesigning the US health care system.[97] Aside from the enormous cost, a huge question remains: how can health care be provided for an additional 50 million citizens without an immediate increase in the number of physicians, nurses, and other health care providers?[98]

A few months before he was appointed in July 2010 to be head of the Centers for Medicare and Medicaid Services (CMS), Donald Berwick, MD said, "...in an era of financial meltdown, vast federal debt, powerful fiscal hawks like the Congressional Budget Office and the Office of Management and Budget, and skepticism about any new government program, putting off the math may not work. Universal coverage will come packaged with affordability, or it may not come at all."[99]

J. James Rohack, MD, in leading the American Medical Association in support of health care legislation said, "Without a doubt, we must reform the health system so that every American has affordable, high-quality health care coverage. ...There is a clear understanding that if we don't slow the rate of growth on health care costs, it will be near impossible to achieve the vision of affordable, quality health care and coverage for all."[100]

Some physicians feel that one crucial point is being left out of the debate. The cost of malpractice insurance in the US is astronomical. In Denmark, Germany, and Sweden there is little litigation and physicians generally do not carry malpractice insurance. The American Medical Association did not press this point when offering support for President Obama's health plan. In addition to the high cost of malpractice insurance, the low level and delay of reimbursement to physicians for the care of Medicare and Medicaid patients by the US government and many state agencies contributes to economic pressure on physicians and pricing schemes that are impossible for the public to understand.

Physician-writer Atul Gawande studied the difference in health care costs across the country and wrote a thought-provoking article in *The New Yorker*.[101] He compared widely disparate Medicare per capita expenditures in communities such as McAllen Texas, Grand Junction, Colorado and Miami, Florida. His observations illuminate how the mode of thinking by physicians in a community can influence health care expenditures and the quality of care. He predicts that it will take at least a decade to change the culture of medicine "to increase prevention and the quality of care, while discouraging overtreatment, undertreatment, and sheer profiteering." Unless we figure out how to bring costs down in this, the most expensive health care system in the world, he predicts that reform will fail.

Conclusion

What Can the US Learn from Denmark, Germany and Sweden?

The Key Role of Expectations

In the thirty case studies presented in this book, the students who participated in the US-EU-MEE program demonstrated that they learned not
only the basic organization of the health care systems in their host countries, but also perceived the strong connections binding culture, ethics,
politics and health care. The expectations of the people in Denmark,
Germany and Sweden have been shaped over many years by prevailing
political philosophy and long-standing health care practices. The citizens
expect health care to be provided or highly regulated by the government
and although they may complain, polls show they are generally satisfied
with the level of care they receive.[102] Likewise, they have for many years
accepted the high taxes necessary to support their health care systems and
the limitations this imposes on the control of their own earnings. How are
expectations different in the US?

The Importance of Primary Care

From all three European countries the US can learn the importance of
primary care and accessibility to a personal physician. To make this possible Sweden and Denmark, for example, have at times attempted to
equalize the geographic distribution of physicians. In Denmark a patient
is assigned a primary care physician within a prescribed distance and this
physician serves as a gatekeeper to specialist care. Primary care physicians in Sweden do not have the gatekeeper role but most health centers
and hospitals are owned by county councils and staffed by salaried physicians and other health care providers. The German Statutory Health
Insurance (SHI) provides for patient choice of primary care physicians
and specialists. To maintain the level of primary care practitioners,
Denmark, Germany and Sweden will have to find ways to curb the rising
proportion of specialists, as will the US.[103]

The Economics of Health Care

The US can learn a great deal about the economics of health care from Denmark, Germany and Sweden. All three countries have found it difficult to maintain the level of free care expected by their people. Germany instituted stringent measures to control costs when they saw their yearly health care deficit rise to three and four billion Euros per year.[104] Sweden took action to counteract the tendency of their generous sick leave and disability policies to result in too large a proportion of their able-bodied workforce choosing leisure over work.[105] All three countries are adopting more free-market features such as competition among insurance providers, more cost sharing by patients and limited coverage beyond basic health care.

Expectations for US Health Care

To be sure, Denmark, Sweden and Germany are smaller and less diverse countries in both geography and population than the US but they can offer us valuable lessons. What sort of health care system will meet the expectations of the US people? Will the straightforward responsibilties of state, regional and local governments in Sweden, the annual budget restrictions of Denmark, or the long-standing and highly organized system of sickness funds in Germany serve as models for a better health care system in the US? Can costs be lowered by more attention to good nutrition, exercise and healthy lifestyle choices rather than increasing reliance on pharmaceuticals and expensive tests and procedures?

The health care dilemma for the US is to maintain excellence in acute care and the high level of entrepreneurial effort to find new treatments for serious disease while reducing costs and offering an acceptable level of choice of care for all citizens. As US-EU-MEE participant Jon Duke observed during his sojourn as an exchange student in Denmark, "There is no perfect health care system."

References

Preface

1. Armstrong EG, Fischer MR. Comparing health care delivery systems —
   initiating a student exchange project between Europe and the United States.
   Med Ed 2001;35:695–701.
2. United States Europe Medical Educational Exchange Project. *Passport*
   2004.
3. PricewaterhouseCooper. HealthCast 2020: creating a sustainable future.
   Executive Summary, 2005. www.pwc.com/healthcare. Accessed 8/8/08.
4. PricewaterhouseCooper. You get what you pay for: a global look at balancing
   demand, quality, and efficiency in healthcare payment reform, 2008.
   http:// www.pwc.com/extweb/pwcpublications.nsf/docid/ BC589DEBA59D9
   B228525746500600790. Accessed 8/6/08.

Chapter 1. Danish and US Health Care Systems Compared

1. Duke J. Experiencing '*hygge*'. US-EU-MEE case report, 1999.
2. Gram, Niels, Copenhagen Hospital Corporation Chief Financial Officer.
   Quoted by US-EU-MEE student, Jon Duke, from personal interview,
   1999.

3. Dogonowski AM. Health Care Contrast In New York. US-EU-MEE case report, 2003

4. Medicare and Medicaid. http://www.cms.hhs.gov/history. Accessed July 9, 2009.

5. US Census Bureau. http://www.census.gov/ Accessed June 30, 2009.

6. Kaiser Family Foundation. The Uninsured: A Primer, October 2008. Kaiser Family Foundation Health Coverage & the Uninsured. http://www.kff.org/ uninsured/upload/7613.pdf. Accessed July 12, 2009.

7. WHO Information: Denmark http://www.who.int/countries/dnk/en/. Accessed April 29, 2007.

8. Health Care in Denmark. http://www.im.dk/publikationer/healthcare_in_dk/ all.htm#c1-3. Accessed Nov. 15, 2006.

9. The local government reform in brief. Chapter 2: A new map of Denmark. http://www.im.dk/publikationer/government_reform_in_brief/kap02.htm. Accessed Nov. 15, 2006.

10. Ministry of the Interior and Health, Ministry of Social Affairs. Report on health and long-term care in Denmark. April 2005. 1. Local government reform in Denmark. http://eng.social.dk/index.aspx?id=6c69ba60-5ac5-49c7-bda8-c719fcaf5230. Accessed Dec. 1, 2006. (No page numbers in this excellent report).

11. Pederson KM, Christiansen T, Bech M. *Health Econ*, 2005 Sep. 14(Suppl 1): 541–557.

12. Vallgårda S, Krasnik A, Vrangbæk K. Health Care Systems in Transition: Denmark. Thomson S, Mossialos E (eds). Organizational Structure and Management, p. 20. http://www.euro.who.int/document/e72967.pdf. Accessed Nov. 16, 2006.

13. Ministry of the Interior and Health, Ministry of Social Affairs. Report on health and long-term care in Denmark, April 2005. 2.1: The National Health Service. http://eng.social.dk/index.aspx?id=6c69ba60-5ac5-49c7-bda8-c719fcaf5230. Accessed Nov. 12, 2006.

14. Duke J. Experiencing '*hygge*'. US-EU-MEE case report, 1999.

15. Chan B. A Foreigner with Tuberculosis. US-EU-MEE case report, 2003.

16. Eichbaum Q. In the Same Boat. US-EU-MEE case report, 2001.

17. Ministry of the Interior and Health, Ministry of Social Affairs. Report on health and long-term care in Denmark, April 2005. 3.1 The health area: Freedom of choice in the health area. http://eng.social.dk/index.aspx? id=6c69ba60-5ac5-49c7-bda8-c719fcaf5230. Accessed Nov. 12, 2006.

18. Ministry of the Interior and Health, Ministry of Social Affairs. Report on health and long-term care in Denmark, April 2005. 3.1 The health area: Freedom of choice in the health area. http://eng.social.dk/index.aspx?id=6c69ba60-5ac5-49c7-bda8-c719fcaf5230. Accessed Nov. 12, 2006.

19. *Indenrigs-og Sundhedsministeriet.* Transparency and Quality Management — the Danish Model. Sept. 11, 2005, http://www.im.dk/im/site.aspx?p=2246&ArticleID=4168. Accessed Nov. 13, 2006.

20. Health service/health insurance in Denmark. The state-run health system. March 2005. http://www.ess-europe.de/en/denmark.htm. Accessed Nov. 13, 2006.

21. Ministry of the Interior and Health, Ministry of Social Affairs. Report on health and long-term care in Denmark, April 2005. 3.1 The health area: Freedom of choice in the health area. http://eng.social.dk/index.aspx?id=6c69ba60-5ac5-49c7-bda8.

22. Hurst J, Siciliani L. Tackling excessive waiting times for elective surgery: A comparison of policies in 12 OECD countries. OECD Health Working Papers, 2003 (6). http://www.oecd.org/dataoecd/24/32/5162353.pdf. Accessed Nov. 29, 2007.

23. Ministry of the Interior and Health, Ministry of Social Affairs. Report on health and long-term care in Denmark, April 2005. 3.1 The health area: Freedom of choice in the health area. http://eng.social.dk/index.aspx?id=6c69ba60-5ac5-49c7-bda8-c719fcaf5230. Accessed Nov. 12, 2006.

24. OECD Economic Survey: Denmark, October 2008, p. 145.

25. OECD Economic Survey: Denmark, October 2008, p. 147.

26. OECD Economic Survey: Denmark, October 2008, p. 136.

27. The Local Government Reform in Brief, Chapter 3. http://www.im.dk/publikationer/government_reform_in_brief/kap03.htm. Accessed Nov. 9, 2006.

28. National Health Service Corps. http://bhpr.hrsa.gov/. Accessed Nov. 9, 2006.

29. Frontier Nursing Service. http://www.frontiernursing.org/. Accessed Nov. 9, 2006.

30. Infertility insurance: making companies pay. http://americanradioworks.publicradio.org/features/fertility_race/part9/section4.shtml. Accessed July 14, 2009.

31. Centers for Disease Control. Cigarette smoking among adults — United States 2004. http://www.cdc.gov/mmwr/preview/mmwrhtml/mm5444a2.htm. Accessed April 22, 2007.

32. Inventive Parent. Car Seat Laws. http://www.inventiveparent.com/state-laws.htm. Accessed April 22, 2007.

33. Kearney PM, Whelton M, Reynolds K, Muntner P, Whelton PK, He J. Global burden of hypertension: Analysis of worldwide data. *Lancet*, 2005 Jan 15–21;365(9455):217–223.

34. Vidt DG. Pathogenesis and treatment of resistant hypertension. *Minerva Med*, 2003 Aug;94(4):201–14.

35. Dall, Michael. Chairman, Research and Educational Committee, The Danish Medical Association. Personal communication, April 28, 2008.

36. Blume D. Engaging citizens in the Danish health care sector. Organisation for Economic Co-operation and Development, 2001. http://www.oecd.org/dataoecd/53/44/2536455.pdf. Accessed April 22, 2007.

37. OECD Health Working Paper No. 22. Health Care Quality Indicators Project. Initial Indicators Report. 9 March 2006. Soeren Mattke, Edward Kelley, Peter Scherer, Jeremy Hurst, Maria Louisa Gill Lapetra, and the HCQI Expert Group Members led by Arnie Epstein, Harvard University. http://www.oecd.org/dataoecd/1/34/36262514.pdf. Accessed April 14, 2007.

38. US Bureau of Labor Statistics. Volunteering in the United States, 2006. http://www.bls.gov/news.release/volun.nr0.htm. Accessed May 20, 2007.

39. *Indenrigs-og Sundhedsministeriet*. Health Care in Denmark. Patients' rights. http://www.im.dk/publikationer/healthcare_in_dk/c7.htm. Accessed April 14, 2007.

40. *Indenrigs-og Sundhedsministeriet*. Health Care in Denmark. Research and Ethics. Accessed April 14, 2007.

41. The Danish Council of Ethics. http://www.etiskraad.dk/sw295.asp. Accessed May 20, 2007.

42. Eichbaum Q. In the Same Boat. US-EU-MEE case report, 2001.

43. Budetti, Peter P. Medical Malpractice Law in the United States. Kaiser Family Report, May 2005, p. 28. http://www.kff.org/insurance/upload/Medical-Malpractice-Law-in-the-United-States-Report.pdf. Accessed Nov. 28, 2007.

44. Standing Committee of the Hospitals of the European Union. Insurance and Malpractice. April 12, 2004. http://www.hope.be/07publi/07newpublics/HOPE%20MALPRACTICE%20REPORT%20APRIL%202004.pdf. Accessed April 22, 2007.

45. Csillag C. Danish doctors want a new system to report medical errors. *Lancet* 360 (9336):858, Sept. 14, 2002.

46. Corrigan J, Kohn LT, Donaldson MS, Eds. *To Err is Human: Building a Safer Health System*. Institute of Medicine, 1999.

47. Spath PL. Error reduction in health care: a systems approach to improving patient safety. Health Forum, John Wiley, New York, 2000. Based on work of Donald Berwick and the Institute for Healthcare Improvement.

48. Ostergaard HT, Ostergaard D, Lippert A. Implementation of team training in medical education in Denmark. Postgrad Med J 2008 Oct;84(996):507–511.

49. Duke J. Experiencing '*hygge*'. US-EU-MEE Case Report, 2000.

50. Tax in Denmark: How is income taxed? http://www.skm.dk/foreign/english/taxindenmark2008/section2howisincometaxed/. Accessed Nov. 9, 2006. Denmark has a progressive tax, i.e. higher income is taxed more.

51. The Local Government Reform in Brief. Chapter 4. http://www.im.dk/publikationer/government_reform_in_brief/kap04.htm Accessed Nov. 9, 2006.

52. OECD Health Data 2007.

53. Krakower D. The Silent Killer. US-EU-MEE case report, 2004.

54. Price, quality and access to treatment in private hospitals, June 2009. Accessed July 12, 2009. http://www.rigsrevisionen.dk/composite-2091.htm

55. *Sygeforsikringen* "danmark" — English summary. http://www.sygeforsikring.dk/Default.aspx?ID=229. Accessed Nov. 29, 2006.

56. Vallgårda S, Krasnik A, Vrangbæk K. Health Care Systems in Transition: Denmark. Thomson S, Mossialos E (eds). Out-of-pocket payments, p. 30. http://www.euro.who.int/document/e72967.pdf. Accessed Nov. 18, 2006.

57. Krakower D. The Silent Killer. US-EU-MEE case report, 2004.

58. Amgros. Public Procurement Network. http://www.ks.dk/english/procurement/guide/cpo-countries/amg-dk/amg-bas/. Accessed Nov. 17, 2007.

59. European Observatory on Health Care Systems. Health Care Systems in Transition: Denmark p. 30. Out-of-pocket payments http://www.euro.who.int/document/e72967.pdf. Accessed Nov. 17, 2007. Reimbursement scheme in detail.

60. Kanavos P. Overview of Pharmaceutical Pricing and Reimbursement Regulation in Europe. LSE health and social care. 4.9 Generics and generic Policy: a part of the demand side. 2000. http://ec.europa.eu/enterprise/phabiocom/docs/synthesis.pdf. Accessed May 31, 2007.

61. Vallgårda S, Krasnik A, Vrangbæck K. Health Care Systems in Transition: Denmark. Thomson S, Mossialos E (eds). 2001. http://www.euro.who.int/document/e72967.pdf. Accessed April 20, 2007.

62.   Miller K. Hobart-Smith College exchange student in Denmark. Personal communication.

63.   Krakower D. The Silent Killer. US-EU-MEE case report, 2004.

64.   Background Briefing; Health Care Lessons from Denmark (2002). www. civitas.org.uk/pdf/Denmark.pdf. Accessed January 10, 2007. Cost-sharing by more private expenditure especially as co-pays for adult dental care & drugs.

65.   Chan B. A Foreigner in Denmark. US-EU-MEE case report, 2003.

66.   Thyssen J. A Doctor as Patient at Lemuel Shattuck Hospital. US-EU-MEE case report, 2003.

67.   OECD in Figures 2006-2007. Economic Survey of Denmark 2005, pp. 8, 9.

68.   Simoens S, Villeneuve M, Hurst J. Tackling Nurse Shortages in OECD Countries. OECD Health Working Papers #19, 2005. http://www.oecd.org/ dataoecd/11/10/34571365.pdf. Accessed May 22, 2007.

69.   Vallgårda S, Krasnik A, Vrangbæck K. Health Care Systems in Transition: Denmark. Thomson S, Mossialos E (eds). 2001. Changes in the financing and budgeting of hospitals, p. 79. http://www.euro.who.int/document/e72967. pdf. Accessed May 22, 2007.

70.   Helleberg CM. Strengthening the right incentives: DRG budgeting inside a university hospital. Accessed May 22, 2007. Detailed description of DRG system.

71.   OECD Working Papers #21. The Supplies of Physician Services in OECD Countries. Stephen Simoenes, Jeffery Hurst. January 2006. http://www. oecd.org/dataoecd/27/22/35987490.pdf. Accessed May 24, 2007.

72.   OECD Economic Survey of Denmark 2005, p. 3. http://www.oecd.org/ dataoecd/51/28/34422696.pdf. Accessed July 7, 2009.

73.   US Social Security and Medicare Boards of Trustees. Status of the Social Security and Medicare Programs: A Summary of the 2007 Annual Reports. http://www.ssa.gov/OACT/TRSUM/trsummary.html. Accessed May 31, 2007.

74.   Bok, D. The great health care debate of 1993-94. Public Talk. Online Journal of Discourse Leadership. http://www.upenn.edu/pnc/ptbok.html. Accessed March 20, 2007.

75.   Calikoglu S.Trends in the distribution of health care financing across developed countries: The role of political economy of states. *Int J Health Serv* 2009;39(1):59–83.

76. OECD. Health Care Quality Indicators Project. http://www.oecd.org/ health/hcqi. Accessed May 15, 2007. Project since 2001 to establish comparable data across countries.

77. Vallgårda S, Krasnik A, Vrangbæck K. Health Care Systems in Transition: Denmark. Thomson S, Mossialos E (eds). 2001. Improvement in Life Expectancy, Chart, p. 7. http://www.euro.who.int/document/e72967.pdf. Accessed May 22, 2007.

78. Denmark Ministry of Health. Lifetime in Denmark. Second report from the Life Expectancy Committee of the Ministry of Health, 1994. http:// www.eva-phr.nrw.de/abstracts/dk/dk_650717.html. Accessed May 31, 2007.

79. National Center for Health Statistics. http://www.cdc.gov/nchs/products/ pubs/pubd/lftbls/life/1966.htm. Accessed May 7, 2007.

80. OECD in Figures 2006-2007, OECD Observer 2006/Supplement 1, pp. 10, 11.

81. Background Briefing: Health Care Lessons from Denmark (2002). Patient Satisfaction. p. 3. http://www.civitas.org.uk/pdf/denmark.pdf. Print copy, January 10, 2007.

82. Eichbaum Q. In the Same Boat. US-EU-MEE case report, 2001.

83. Thyssen JP, Meyer U, Olsen CH, Thielke D, Winding O, Andersen S, Michelsen N, Jaszczak P. USEUMEE — A comparison of the Danish and American health care systems. *Ugeskr Laeger.* 2005 Apr. 11;167(15): 1635–1637.

Note: Historic currency exchange in this chapter calculated by www.XE. com and www.x-rates.com

Chapter 4. German and US Health Care Systems Compared

1. Organisation for Economic Co-operation and Development. OECD Health Data 2009, June 2009. US, Switzerland, Germany among the most expensive health care.

2. *Deutsche Socialversicherung.* Health insurance history. http://www. deutsche-sozialversicherung.de/en/health/history_print.html. Accessed March 9, 2007.

3.   Centers for Medicare and Medicaid. Medicare & You 2009. CMS Publication 10050–46, September 2008.

4.   OECD in Figures 2006–2007, p. 83. US public spending for health care higher than many EU and Asian countries.

5.   Huber M. Health at a glance. OECD Indicators 2003, October 16. 2003. http://www.oecd.org/dataoecd/15/30/16782333.pfd. Accessed March 4, 2007. Pharmaceuticals are a substantial part of the US health care cost.

6.   Freking K. Health care expenses to double in 10 years. ABC Health News. http://abcnews.go.com/Health/wireStory?id=2891537&CMP=OTC-RSSFeeds0312. Accessed March 4, 2007.

7.   Kalayoglu M. 64-Slice CT and the new age for cardiac diagnostics. Medcompare. http://www.medcompare.com/spotlight.asp?spotlightid=147. Accessed March 4, 2007. Health care technology and escalating costs.

8.   US Social Security Online. Frequently Asked Questions. http://www.ssa.gov/pubs/10055.html. Accessed August 22, 2007. Fewer US workers to support retirees.

9.   Lutz W. European demographic data sheet 2006. Vienna Institute of Demography, International Institute for Applied Systems Analysis and Population Reference Bureau, Vienna and Washington, DC. 2006. http://www.prb.org. Accessed August 17, 2006. Germany also facing shortage of workers to support retirees.

10. US Census Bureau Reports. Health insurance, what's new? http://www.census,gov/. Accessed June 23, 2009.

11. James K. German health system not quite in intensive care. *Deutsche Welle*. http://www.dw-world.de/popups/popup_printcontent/0.1973312,00.html. Accessed March 4, 2007. Germany's uninsured have been largely taken care of by 2007 and 2009 health insurance reforms.

12. Matz-Townsend. Health Insurance Options in Germany (2009). http://www.howtogermany.com/pages/health.insurance2.htm. Accessed June 23, 2009.

13. US Census Bureau. http://www.census/gov/population/www/popclockus.html. Accessed July 1, 2009.

14. Expenditure on health percent Gross Domestic Product. OECD Health Data 2009. Version released November 2009. Public and private expenditures for health care in US and Germany.

15. Expenditure on health percent Gross Domestic Product, Germany and the US 1987–2007. OECD Health Data 2009. Version released November 2009. Rise in expenditure as percent of GDP.

16. Total public expenditure on health percent total expenditure on health, Germany and the US 1987–2007. OECD Health Data 2009. Version released November 2009. Rise in expenditure as percent of GDP.

17. Total expenditure on health per capita USD Purchasing Power Parity. OECD Health Data 2009. Version released November 2009. Tables 1970–2007.

18. Social Security Online. History archives. Otto von Bismarck. http://www. ssa.gov/history/ottob.htm. Accessed March 11, 2007.

19. Inglehart JK. Germany's health care system (Part I). *N Engl J Med* 324(7); Feb. 1991:503–508.

20. Braun M. German health care reform. May 26, 2009. http://www.mercer.com/ referencecontent.htm?idContent=1346005. Accessed June 23, 2009. Historical notes.

21. Matz-Townsend C. Health insurance options in Germany 2009. http://www.howtogermany.com/pages/healthinsurance2.html. Accessed June 23, 2009. Government contribution from taxes.

22. *Bundesministerium fuer Besundheit, Gesetzliche Krankenversicherung, Kennzahlen und Faustformeln, Tabelle:KF06Bund, Stand: 1.März* 2007. Number of *Krankenkassen* reduced to 242 by 2007.

23. Health Insurance Options in Germany 2009. http://www.howtogermany.com/ pages/healthinsurance2.html. Accessed June 24, 2009. Number of *Krankenkassen* reduced to around *200* by 2009.

24. BKK *Bundesverband* (German Federal Assn. of Company Health Insurance Funds). *Aerzte Zeitung*, 11.04.2007. Redistribution of funds for risk adjustment.

25. German Ministry of Health, www.bmg.bund.de. Accessed January 10, 2008. Sickness fund contributions according to salary.

26. Germany — Health Insurance, August 1995. http://www.germanculture.com. ua/library/facts/bl_health_insurance.htm. Accessed March 8, 2007. Health care for German state and federal employees.

27. Rohde C. *Nie Krank*. US-EU-MEE case report, 2000.

28. German Ministry of Health, www.bmg.bund.de. Accessed January 10, 2008.

29. Altin SE. A Ray of Hope. US-EU-MEE case report, 2005.

30.   German Culture. Health insurance in Germany, p. 2, http://www.
germanculture.com.ua/library/facts/bl_health_insurance.htm. Accessed
March 8, 2007.

31.   *Zahlenbericht der privaten Krankenversicherung* 2006/2007, *Verband der
privaten Krankenversicherung e.V.*, pp. 9 and 27. Berlin, Germany.

32   *Zahlenbericht der privaten Krankenversicherung* 2006/2007, *Verband der
privaten Krankenversicherung e.V.*, p. 32. Berlin, Germany.

33.   Busse R. Health care systems in eight countries: trends and challenges.
Germany. http://www.euro.who.int/document/OBS/hcs8countries.pdf.
Accessed March 5, 2007.

34.   Shu A. Frau Baumgartner and Herr Schneider. US-EU-MEE case report, 2002.

35.   Busse R, Riesberg A. Health Care Systems in Transition: Germany. 2004.
http://www.euro.who.int/document/OBS/he58countries.pdf.   Accessed
March 5, 2007. pp. 39, 40, 46. The Social Code Book.

36.   Wikipedia. Federal Ministry for Health and Social Security (Germany)
January 2007. http://en.wikipedia.org/wiki/. Accessed March 5, 2007. German
ministry changes.

37.   Busse R, Riesberg A. Health Care Systems in Transition: Germany, 2004,
p. 47. Role of the German Federal Joint Committee (G-BA).

38.   American & German Healthcare 2009: Healthcare Reform and Progress
http://www.cges.umn.edu/docs/Dietz_090428_KeyElementsofReform.pdf.
Accessed June 23, 2009.

39.   Jackson J. The German Health System: Lessons for Reform in the
United States. *Arch of Int Med*, Jan. 27, 1997;157(2):155–160.

40.   *Gemeinsamer Bundesausschuss*. http://www.g-ba.de/cms/front_content.php?
idcatart=207&lang=1&client=1. Accessed March 6, 2007.

41.   Wahner-Roedler DL, *et al*. The German health-care system. *Mayo Clinic
Proceedings*, 72(11); November 1997:1061–1068.

42.   Busse R, Riesberg A. Health Care Systems in Transition: Germany, 2004.
Reunification challenge to the German health care system.

43.   Germany Online: Information Services. This week in Germany: politics.
July 25, 2003. http://www.germany.info/relaunch/info/publications/week/
2003/030725/politics2.html. Accessed March 8, 2007. Agenda 2010. "Day
Fare"

44.   Camerra-Rowe Pamela. Agenda 2010: Redefining German social democracy.
Questia Journal. German Politics and Society, 22, 2004.

45. Wallace Charles P. Risking his own welfare. *Time on CNN, October 26, 2003.* http://www.time.com/time/magazine/article/0,9171, 901031103-526378,00.html. Accessed March 10, 2007.

46. Beck E. Tough Love: German health care reform. *Pharmaceutical Marketing Europe,* Winter 2003.

47. *Zahlenbericht der privaten Krankenversicherung* 2006/2007, *Verband der privaten Krandenversicherung e.V.,* pp. 9 and 27, Berlin, Germany.

48. Health Policy Monitor. Health fund now operational. http://www.hpm.org/en/ Surveys/TU_Berlin_-_D/13/Health_Fund_now_operational.html. Accessed July 12, 2009.

49. James K. German health care reform: mission impossible? *Deutsche Welle.* http://www.dw-world.de/popups/popup_printcvontent/0,,2117345.00.html. Accessed February 19, 2007.

50. Acute care beds. OECD in Figures 2006–2007, p. 8.

51 Busse R, Germany opts for Australian Diagnosis-Related Groups *WHO Euro Observer,* Autumn 2000;2(3):2-3. http://www.euro.who.int/document/ OBS/EuroObserver2_3.pdf. Accessed March 5, 2007.

52. Shu A. Frau Baumgartner and Herr Schneider. US-EU-MEE case report, 2002.

53 National Coalition on Health. German Health Ministry. http://www.nchc. org/facts.Germany.pdf. Accessed February 19, 2007.

54. James K. German health care reform: mission impossible? *Deutsche Welle.* http://www.iht.com/articles/2006/09/07/news/germany.php. Accessed February 18, 2007.

55. German doctors to step up strike. BBC News Europe. http://newsvote.bbc. co.uk/mpapps/pagetools/print/news.bbc.co.uk/2/hi/europe/5072386.stm. Accessed February 26, 2007.

56. Cremer A. German Parliament backs plan to cut health costs: main points. Bloomberg News http://www.bloomberg.com/apps/news?pid=newsarchive& sid=aFMxwWag1eFk. Accessed February 19, 2007.

57. Armitage T. German health reform clears final hurdle. Reuters News Service. http://www.pamf.org/health/healthinfo/reutershome_top.cfm?fx=article& id=34835. Accessed February 19, 2007.

58. German health reform bill clears final hurdle. Earthtimes Online World News. http://www.earthtimes.org/articles/show/31321.html. Accessed March 12, 2007. Will features be dismantled before the new plan is fully implemented?

59. Cremer A. German Parliament backs plan to cut health costs: main points of 2007 reform. Bloomberg News Service. http://www.bloomberg.com.apps/news?pid=newsarchive?sid=aFMxwWag1eFk. Accessed February 19, 2007.

60. Cremer A. German Parliament backs plan to cut health costs: main points, can raise premium no more than 1% of household income. Bloomberg News Service. http://www.bloomberg.com.apps/news?pid=newsarchive?sid=aFMxwWag1eFk. Accessed February 19, 2007.

61. Cremer A. German Parliament backs plan to cut health costs: main points, will provide insurance for 200,000 uninsured. (Update 2), Bloomberg News http://www.bloomberg.com/apps/news?pid=newsarchive&sid=aFMxw Wag1eFk. Accessed February 19, 2007.

62. Cremer A. German Parliament backs plan to cut health costs: main points. Bloomberg News Service. http://www.bloomberg.com.apps/news?pid=new sarchive?sid=aFMxwWag1eFk. Accessed February 23, 3008. Contributions raised 0.5 percent in January 2007 to fund changes and wipe out existing debt.

63. Cremer A. German Parliament backs plan to cut health costs: main points. Bloomberg News Service. http://www.bloomberg.com.apps/news?pid=new sarchive?sid=aFMxwWag1eFk. Accessed March 8, 2008. Children's health care costs covered by general tax revenue. Pharmaceutical constraints dropped.

64. Cremer A. German Parliament backs plan to cut health costs: main points. (Update 2), Bloomberg News http://www.bloomberg.com/apps/news? pid=newsarchive&sid=aFMxwWag1eFk. Accessed February 19, 2007. Ulla Schmidt quote.

65. Wesbury B. Is the German boom a mirage? MSNBC Newsweek International Edition. http://www.msnbc.co/id/17435372/site/newsweek/. Accessed March 18, 2007.

66. Cremer A, Rach C. German Upper House passes health bill ending yearlong wrangle. Bloomberg News Service. http://www.bloomberg.com/apps/news? pid=newsarchive?sid=aFMxwWag1eFk. Accessed February 19, 2007. Edmund Stoiber quote.

67. James K. German health care reform: mission impossible? *Deutsche Welle*. http://www.iht.com/articles/2006/09/07/news/germany.php. Accessed February 18, 2007. Germans divided on new health plan.

68. German health care reform approved. Business Insurance. http://www.businessinsurance.com/cqi.bin/news.pl?news/d=9555. Accessed February 19, 2007.

69. German JK. Health care reform: mission impossible? *Deutsche Welle*. http://www.iht.com/articles/2006/09/07/news/germany.php. Accessed February 18, 2007. Barbara Marnach quote.

70. Cremer A, Rach C. German Upper House passes health bill ending year-long wrangle. Bloomberg News Service. http://www.bloomberg.com/apps/news?pid=newsarchive?sid=aFMxwWag1eFk. Accessed February 19, 2007. Walter Hirche quote.

71. German JK. Health care reform: mission impossible? *Deutsche Welle*. http://www.iht.com/articles/2006/09/07/news/germany.php. Accessed February 18, 2007. Sophia Schlette quote.

72. German JK. Health care reform: mission impossible? *Deutsche Welle*. http://www.iht.com/articles/2006/09/07/news/germany.php. Accessed February 18, 2007. Protests.

73. Cremer A. German Parliament backs plan to cut health costs: main points. Bloomberg News http://www.bloomberg.com/apps/news?pid=newsarchive&sid=aFMxwWag1eFk. Accessed February 19, 2007. Marlies Volkmer quote.

74. Cremer A. German house backs health bill amid coalition dissent (Update 2). Bloomberg News Service. http://www.bloomberg.com/apps/news?pid=2067000/&refer=germany&sid=a4h.JuizUh&8k. Accessed February 19, 2007. Guido Westerwelle quote.

75. German JK. Health system not quite in intensive care. *Deutsche Welle*. http://www.dw-world.de/popups/popup.printcontent/0,,1973312.00,00, html. Accessed March 4, 2007.

76. German JK. Health care reform: mission impossible? *Deutsche Welle*. http://www.iht.com/articles/2006/09/07/news/germany.php. Accessed February 19, 2007. Running possible shortfall up to €7 billion each year.

77. German JK. Health system not quite in intensive care. *Deutsche Welle*. http://www.dw-world.de/popups/popup.printcontent/0.1973312.00,00, html. Accessed March 4, 2007. Survey results.

78. German JK. Health system not quite in intensive care. *Deutsche Welle*. http://www.dw-world.de/popups/popup.printcontent/0.1973312.00,00,html. Accessed March 4, 2007. Germans have not had long waiting times.

79. German JK. Health system not quite in intensive care. *Deutsche Welle*. http://www.dw-world.de/popups/popup.printcontent/0,,1973312.00,00,html. Accessed March 4, 2007. Jeanne Arenz quote.

Chapter 7. Swedish and US Health Care Systems Compared

1. Smorgasbord. Sweden. Parliamentary System. http://www.sverigeturism.se/ smorgasbord/smorgasbord/society/government/parlament.html. Accessed Sept. 30, 2007.

2. The World Factbook. Sweden. https://www.cia.gov/library/publications/ the-world-factbook/print/sw.html. Accessed Sept. 30, 2007. Literacy rate 99%: of population over 15 years of age, 99% can read and write.

3. The World Factbook. Sweden. https://www.cia.gov/library/publications/ the-world-factbook/print/sw.html. Accessed Sept. 30, 2007. Estimated unemployment rate (2006) 5.6%.

4. EIRO online (European Industrial Relations Observatory). http://www. eurofound.europa.eu/eiro/2007/08/articles/se0708039i.html. Accessed Sept. 30, 2007.

5. Global income per capita. World Development Indicators Database. World Bank. July 1, 2007. http://siteresources.worldbank.org/DATASTATISTICS/ Resources/GNIPC.pdf. Accessed Sept. 8, 2007.

6. US Dept. of State. Background note: Sweden. http://www.state.gov/r/pa/ ei/bgn/2880.htm. Accessed Sept. 8, 2007.

7. Earthtrends: The Environmental Information Portal. http://earthtrends.wri.org/ text/population-health/country-profile-173.html. Accessed Sept. 13, 2007. Statistical Yearbook of Sweden 2007. http://www.scb.se/templates/Product 30937.asp. Accessed Sept. 9, 2007.

8. Population Distribution 2005. US Census Bureau. Population Profile of the US Dynamic Version, p. 3. http://www.census.gov/population/pop-profile/ dynamic/PopDistribution.pdf. Accessed Sept. 8, 2007. Los Angeles County Online. Statistical data. http://www.lacounty.info/statistical_information.htm. Accessed Sept. 8, 2007.

9. US Dept. of State. Background note: Sweden.http://www.state.gov/r/pa/ei/ bgn/2880.htm. Accessed Sept. 8, 2007. The Swedish System of Government.

10. Swedish Institute Fact Sheet FS55z, March 2007. www.sweden.se. Accessed Sept. 10, 2007.

11. US Dept. of State Background Note: Sweden. History, p. 5. Bureau of European and Eurasian Affairs. August 2007.

12. Dahring W. Swedish Culture. http://www.mnsu.edu/emuseum/cultural/ oldworld/europe/sweden.html. Accessed Sept. 10, 2007.

13. Skans O. School to Work Transition in Sweden. p. 91. http://www.jil. go.jp/english/documents/JILPTRNo5_skans.pdf. Accessed Sept. 10, 2007.

14. Institutions of Higher Learning. http://www.sweden.se/eng/Home/Education/ Research/Facts/Higher-education-and-research-in-Sweden/#edx_3. Accessed June 15, 2010.

15. US Dept. of State. Background note: Sweden. http://www.state.gov/r/pa/ ei/bgn/2880.htm. Accessed Sept. 8, 2007.

16. Health-EU. The Public Health Portal of the European Union. http://ec. europa.eu/health-eu/care_for_me/long_term_care/ms_se_en.htm. Accessed 7/17/09.

17. Government Offices of Sweden. Health and medical care in Sweden. Ministry of Health and Social Affairs. Fact sheet No. 16, August 2007.

18. Health-EU. The Public Health Portal of the European Union. http://ec.europa. eu/health-eu/care_for_me/long_term_care/ms_se_en.htm. Accessed 7/17/09.

19. Tang P. An Up and Down Course, US-EU-MEE Case 26. Lund University Hospital, Lund, Sweden, 2000.

20. Government Offices of Sweden. Health and medical care in Sweden. Ministry of Health and Social Affairs Fact Sheet No. 16, August 2007, p. 2 http://www.sweden.gov.se.

21. OECD Health Data: Specialists outnumber GPs in most OECD countries. http://www.oecd.org/document/10/0,3343,en_2649_201185_38976778_1_ 1_1_1,00.html. Accessed July 18, 2007.

22. Integrated care. Swedish Institute. Swedish health care, Management. Fact Sheet FS 76z, January 2007, p.1. http://www.sweden.se/templates/cs/ FactSheet____15865.aspx

23. Swedish Institute. Patient fees. Swedish health care, Fact Sheet FS 76z, January 2007, p. 2. http://www.sweden.se/templates/cs/FactSheet____ 15865.aspx

24. Financing. Swedish Institute. Swedish health care, Financing. Fact Sheet FS 76z, January 2007, p. 2. http://www.sweden.se/templates/cs/ FactSheet____15865.aspx

25. European Observatory on Health Systems and Policies, "HiT Summary, Sweden 2005 Copenhagen, Denmark.

26. OECD Health Data 2009: How does Sweden compare? http://www.oecd.org/ dataoecd/46/6/38980334.pdf. Accessed 12/15/09.

27. OECD Health Data 2009. June 2009. Public/private comparison, Sweden and US.

28. Angeles J. Improving Medicaid as part of building on the current system to achieve universal coverage. Center on Budget and Policy Priorities. Feb. 24, 2009. http://www.cbpp.org/cms/index.cf?fa=view&id=2664. Accessed July 9, 2009.

29. Sweden Health and Medical Services Act of 1982. http://www.sweden.gov.se/content/1/c6/02/31/25/a7ea8ee1.pdf. Accessed August 22, 2007.

30. Government Agencies. Health and medical care in Sweden. Ministry of Health and Social Affairs. Fact sheet No. 16, August, 2007.

31. County Councils. Health and medical care in Sweden. Ministry of Health and Social Affairs. Fact sheet No. 16, August 2007. Responsibilities of the county councils.

32. Swedish Institute. Sweden's regional hospitals. Fact Sheet 76z, January 2007, p. 2.

33. Swedish Institute. The organization of Swedish health services. Fact Sheet 76z, January 2007, p. 2.

34. County Councils. Health and medical Care in Sweden. Ministry of Health and Social Affairs. Fact sheet No. 16, August, 2007. Expenditure on purchase of health and medical care services from private companies.

35. Swedish Institute. Management. Swedish health care. Fact Sheet FS 76z. January 2007. Number of municipalities. Responsibilities of municipalities for health care.

36. Municipalities. Health and medical care in Sweden. Ministry of Health and Social Affairs. Fact sheet No.16, August 2007. Responsibility for care of elderly and disabled people living at home.

37. The Swedish Institute. The health care system in Sweden. Fact Sheet September 2003. www.si.se and www.sweden.se. Accessed August 22, 2007.

38. Health and medical care in Sweden. Ministry of Health and Social Affairs. Fact sheet No. 16, August 2007. The role of the Swedish Assn. of Local Authorities and Regions.

39. The Swedish Medical Association. 2005. http://www.slf.se/upload/Lakar-forbundet/In%20English/rekrytfolder_eng_200.pdf. Accessed Sept. 9, 2007.

40. McCants Carr R. US-EU-MEE case report. Lund University, Sweden, Spring 2001. A Day at Vardcentral.

41. Report on key learnings: study visit to Sweden. The Change Foundation, 2003. http://changefoundation.com/tcf/tcfbul.nsf/faf9f5c4d4ab768605256b8e

00037216/145dd9b791097e5085256e1500541438/$FILE/Sweden%202003 %20Final.pdf. Report on Key Learnings.

42. OECD Health Data 2007. Percentage decrease 2004–2006 physicians and nurses per 1000 population in Sweden and Denmark.

43. Swedish Institute. Financing. Swedish health care. Fact Sheet FS 76z, January 2007.

44. Swedish Institute. Patient Fees. Swedish health care. Fact Sheet FS 76z, January 2007.

45. Guinness World Records. http://www.libraryspot.com/know/highesttax.htm

46. Swedish Institute. Efficacy and Improvement. Swedish health care. Fact Sheet FS 76z, January 2007.

47. Sanandaji N. Taxes still too high in Sweden. http//www.thelocal.se/17964/20090303/. 3 March 2009.

48. Udompanyanan K, MD. US-EU-MEE case report, Lund University, Sweden, May 2002. Younger population perspective on taxes. System not sustainable without raising taxes.

49. Center for Freedom & Prosperity. June 2006. http://www.freedomand prosperity.org/Papers/sweden/sweden.shtml. Accessed Sept. 20, 2007. The effect of high Swedish taxes on the economy. Wealthy sheltering money.

50. OECD Health Data 2009, June 2009. Macro-economic references. Public Revenue percent of GDP.

51. Sanandaji N. Sweden's entrepreneurs face an uphill struggle, Feb. 19, 2007. http://www.thelocal.se/6463/20070219/. Accessed Sept. 20, 2007.

52. Sanandaji N. Sweden needs a better business climate. http://www.thelocal.se/8667/. Accessed October 4, 2007.

53. Farrell D. Sweden's balancing lessons for Europe. *BusinessWeek* online. http://www.businessweek.com/print/globalbiz/content/sep2006/gb2006092 2_333746.htm. Accessed September 27, 2007.

54. Parental Benefit. *Försäkringskassan.* http://www.forsakringskassan.se/sprak/eng/foralder/. Accessed Oct. 3, 2007.

55. Ministry of Health and Social Affairs, Government Offices of Sweden. Social insurance in Sweden. Fact Sheet No. 8, March 2007.

56. Normann G, Mitchell DJ. Pension reform in Sweden: Lessons for American policymakers. http://www.heritage.org/Research/SocialSecurity/bg1381.es.cfm, June 29, 2000. Accessed November 4, 2007.

57. Sudén A. How do individual accounts work in the Swedish pension system? Center for Retirement Research at Boston College. August 2004. http://www.bc.edu/centers/crr/issues/ib_22.pdf. Accessed Oct. 30, 2007.

58. Government Offices of Sweden. Social insurance in Sweden. The public pension system. Fact Sheet No. 8, March 2007. Percentage paid by employers and individuals.

59. Sudén A. How do individual accounts work in the Swedish pension system? Center for Retirement Research at Boston College. August 2004. http://www.bc.edu/centers/crr/issues/ib_22.pdf. Accessed Oct. 30, 2007.

60. Sundström K. OECD Observer. Can governments influence population growth? Dec. 2001. http://www.oecdobserver.org/news/fullstory.php/aid/563/Can_governments_influence_population_growth_.html

61. Gender Equality in Sweden. Fact Sheet FS82 q. October 26, 2007. http://www.sweden.se/templates/cs/FactSheet____17932.aspx. Accessed Nov. 13, 2007

62. Westerberg S. The folly of Sweden's state controlled families. Speech in London to the Nordic Committee for Human Rights, 1999. http://www.nkmr.org/siv_westerbergs_london_lecture.htm. Accessed October 16, 2007.

63. Normann G. Pension Reform in Sweden: Lessons for American Policymakers. June 29, 2000. http://www.heritage.org/Research/Social Securitylog1381.ex.cfm. Accessed November 4, 2007.

64. Persson K. Economic Conditions and welfare in Sweden and the Nordic countries. Speech at the Union Conference of the Nordic Teachers' Council, October 23, 2003. http://www.riksbank.com/templates/speech.aspx?id=8464. Accessed October 2, 2007.

65. OECD Summary Chapter 3, The Economic Survey of Sweden 2005. Best practice for reducing sickness and disability absences, June 9, 2005. http://www.oecd.org/documentprint/0,3455,en_2649_201185_34971821_1_1_1_1,00.html Accessed November 4, 2007.

66. Statistical Yearbook of Sweden, 2007. http://www.scb.se/templates/Product____30937.asp.

67. OECD Economics. Review of Sweden 2005.

68. Sweden aims to halve sick leave. August 7, 2005. http://www.thelocal.se/article.php?ID=1851. Accessed November 6, 2007. Bertil Thorslund quote.

69. Rives K. A stressful situation: plans to rein in sick leave spur a backlash in Sweden. *Newsweek,* October 9, 2007. http://www.newsweek.com/id/42511/output/print. Accessed November 4, 2007.

70. Sweden aims to halve sick leave. August 7, 2005. http://www.thelocal.se/article.php?ID=1851. Accessed November 6, 2007.

71. Government Offices of Sweden. The public pension system. Social insurance in Sweden. Fact Sheet No. 8. March 2007.

72. OECD Summary Chapter 3, The Economic Survey of Sweden 2005. Best practice for reducing sickness and disability absences, June 9, 2005. http://www.oecd.org/documentprint/0,3455,en_2649_201185_34971821_1_1_1_1,00.html. Accessed Nov. 4, 2007.

73. OECD Health Data 2007, July 2007. Average length of stay and acute care beds.

74. Kowalczyk L. State signals it is open to retail medical clinics. Boston.com. White Coat Notes, July 17, 07. http://www.boston.com/yourlife/health/blog/2007/07/state_signals_i.html. Accessed November 27, 2007.

75. OECD Health Working Papers No. 28. Pharmaceutical pricing and reimbursement policies in Sweden, July 26, 2007. http://www.oecd.org/dataoecd/63/17/39020934.pdf. Accessed Sept. 27, 2007.

76. Farrell D. Sweden's balancing lessons for Europe. *BusinessWeek*, Sept. 22, 2006. http://www.businessweek.com/print/globalbiz/content/sep2006/gb2006092_333746.htm. Accessed September 27, 2007.

77. Reinfeldt F. The New Swedish Model: a reform agenda for growth and the environment. Speech at the London School of Economics and Political Science, Feb. 26, 2008. http://www.sweden.gov.se/sb/d/10296/a/99193. Accessed 12/8/09.

Note: Historic currency exchange in this chapter calculated by www.XE.com and www.x-rates.com

Chapter 10. The US Health Care System

1. Carr S. A quotation with a life of its own. *Patient Safety and Quality Healthcare*. http://www.psqh.com/julaug08/editor/html. Accessed May 14, 2010.

2. Modern History Sourcebook: William Bradford, *History of Plymouth Plantation c1650*. http://www.fordham.edu/halsall/mod/1650bradford.html. Accessed July 18, 2009.

3. The history of health insurance in the United States. Northern California Neurosurgery Medical Group, 2007. http://www.neurosurgical.com/medical_history_and_ethics/history/history_of_health_insurance.htm. Accessed July 17, 2009.

4. French R. World War II created health insurance perk. *The Detroit News*, Oct. 25, 2006. http://www.detnews.com/apps/pbcs.dll/article?AID=/20061025/AUTO01/101220010/1040/LIFESTYLE03. Accessed July 18, 2009.

5. OECD Health Data 2008. Released June 2008.

6. OECD in Figures 2006–2007, p. 83. U.S. public spending for health care higher than many EU and Asian countries.

7. Medicare and Medicaid: history overview. http://www.cms.hhs.gov/history/. Accessed July 18, 2009. Origin of Title XVIII and XIX in 1965.

8. Medicare at a Glance. Fact Sheet. Kaiser Family Foundation, November 2008. http://www.kff.org/medicare/upload/1066_11.pdf. Accessed July 18, 2009.

9. Centers for Medicare and Medicaid Services. *Medicare & You 2009*. US Department of Health and Human Services, p. 82.

10. National Health Expenditure Data 2007. http://www.cms.hhs.gov/NationalHealthExpendData/. Accessed July 18, 2009.

11. Brief Summaries of Medicare and Medicaid as of November 2009. http://www.cms.gov/medicaremedicaidstasupp/downloads/2009BriefSummaries. Accessed June 2, 2010.

12. US Office of Personnel Management. http://www.upm.gov/insure/index.aspx. Accessed July 12, 2009.

13. Indian Health Service. http://www.ihs.gov/index.cfm?module=Medical. Accessed July 18, 2009.

14. US Office of Personnel Management. http://www.upm.gov/insure/index.aspx. Accessed July 12, 2009. Federal Insurance Contribution Act (FICA).

15. Centers for Medicare and Medicaid Services. *Medicare & You 2009*. US Department of Health and Human Services, p. 16. Medicare Part A.

16. Centers for Medicare and Medicaid Services. *Medicare & You 2009*. US Department of Health and Human Services, p. 21. Medicare Part B.

17. Centers for Medicare and Medicaid Services. *Medicare & You 2010*. US Department of Health and Human Services, p. 23. Penalty for not signing up for Part B on time.

18. Thyssen JP, Meyer U, Olsen CH, Thielke D, Winding O, Andersen S, Michelsen N, Jaszczak P. US-EU-MEE — A comparison of the Danish and American health care systems. *Ugeskr Laeger.* 2005 Apr. 11;167(15):1635–7.

19. Centers for Medicare and Medicaid Services. *Medicare & You 2009.* US Department of Health and Human Services, p. 124.

20. Centers for Medicare and Medicaid Services. *Medicare & You 2009.* US Department of Health and Human Services, p. 50.

21. Centers for Medicare and Medicaid Services. *Medicare & You 2009.* US Department of Health and Human Services, p. 63.

22. Centers for Medicare and Medicaid Services. *Medicare & You 2007.* US Department of Health and Human Services, p. 45. Drug coverage gap; "donut hole".

23. Medicaid Program: General Information. http://www.cms.hhs.gov/MedicaidGenInfo/. Accessed July 12, 2009.

24. Centers for Medicare and Medicaid Services. *Medicare & You 2009.* US Department of Health and Human Services, p. 33.

25. Centers for Medicare and Medicaid Services. http://www.cms.hhs.gov/NationalCHIPPolicy/. Updated April 2, 2009. Accessed July 12, 2009. Description of SCHIP. New Obama policies.

26. Kaiser Family Foundation Commission on Medicaid and the Uninsured. CHIP Tips. http://www.kff.org/medicaid/upload/7910.pdf. June 2009. Accessed July 10, 2009.

27. Ludmerer KM. *A Time to Heal.* Oxford University Press, New York, NY, 1999. pp. 221–223.

28. Cohen J. Too many doctors: a prescription for bad medicine. *Acad Med* 71:654, 1996.

29. Ludmerer KM. *A Time to Heal.* Oxford University Press, New York, NY, 1999, p. 351. HMOs.

30. Ludmerer KM. *A Time to Heal.* Oxford University Press, New York, NY, 1999, p. 351. DRGs

31. Patient information. Mount Auburn Hospital, Cambridge, MA, September, 1997.

32. Ludmerer KM. *A Time to Heal.* Oxford University Press, New York, NY, 1999, p. 359.

33. Ludmerer KM. *A Time to Heal.* Oxford University Press, New York, NY, 1999, p. 353.

34. Cohen J. Time to stanch the flow of residents. *Acad Med* 69:464, 1994.
35. Ludmerer KM. *A Time to Heal.* Oxford University Press, New York, NY, 1999, p. 354.
36. Bulger R. Responding to incentives in academic health centers. *Health Affairs*, Winter 1992, p. 262. Effect of speed on patient-doctor relationship.
37. Bowman K. The 1993–1994 debate on health care reform: Did the polls mislead the policy makers? American Enterprise Institute, 1995, p. 30.
38. Bok D. The great health care debate of 1993-94. Public Talk. Online Journal of Discourse Leadership. http://www.upenn.edu/pnc/ptbok.html. Accessed March 20, 2007. (No page numbers). Demise of the Clinton plan.
39. Bowman K. The 1993–1994 debate on health care reform: did the polls mislead the policy makers? American Enterprise Institute, 1995, p. 31.
40. Bok D. The great health care debate of 1993–94. Public Talk. Online Journal of Discourse Leadership. http://www.upenn.edu/pnc/ptbok.html. Accessed March 20, 2007. (No page numbers). Concerns that the Clinton plan would cost too much and there would be fraud and abuse. Dissatisfaction with the way the plan was crafted.
41. Bok D. The great health care debate of 1993–94. Public Talk. Online Journal of Discourse Leadership. http://www.upenn.edu/pnc/ptbok.html. Accessed March 20, 2007. (No page numbers). Twenty-seven alternate plans presented by members of congress.
42. Bowman K. The 1993–1994 debate on health care reform: did the polls mislead the policy makers? American Enterprise Institute, 1995, p. 31.
43. Hiebert-White J. Costs: health spending to double by 2016: government share to possibly reach 50 percent. http://www.healthaffairs.org. Accessed March 8, 2007.
44. Facing up to the nation's finances. http://www.facingup.org/why-it-matters/facts-figures. Accessed July 24, 2009.
45. Kaiser Family Foundation. Trends in health care costs and spending. September 2007. http://www.kff.org/insurance/upload/7692.pdf. Accessed Nov. 7, 2007.
46. Freudenheim M. Health care costs rise twice as much as inflation. *New York Times.* September 27, 2006.
47. OECD Health Data 2009. Total health spending as percent of GDP. Released November 2009.

48. OECD Health Data 2009. Total health spending per capita. Released November 2009.

49. Leape L, Berwick D. Five years after *To Err is Human*. *JAMA* 1005; 293:2384–2390.

50. Dept. of Health and Human Services Fiscal Year 2008. Citizen's Report. http://www.hhs.gov/asrt/ob/docbudget/citizensreport.pdf. Accessed July 24, 2009.

51. A New Era of Responsibility: the 2010 Budget. US Office of Management and Budget. http://www.whitehouse.gov/omb/. Accessed July 4, 2009. President Obama's statements.

52. The Patient Protection and Affordable Care Act and the Health Care and Education Reconciliation Act. Full Text. http://dpc.senate.gov/dpcdoc-sen_health_care_bill.cfm.

53. Warner J. Boomer health care dilemma. Reviewed by Brunilda Nazario, MD, WebMD Medical News, CBS News. http://www.cbsnews.com/stories/2004/09/29/health/webmd/printable646306.shtml. Accessed March 4, 2007 (David Cutler interview).

54. Kaiser Family Foundation. How changes in medical technology affect health care costs. Snapshots: health care costs, March 2007. http://www.kff.org/insurnce/snapshot/chem030807oth.cfm. Accessed March 19, 2007.

55. US Census Bureau. http://www.census.gov. Accessed June 30, 2009.

56. US Census Bureau overstated number of uninsured residents by nearly 2M people because of computer programming error. Reprinted by permission from Kaisernetwork.org, a free service of the Henry J. Kaiser Family Foundation. http://www.medicalnewstoday.com/medicalnews.php?mewsod=66207. Accessed May 31, 2007.

57. Kaiser Commission on Medicaid and the Uninsured. The uninsured and the difference health insurance makes. Fact Sheet. September 2008. http://www.kff.org/uninsured/upload/1420-10.pdf. Accessed July 30, 2009.

58. Fact Sheet: Medicare two-year waiting period for people with disabilities. http://www.medicarerights.org/pdf/two_year_waiting_period_fact_sheet.pdf. Accessed July 7, 2009.

59 DeNavas-Walt C, Proctor BD, Smith JC. US Census Bureau, Current population report P60-235, Income, poverty, and health insurance coverage in the United States, 2007. US Government Printing Office, Issued

August 2008. http://www.census.gov/hhes/www/hlthins/hlthin07/p60no235_table6.pdf. Accessed July 30, 2009.

60. Kaiser Family Foundation. Covering the uninsured: options for reform. Sept. 17, 2008. http://www.kff.org/uninsured/h08_7813.cfm. Accessed July 30, 2009.

61. Dorn S, Kenney GM. Automatically enrolling eligible children and families Into Medicaid and SCHIP: opportunities, obstacles, and options for federal policymakers, Vol. 26, June 13, 2006. http://www.commonwealthfund.org/publications/publications_show.htm?doc_id=376814. Accessed November 18, 2007. Many eligible for Medicaid and SCHIP are not enrolled.

62. Holohan J, Cook A, Dubay L. Characteristics of the uninsured: Who is eligible for public coverage and who needs help affording coverage? Kaiser Commission on Medicaid and the uninsured. February 2007, p. 14. http://www.kff.org/uninsured/upload/7613.pdf accessed March 18, 2007.

63. Nordin U. Health care for the hidden. *The Magazine of the International Red Cross and Red Crescent Program.* 2007. http://www.redcross.int/en/mag/magazine2007_1/14-15.html, Accessed October 29, 2007.

64. Rand Corporation. Rand study finds undocumented immigrants most likely to be uninsured. News Release, November 10, 2005. http://www.rand.org/news/press.05/11.10.html, Accessed November 18, 2007.

65. Wulsin L. Covering 800,000 undocumented workers. Insure the Uninsured Project, September 5, 2007. http://lahealthaction.org/library/Covering_undocumented_wor.pdf. Accessed November 20, 2007.

66. CBS News October 2, 2007. Los Angeles County health care costs for illegal immigrants.

67. Wagner D. Mexicans go to Arizona for medical help. *USA Today,* May 17, 2005. http://www.usatoday.com/news/nation/2005-05-17-arizona-exicans_x.htm. Accessed November 20, 2007.

68. Federal Statutory EMTLA Regulations. http://www.emtla.com/law/index.html. Accessed July 15, 2009.

69. Scott MK. Health care in the express lane: the emergence of retail clinics. California Health Care Foundation, July 2006, http://www.chcf.org/documents/policy/HealthCareInTheExpressLaneRetailClinics.pdf. Accessed March 22, 2007.

70. Taylor S. The underinsured in America. *Healthbeat,* funded by the Robert Wood Johnson Foundation. April 6, 2007. http://www.pbs.org/newshour/

indepth_coverage/health/uninsured/underinsured.html. Accessed Nov. 24, 2007.

71. Wallack V. New Dirigo insurer 'better arrangement'. *Lakes Region Weekly,* September13, 2007.

72. Miller T. Maine looks to expand reach of health care program. *Healthbeat,* April 6, 2007. http://www.pbs.org/newshour/indepth_coverage/health/uninsured/maine.html

73. Seattle Post-Intelligencer. Fewer employers offering health plans. February 13, 2007. http://seattlepi.nwsource.com/business/303408_healthinsurance13.html. Accessed February 14, 2007.

74. Rowland D. Health care: squeezing the middle class with more costs and less coverage. Testimony before the U.S. House of Representatives Ways and Means Committee, January 31, 2007. Henry J. Kaiser Family Foundation. http://www.kff.org/uninsured/upload/7612.pdf. Accessed March 20, 2007.

75. Health Savings Accounts. U.S. Department of the Treasurery. http://www.ustreas.gov/offices/public-affairs/hsa/ Accessed March 19, 2007.

76. SHPS, Inc. Making consumerism work: a practical guide for transforming healthcare, 2006. http://www.shps.com/corp/news/6_6_06.stm. Accessed November 28, 2007.

77. Hospital Corp. of America posts cost of services for uninsured online. http://www.medicalnewstoday.com/articles/64667.php. Accessed March 8, 2007.

78. Commonwealth Choice: How much is the penalty for no insurance? http://www.massresources.org/pages.cfm?contentID=85&pageID=13&Subpages=yes#individuals. Accessed December 29, 2009.

79. Cover Tennessee. Enrollment suspended effective 12/1/09; reached budget capacity. http://www.covertn.gov. Accessed December 29, 2009.

80. Families USA. A closer look at CoverTN, Tennessee's barebones health plan: A case study. Detailing shortcomings of Gov. Bredesen's CoverTN health insurance. http://www.familiesusa.org/assets/pdfs/covertn-a-closer-look.pdf. Accessed Dec. 29, 2009.

81. No Maine miracle cure. *Wall Street Journal* August 21, 2009. http://online.wsj.com/article/SB10001424052970204619004574322401816501182.html Problems with DirigoChoice, the Maine experiment in universal coverage.

82. Fetters E, Luke R. Retail-based clinics: Passing fad or here to stay? NEWS browser, February 2007. http://www.healthleadersmedia.com/print.cfm?content_id=87008&parent=105. Accessed February 20, 2007.

83. Kowalczyk L. State signals it is open to retail medical clinics. Boston.com, White Coat Notes, July 17, 07. http://www.boston.com/yourlife/health/blog/2007/07/state_signals_i.html. Accessed November 27, 2007.

84. Schmit J. Could walk-in retail clinics help slow rising health costs? *USA Today*.com. http://usatoday.printthis.clickability.com/pt/cpt?action=cpt&title=USATODAY.com+-+Co. Accessed August 24, 2006.

85. Turner GM. Customer Health Care. *Wall Street Journal.* May 14, 2007.

86. Holstein WJ. For better care, work across lines. *The New York Times*.com. http://www.nytimes.com/2006/12/31/jobs/31advi.html?ei=5070&en=00ac448335e34ed9&e. Accessed January 7, 2007. Clayton Christesen's disruptive technologies.

87. Christensen C. Health care: the simple solution. Bloomberg Business Week. http://www.businessweek.com/print/magazine/content/10_11/b4170072386095.html. Accessed April 24, 2010.

88. OECD Health Data 2009, July 2009. Life expectancy comparison.

89. Hughes, Samuel. Diagnosing health care. *The Pennsylvania Gazette*, Nov/Dec, 2007, p. 56.

90. Ohsfeldt R, Schneider J. *The Business of Health: The Role of Competition, Markets, and Regulation.* Washington: AEI Press, October 2006.

91. O'Neill JE, O'Neill DM. Health status, health care and inequality: Canada vs. the US National Bureau of Economic Research. http://www.nber.org/papers/w13429, September 2007. Accessed November 25, 2007.

92. OECD 2009 Health Data. Infant Mortality. July 2009.

93. Giuliani RW. A Free-market cure for US healthcare system. *The Boston Globe*, August 3, 2007. Accessed on Boston.com October 29, 2007.

94. Leape L, Berwick D. Five years after *To Err is Human. JAMA* 2005; 293: 2384–2390.

95. Inglehart JK. More checks than balances in the struggle for health care reform. *New Eng J Med.* www.http://healthcarereform.nejm.org/?p=922uery=TOC. Accessed July 15, 2009.

96. Curfman GD, Morrissey S, Malina D, Drazen JM. Health care reform 2009. healthcarereform.nejm.org. *New Eng J Med* online. Accessed July 30, 2009.

97. Brett AS. "American values" — a smoke screen in the debate on health care reform. *New Engl J Med.* www.http://healthcarereform.nejm.org/?p=1245? query=TOC. Accessed July 30, 2009.

98. Whelan D. Is there another doctor in the house? www.http:// members.forbes.com/forbes/2007/0326/046a_print.html. Accessed March 17, 2007.

99. Berwick DM. America's health care priorities II: doctors, hospitals and the quality of care. Changing and improving care. www.http://economix. blogs.nytimes.com/2009/06/23/americas-health-care-priorities-ii-doctors-html. Accessed July 25, 2009.

100. Rohack JJ. America's health care priorities II: doctors, hospitals and the quality of care. Expanding coverage and controlling costs. www.http:// economix.blogs.nytimes.com/2009/06/23/americas-health-care-priorities-ii-doctors-html. Accessed July 25, 2009.

101. Gawande A. The cost conundrum. *The New Yorker.* June 1, 2009: 36–44.

102. Brown JT, Khoury C. In OECD countries, universal healthcare gets high marks. Aug. 20, 2009. http://www.gallup.com/poll/122393/oecd-countries-universal-healthcare-gets-high-marks.aspx. Accessed. Jan. 12, 2010.

103. OECD Health Data. Specialists outnumber GPs in most OECD countries. July 18, 2007.

104. German health insurance funds face 4-bil. Euro deficit in 2010: contributions to rise. HIS Global Insight Same Day Analysis. http://www. ihsglobalinsight.com/SDA/SDADetail17992.htm. Accessed Jan. 13, 2010.

105. Reinfeldt F. "The New Swedish Model: A reform agenda for growth and the environment." Speech at the London School of Economics and Political Science, Feb. 26, 2008. http://www.sweden.gov.se/sb/d/10296/a/99193. Accessed Jan. 4, 2010.

Index